Imperial College London
2407606171

AF606572

CANCER ETIOLOGY, DIAGNOSIS AND TREATMENT

GLIOBLASTOMA: RISK FACTORS, DIAGNOSIS AND TREATMENT OPTIONS

Cancer Etiology, Diagnosis and Treatment

Additional books in this series can be found on Nova's website under the Series tab.

Additional E-books in this series can be found on Nova's website under the E-book tab.

CANCER ETIOLOGY, DIAGNOSIS AND TREATMENT

GLIOBLASTOMA: RISK FACTORS, DIAGNOSIS AND TREATMENT OPTIONS

MARCELO F. BEZERRA AND
CLAUDIO R. ALVES
EDITORS

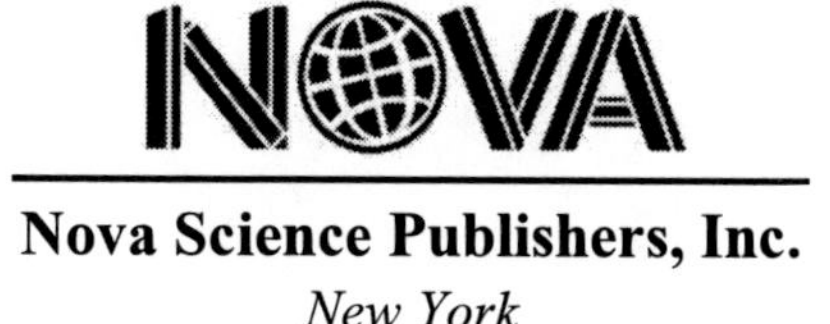

Nova Science Publishers, Inc.
New York

For permission to use material from this book please contact us:
Telephone 631-231-7269; Fax 631-231-8175
Web Site: http://www.novapublishers.com

Additional color graphics may be available in the e-book version of this book.

LIBRARY OF CONGRESS CATALOGING-IN-PUBLICATION DATA

Glioblastoma : risk factors, diagnosis, and treatment options / editors, Marcelo F. Bezerra and Claudio R. Alve.

p. ; cm.
Includes bibliographical references and index.
ISBN 978-1-62100-858-3 (hardcover)
I. Bezerra, Marcelo F. II. Alve, Claudio R.
[DNLM: 1. Glioblastoma. QZ 380]
616.99'481--dc23 2011038715

Published by Nova Science Publishers, Inc. † New York

CONTENTS

PREFACE

Glioblastoma is the most common and lethal primary brain tumor which exhibits clinical, radiological and pathological heterogenity. Despite advances in standard therapy, including surgical resection, radiotherapy and chemotherapy, the prognosis for patients remains poor. In this book, the authors present topical research on the risk factors, diagnosis and treatment options for glioblastoma. Topics discussed include the therapeutic potential of scorpion toxins against glioblastoma; co-amplified oncogenes in glioblastoma; mesenchymal stem cells as a novel therapeutic delivery vehicle for glioblastoma; targeting fibroblast growth factor (FGF) signals and how to stop glial neoplastic brain development.

Chapter 1 - Glioblastoma (GBM) , also known as glioblastoma *multiforme*, is the most common and lethal primary brain tumor which exhibits clinical, radiological and pathological heterogeneity. Based on the fact that the incidence has been documented to be constant in various reports, genetic variation is more likely to play a major role in developing GBM than environmental, geographical and nutritional factors. MRI with contrast enhancement is the most commonly used method in the initial evaluation and follow-up after treatment. The typical finding of GBM is ring enhanced white matter lesion with central necrosis and perilesional edema on MRI. Microvascular proliferation and necrosis have been used as the most critical factor in pathological confirmation. Recently, some biomarkers such as O^6-methylguanine-DNA methyltransferase (MGMT) methylation, BRAF fusions, and IDH1 mutations have been suggested as possible prognostic and grading factors. Standard therapy includes microsurgical resection and a multimodal treatment of concomitant radiotherapy and chemotherapy, followed by adjuvant chemotherapy with temozolomide. In addition to functional or diffusion tensor MRI with navigation system or intraoperative MRI, fluorescence-guided resection helps surgeons to increase safety and accuracy in GBM surgery. MR spectroscopy and positron-emission tomography (PET) scans may provide useful information in differential diagnosis and making treatment plans. Anti-angiogenic therapy with antivascular endothelial growth factor antibodies (bevacizumab) is on its way into clinical practice. In this article, the authors discuss and highlight the advances in diagnosis and treatment of GBM with relevant reviews.

Chapter 2 - Despite advances in standard therapy, including surgical resection, radiotherapy and chemotherapy, the prognosis for patients with glioblastoma remains poor. A unique feature contributing to the disease aggressiveness is the ability of malignant glioma cells to actively migrate along brain vasculature instead of passive metastasis through vascular circulation. During the last decade, different ion channel types have been found to be overexpressed in a variety of tumors, thus emerging as possible tumoral markers. Ion channels may be considered as a suitable pharmacological target for glioblastoma therapy. Because scorpion toxins have well defined structures, constrained by disulfide bridges, and interact with ionic channels (their targets) through multiple contacts, they bind with much higher affinity and specificity than most other ionic channel blockers available to date. Scorpion toxins represent thus promising agents for treatment and early detection of malignant glioma brain tumors. In this review we present the main results of years of research involving glioma ionic channels and scorpion toxins that have anti-glioblastoma activity on the basis of recent publications and our experience.

Chapter 3 - Glioblastomamultiforme (GBM) is the most common central nervous system malignancy. Why patients develop GBM is still unknown. These aggressive tumors may present in a number of ways, depending on such factors as growth rate and anatomic location. While standard histopathology and epidemiology studies have helped us categorize patients with GBM into risk groups, treatment results for most patients remain unsatisfactory. An improved epidemiological understanding in conjunction with continued advances in the use of molecular markers will hopefully lead to better treatment and prevention strategies. This chapter serves as an introduction into the epidemiology of GBM and its associated risk factors. Also presented are the neurological signs and symptoms that a GBM may cause, and the prognostic factors used for estimating survival. Lastly, there is a brief review of standard and experimental treatment options.

Chapter 4 - It is well-established that *epidermal growth factor receptor* (*EGFR*) is often amplified in glioblastomas. Other oncogenes can be co-amplified with *EGFR* or amplified without its amplification. Many varieties of oncogene co-amplifications exist, including those involving genes within the same amplicon or in multiple amplicons. Many amplified oncogenes, including *EGFR*, are also frequently rearranged or mutated. Various functions in tumor cells are enhanced according to the specific combinations of genes amplified and/or mutated. Oncogenes mediate cell proliferation, protection from apoptosis, metabolic enhancements, etc. Elucidation of mechanisms that favor oncogene amplifications in the cancer cell genome is greatly needed to further understand malignancy. Also, application of multiplex techniques to detect oncogene amplifications in individual tumors is putatively an emerging need for selecting treatment combinations for patients with glioblastomas in clinical trials. This review highlights traditional oncogenes known to be amplified in glioblastomas. A focused view of copy number gains in known oncogenes provides a simplified approach to understand an important aspect of the complex genomic changes occurring in glioblastomas. Importantly, established amplified oncogenes are within the scope of potential cancer targets for the pharmaceutical industry to consider when designing cocktails of drugs to treat tumors in individual patients.

Chapter 5 - Each year 40,000 people are diagnosed with primary brain tumors, the majority of which are glioblastoma (GB) .[1]Glioblastoma is the most common brain tumor in adults and is the most malignant subtype. Despite best treatments with maximum surgical resection, radiation and chemotherapy, long-term survival of GB patients is rare (median survival is 14.6 months) .[2-4]Complete surgical resection is a challenge due to the diffusely infiltrative growth pattern of GB, and systemic therapy is limited by the selectivity of the blood brain barrier. Experimental evidence suggests that a subpopulation of cells called brain tumor stem cells (BTSCs) retain tumor initiating ability and are responsible for the invasive and chemo/radioresistant nature of malignant gliomas. [5-12]It is believed that BTSCs infiltrate into normal brain tissue of patients, resulting in distant disease recurrence and death.[13]As a result there is an increased impetus to find novel methods to eradicate the BTSC population. The use of mesenchymal stem cells (MSC) has become an attractive option.[14] MSCs are attractive for clinical use because they possess a natural affinity for tumors, can be easily isolated and expanded to the numbers required for application, and can be genetically modified through various means. Bone marrow-derived mesenchymal stem cells (BM-MSCs) can selectively home to gliomas as well as track disseminated nests of

BTSCs in animal models.[15] Therefore, MSCs can serve as vehicles to deliver chemotherapeutic agents such as cytokines and oncolytic viruses to tumors.

Chapter 6 - Glioblastoma multiforme (GBM) is the most malignant form of human astrocytoma with a survival for the majority of patients less than two years. Glioblastoma exhibits a rapid, progressive and infiltrative growth, which renders the tumor unressectable at the time of diagnosis. Current treatment modalities include maximal surgical debulking, followed by focal radiotherapy and adjuvant chemotherapy. Glioblastoma is highly vascularized and, therefore, antiangiogenic agents aimed to the inhibition of vascular endothelial cell growth factor (VEGF) signalling are increasingly being explored as therapeutic options. However, patients succumb in a very high number of cases because of chemoresistance development and the appearance of mechanisms circumventing the effects of VEGF-targeted antiangiogenic drugs. The fibroblast growth factor (FGF) signalling network plays a key role in glioma growth. In addition, FGF plays an important role in the overcoming of chemotherapy and the failures of anti-VEGF therapies. This review summarizes laboratory and clinical research on glioblastoma angiogenesis and discusses the potential use of new safe and efficient FGF inhibitors for the treatment of glioblastoma.

Chapter 7 - Antisense technique was particularly used to target tumour antigens, which arrest of expression was not efficiently stopped using antibodies or other inhibitors. Antisense is working not only as an anti – gene stopping tool, but especially indirectly by inducing apoptosis and a strong immune in vitro and in vivo anti tumour response, verified in murine models i. e. of glioma or teratocarcinoma containing neuro-glial derivatives. Antisense strategy targeting principal growth factors as IGF-I, TGFbeta and their receptors, but also their downstream signalling effectors, particularly glycogenesis, has given satisfactory experimental results for treatment of different malignant tumours including human glial tumour - glioblastoma.

Chapter 8 - It has been reported that the therapeutic response to certain drugs such as temozolomide and nimustine hydochloride (ACNU) correlates with the expression of the O6-methylguanine-DNA methyltransferase (MGMT) protein. Studies further indicate that MGMT expression may be suppressed by various anticancer agents or interferon-beta (IFN-β) . We examined a cohort of patients with malignant glioma to determine the influence of chemotherapy on MGMT expression. Tissue samples from 24 patients were collected, each documenting a recurrence of tumor following chemotherapy. The histologic diagnoses recorded prior to chemotherapy were anaplastic oligodendroglioma (3 cases) , anaplastic astrocytoma (5 cases) , and glioblastoma (16 cases) . Biopsy confirmation of a second recurrence, unchanged in type, was also obtained from four patients with diagnoses including anaplastic oligodendroglioma (2 cases) , anaplastic astrocytoma (1 case) , and glioblastoma (1 case) . As initial chemotherapy, the patients received one of three treatments: IAV combination treatment (IFN-β, ACNU, and vincristine, 17 cases) , IPE combination treatment (IFN-β, cisplatin, and etoposide, 3 cases) , or temozolomide monotherapy (4 cases) . All patients underwent irradiation (60 Gy) in addition to initial chemotherapy. Second-line chemotherapy with IPE or temozolomide was administered to two patients each. Expression of MGMT was evaluated histochemically in 52 sequential specimens from 24 tumors. A qualitative decrease in MGMT expression was found in 2 of 17 tumors after treatment with IAV, in 4 of 5 tumors after an IPE regimen, and in 2 of 6 tumors after single-agent temozolomide treatment. These results suggest that expression of MGMT protein in malignant glioma may be suppressed by IPE chemotherapy.

Chapter 9 - Glioblastoma, astrocytoma grade IV, is the most frequent and aggressive primary brain tumor. According to the WHO, it presents two major histological variants: giant cell glioblastoma and gliosarcoma, however it can also exhibit different patterns of differentiation such as small cell, oligodendroglial component and lipidized cells. Due to the aggressive behavior, this tumor has been extensively studied, in order to better understand the phenomena underling the morphological features of neoplastic and microvascular proliferation, necrosis, and so on. The immunohistochemistry is an auxiliary diagnostic tool that has been used for a long time in the routine diagnosis and is being increasingly used to determine patient prognosis and therapeutic response. In the present chapter we will address the main immunohistochemical markers used currently in the differential diagnosis of glioblastoma and its variants, like GFAP, vimentin and galectins 1 and 3. Furthermore, we will discuss the growing role of immunohistochemical markers, for instance EGFR, MGMT, PTEN and CD133, in patient survival and treatment resistance.

Chapter 10 - An association between cancer and thrombosis has long been described. Abnormal elevated expression of tissue factor (TF) , the physiological initiator of blood coagulation, has been well documented in several tumor types, including glioblastoma (GBM) , and seems to be directly correlated with thromboembolic complications in cancer patients. In the last few years, it has become clear that the processes responsible for the progression of cancer are highly dependent on components of the blood coagulation cascade and TF has been pointed as a key determinant of the coagulation/cancer interaction. Actually, TF expression, that has been shown to correlate with the histological grade of malignancy of glioma, is involved in modulation of several intracellular pathways relevant for malignant angiogenesis and tumor growth. GBM is one of the most vascularized malignant tumors and intense angiogenesis is a distinguishing pathological hallmark relative to lower-grade glioma. Moreover, there is a high incidence of thrombotic events throughout the course of malignant glioma. In fact, the prothrombotic properties of GBM cells seem to contribute to the appearance of hypoxic regions within the tumor and, ultimately, to the formation of the GBM-typical necrotic foci that are well-recognized predictors of poor prognosis. Most remarkable, TF is overexpressed in cells around these necrotic foci found in GBM, known as pseudopalisading cells. These regions are highly hypoxic and seem to play a key role in GBM aggressiveness, presenting an increased production of vascular endothelial growth factor (VEGF) , interleukin-8 (IL-8) and metalloproteases. In addition to prothrombotic role, TF enables the activation of the G protein-coupled protease-activated receptors (PARs) . These receptors might be activated through proteolytic cleavage by blood coagulation enzymes thus eliciting the production of several pro-tumoral factors including cytokines, angiogenic factors and metalloproteases among others. Given the importance of coagulation activation in human gliomas, it has been proposed that TF, as well as other clotting proteins, could serve as a therapeutic target. It has already been shown that argatroban, a specific thrombin inhibitor, reduced tumor mass and tumor induced behavioral deficits and prolongs survival time in animal models. We showed that Ixolaris, a potent anticoagulant that does not produce major bleeding when injected subcutaneously in different animal models, potently decreases tumor growth in a human GBM model. Notably, inhibition of tumor growth was accompanied by downregulation of VEGF and vessel density in tumor mass. Our results provide strong evidence that TF may be regarded as an important therapeutic target for GBM.

Chapter 11 - Glioblastomas are the most common and malignant primary central nervous system tumors. The current management of patients with glioblastomas is surgery, followed by concomitant radiotherapy with temozolomide–based chemotherapy. Despite this integrated approach, the prognosis of these patients is very dismal, with a median overall survival of 16 months. Therefore, new and more effective therapeutic options are needed to change this dark scenario. Over the past decade, significant advances have been made in understanding the molecular pathogenesis of malignant gliomas. In general, malignancy results from consecutive genetic mutations and alterations of growth-factor signaling. The increased knowledge of the molecular pathways underlying glioblastomas development is creating a new avenue of potential therapeutic targets. The BRAF protooncogene, codifies a serine/threonine kinase important in the MAPK signaling cascade. A hotspot mutation of BRAF (V600E) , was identified in several tumor types, mainly, in melanomas and papillary thyroid cancer, which leads to hyperstimulation of the MAPK pathway and cellular transformation. Several drugs have been developed to target BRAF oncogene, and recently, exciting results have been achieved in phase I/II clinical trials of metastatic melanoma patients harboring BRAF V600E mutation treated with such class of tyrosine inhibitors. In this chapter we will summarized the current knowledge of BRAF alterations in glioblastomas biology and will address the potential therapeutic impact of the novel BRAF inhibitors in the treatment of these patients.

In: Glioblastoma
Editors: M. F. Bezerra, et.al, pp. 1-41
ISBN: 978-1-62100-858-3

Chapter 1

GLIOBLASTOMA: RISK FACTORS, DIAGNOSIS AND TREATMENT OPTIONS

Kyung-Sub Moon and Maciej S. Lesniak*

The Brain Tumor Center, The University of Chicago Medical Center, Chicago, IL USA

ABSTRACT

Glioblastoma (GBM) , also known as glioblastoma *multiforme*, is the most common and lethal primary brain tumor which exhibits clinical, radiological and pathological heterogeneity. Based on the fact that the incidence has been documented to be constant in various reports, genetic variation is more likely to play a major role in developing GBM than environmental, geographical and nutritional factors. MRI with contrast enhancement is the most commonly used method in the initial evaluation and follow-up after treatment. The typical finding of GBM is ring enhanced white matter lesion with central necrosis and perilesional edema on MRI. Microvascular proliferation and necrosis have been used as the most critical factor in pathological confirmation. Recently, some biomarkers such as O^6-methylguanine-DNA methyltransferase (MGMT) methylation, BRAF fusions, and IDH1 mutations have been suggested as possible prognostic and grading factors. Standard therapy includes microsurgical resection and a multimodal treatment of concomitant radiotherapy and chemotherapy, followed by adjuvant chemotherapy with

* Correspondence to: Maciej S. Lesniak,MD, University of Chicago Brain Tumor Center, 5841 S Maryland Ave, MC 3026, Chicago, IL 60637. E-mail: mlesniak@surgery.bsd.uchicago.edu

temozolomide. In addition to functional or diffusion tensor MRI with navigation system or intraoperative MRI, fluorescence-guided resection helps surgeons to increase safety and accuracy in GBM surgery. MR spectroscopy and positron-emission tomography (PET) scans may provide useful information in differential diagnosis and making treatment plans. Anti-angiogenic therapy with antivascular endothelial growth factor antibodies (bevacizumab) is on its way into clinical practice. In this article, the authors discuss and highlight the advances in diagnosis and treatment of GBM with relevant reviews.

Keywords: diagnosis, glioblastoma, glioma, risk factors, treatment options.

INTRODUCTION

Glioblastoma (GBM) is the most malignant glioma (World Health Organization [WHO] grade IV) with an average life expectancy of 14 months after diagnosis, despite the best standard of care. This dismal disease entity represents various radiological and pathological features. Although majority of the diagnosed patients follow the poor clinical course with rapid recurrence and infiltration into deeper portions of the central nervous system, a small fraction of the patients do much better than the expected. Furthermore, various new treatment strategies based on the tremendous discoveries in basic and translational research have been adopted in recent years. In this chapter, the authors review the recently published articles and discuss the advances in diagnosis and treatment of GBM.

RISK FACTOR

GBM accounts for 12-15% of all brain tumors and 60-75% of astrocytomas. The incidence of GBM is in the range of 3-4 new cases per 100,000 population per year but the poor prognosis makes it a considerable public health issue [1, 2]. The peak incidence is between 45 and 75 years, with a mean age of 61.3 years: more than 80% of patients are older than 50 years [3]. GBM is a relatively frequent intracranial neoplasm in adults (12–20% of all intracranial tumors) [4]. However, it is unusual in pediatric patients and constitutes 7–8.8% of all pediatric brain tumors [5].

Generally, the incidence of primary brain tumors (including gliomas) has been highly reported in developed countries including Western Europe, North

America, and Australia [6]. In population-based studies, the incidence of GBM is fairly constant in United States and Europe [1, 2]. This result may lead one to conclude that environmental, geographical and nutritional factors probably do not play a major role in gliomagenesis, whereas genetics is more likely to tip the scale of etiology [6]. The lower incidence in developing countries can be partly explained by under-estimation, but ethnic differences as a possible factor in glioma development should be considered. According to the data of Central Brain Tumor Registry of the United States, blacks are relatively protected, as their incidence is lower than other ethnic groups such as whites, latinos and Asians [7, 8]. The incidence of GBM is approximately twice as common in whites as in blacks [6]. It is slightly more common in men, with a male to female ratio of 1.3:1 [1]. The reasons for this gender distribution have not been revealed. Some studies suggest a possible relationship between season of birth and risk of GBM. Based on these studies, GBM patients are generally born in winter, particularly in the month of February and January [9, 10]. Perinatal viral origin (infection with an unknown oncovirus, integrating in the genome) has subsequently been put forward, but no hard evidence has yet been found to support it. The association with an oncogenic virus, SV40, remains controversial [11, 12]. Recent study suggests the involvement of host genetic factors in susceptibility to cytomegalovirus-induced GBM [13]. Although most GBMs originate in a sporadic fashion without any known genetic predisposition, several genetic disorders are associated with increased incidence, including tuberous sclerosis, neurofibromatosis type 1 and type 2, von Hippel Lindau disease, as well as some well-known hereditary tumor syndromes (Turcot's syndrome or Li–Fraumeni syndrome) [14, 15].

There is a proven association between GBM and exposure to ionizing radiation or polyvinyl chloride [16, 17]. A large-scale cohort study for childhood cancer patients demonstrated that radiation exposure was associated with increased risk of subsequent glioma and meningioma. Considering the higher risk of subsequent glioma in children irradiated at a very young age, the developing brain may be more susceptible to radiation. Even low-dose therapeutic radiation may result in subsequent development of brain tumors [18]. Long-term exposure to polyvinyl chloride has been reported to cause hepatic angiosarcoma. Moreover, it may also carry a slightly enhanced risk of developing GBM [17]. Polycyclic aromatic hydrocarbons and non-arsenical insecticides were suggested as possible occupational carcinogens associated with an excess risk of brain tumors [19]. Some studies have shown a significant inverse correlation between glioma and allergic conditions such as asthma, eczema and atopy [20, 21]. Based on the observation that total immunoglobulin E levels were lower in glioma patients than control subjects [22] and partly explained by interleukin-13 polymorphism [23], immunological factors may influence glioma development. No definitive links have been found between GBM and smoking, diet, cellular phones or electromagnetic fields [6]. However, recent meta-analysis studies came down on the side of suggesting that there may a possible role of cellular phone use in gliomagenesis [24, 25]. Additionally, a recent study provides evidence of an association between alcohol consumption and risk of GBM. This study also postulates whether the increased risk of GBM associated with alcohol consumption is modified by cigarette smoking, folate intake, or genetic variants in the alcohol-dehydrogenase and acetaldehyde dehydrogenase genes [26].

DIAGNOSIS

Contrast–enhanced multiplanar MRI is the standard assessment technique for GBM, particularly useful in evaluating anatomical location, extension, and characteristics. The mass usually demonstrates low-signal intensity, as a hypodense necrotic central area surrounded by thick, irregularly-enhanced rim, corresponding to the central necrosis with the peripheral cellular vascularized wall, on T_1-weighted images. It conversely appears as high-signal intensity mass on T_2–weighted images. The lesion seems to be much broader and less well defined, overlapping with the perilesional edema. Although it is sometimes difficult to distinguish the lesion from surrounding edema, T_2–weighted images are the best to reveal the surrounding vasogenic edema. GBM generally shows marked and somewhat heterogenous gadolinium enhancement, indicating angiogenesis and vascular permeability. It frequently follows the ring-enhancement pattern, demonstrating enhancement along with the peripheral rim surrounding non-enhanced necrotic portion.

However, these conventional imaging sequences can not fully reflect the complicated biology of infiltrative gliomas [27] and have limited specificity in the identification of features necessary for glioma grading or aggressiveness [28-31]. Basically, GBMs typically show microvascular proliferation and necrosis, in addition to increased cellularity and pleomorphism. New blood vessel formation, essential to maintain high proliferative property, has somewhat different biological features. This disorganized vascular network consists of dilated, tortuous and hyperpermeable vessels induced by oversecretion of proangiogenic cytokines such as vascular endothelial growth factor [32]. It also leads to heterogeneity within tumor blood flow with some areas receiving high blood flow whereas others receiving very little [33]. Under normal conditions, the contrast agent can not leak into the brain across the blood-brain-barrier. However, tumor vasculature is abnormally hyperpermeable, thus gadolinium can leak into the area of the tumor. Although the size of the tumor can be identified by the extent of contrast leakage, this leakage is not consistent within patients and can vary from scan to scan depending on the amount of gadolinium used or the precision of the contrast injection. Some drugs used in glioma patients, such as dexamethasone and antiangiogenic agents can also affect the permeability of the blood-brain-barrier, causing a decrease in the leakage of gadolinium into the brain. However, this decrease in enhancement does not reflect a decrease in tumor cell density or apoptosis [34].

The introduction of physiology-based MRI sequences, such as diffusion and perfusion MRI, overcome the limitation of contrast leakage as a measure of tumor size and response to treatment. These techniques stress the angiogenic features and proliferative ability of tumor cells to distinguish the tumor from surrounding normal tissue [33, 35] and hold promise in the quantitative assessment of aggressiveness [30, 31, 36-41]. Diffusion MRI focuses on cell density and enables the acquisition of images of white matter tracts to evaluate vasogenic edema and tumor infiltration. Perfusion MRI evaluates hemodynamic properties of the tumor such as blood volume or blood flow, oxygenation, vessel size, and vascular permeability [33].

The measuring of the water diffusivity within brain tissue is a fundamental principal of diffusion-weighted imaging. The clinical application using this technique can be divided into apparent diffusion coefficient (ADC) maps for evaluation of cell density and fractional anisotropy maps (diffusion tensor imaging: DTI) for morphology of the white matter track. ADC is calculated to quantitatively measure relative degrees of hydrogen motion within the extracellular space [42]. Less water movement represents low ADC value (dark appearance) and has correlated with increased cellularity and proliferation in pathological studies of gliomas [43-45]. However, similar studies involving mixed-grade gliomas have yielded various results [42, 46-49]. In contrast to the cellular portion, water content can move freely in vasogenic edema, thus this increased movement appears bright on ADC. ADC can be used as a noninvasive biomarker for prediction of treatment response in glioma patients. Increase in tumor diffusion value, particularly in treated area, has been positively associated with subsequent volumetric tumor response and overall survival after treatment [50-52].

White matter tracts (DTI) can be visualized based on the fraction anisotropy value of water molecule in tissue. Isotropy theoretically means that all water molecules diffuse at the same speed and quantity. In nervous tissue, however, water diffusion is imparted in certain directions by white matter fiber bundle. This 'diffusion anisotropy' is significantly decreased when the tumor infiltration destroys white matter fibers [53]. Some studies showed that DTI enables the differentiation of tumor infiltration from purely vasogenic edema [54, 55]. Using this technique, restoration of white matter tracts was confirmed in the patients who responded to the pan-VEGF receptor tyrosine kinase inhibitor, leading to normalization of tumor vasculature and alleviation of vasogenic edema [35]. Serial DTI may thus show resolution of vasogenic edema and potentially the arrest of tumor growth along white matter tracts after GBM treatment. DTI can be successfully combined with neuronavigation for surgical planning and contributes to maximum resection when the tumor is in an eloquent area while minimizing postoperative deficits [56].

Perfusion-weighted MRI is used to quantitatively measure cerebral hemodynamic characteristics [30]. Cerebral blood volume, peak height, and percentage of signal intensity recovery are three imaging measurements previously shown to be clinically useful in predicting glioma histopathologic grade and distinguishing recurrent brain tumors from radiation necrosis [30, 36-38, 41]. Currently, dynamic susceptibility contrast (DSC) MRI has been most widely used to determine cerebral blood volume and flow. It measures the amount of gadolinium that enters into and flushes out from each voxel and this amount is proportional to the cerebral blood volume in the particular region of the brain [33]. The strong correlation between the maximum cerebral blood volume measured in a tumor and the histologic tumor grade has been generally accepted [39, 57]. Regional cerebral blood volume has also been correlated with microvessel density in glioma model and human sample [40, 58, 59]. However, DSC measurements are not considered a valid biomarker of GBM angiogenesis because a direct comparison with tissue specimens obtained through image-guided biopsy has yet to be extensively reported [39, 40, 60, 61].

Although conventional MRI provides the structural information, MR spectroscopy (MRS) provides a qualitative analysis of a number of metabolites within the brain, and a quantitative analysis if a reference of known concentration is used. The principal peaks observed in the brain tumors at 1.5T include branch chain amino acid (0.9-1.0 ppm) , lipid (0.9-1.5 ppm) , lactate (1.3 ppm) , alanine (1.5 ppm) , *N*-acetyl aspartate (NAA; 2.0 ppm) , choline (3.2 ppm) , creatine (3.0 and 3.9 ppm) , and myoinositol (3.6 ppm) [62, 63].

Each metabolite represents the status of neuronal integrity, cell membrane proliferation or degradation, energy metabolism or necrotic transformation of brain or tumor tissue. Through the summation of these spectra data, colorful metabolite map depicting the spatial distribution of the different heights, areas, or peak ratio can be produced. Although the main data assessed from the spectral graphs can limit the clinical diagnostic value, MRS provides information about a number of disease processes and adds another dimension to imaging diagnosis [62]. The typical pattern of glioma spectra is well defined as high choline (metabolism of cell membrane) and low or absent NAA peaks (viable neuron) , with lipid and lactate peaks (necrosis) often seen in GBM [31, 63]. However, numerous investigations have failed to prove the definitive role of MRS in differential diagnosis of tumor types or of tumor from non-neoplastic processes such as demyelination, ischemia, and gliosis [64-67]. The use of MRS for biopsies targeted to the areas with high Choline/NAA ratios has been reported to increase the accuracy of tumor biopsy. It can reduce the false negative rate by targeting metabolically active areas within heterogeneous glioma [68-70].

Conventional MRI has a major limitation to differentiate tumor recurrence from radiation necrosis after GBM treatment. Both lesions generally show various enhancement patterns and degrees possibly with mass effect. Ideally, progressive decrease in NAA and choline peaks and lactate/lipid peaks can suggest necrosis. Significant increase in choline with decrease in NAA can be an indicator of tumor recurrence. However, in most clinical settings, recurrent tumor and necrosis may occur concomitantly and this mixture can make MRS patterns less definitive. In addition to different acquisition on voxel placement or technique, spatial variation of important peaks in individual tumor can be augmented over serial scan time. Some studies stress the Choline/Creatin ratio in mixed tumor recurrence and necrosis [71-73]. A ratio greater than specific value (2.23) with enlargement indicates the predominance of recurrence [71]. This discrimination ability of MRS can be enhanced by the combination with diffusion and/or perfusion MRI [72, 73]. Serial changes in MRS findings of gliomas after treatment have shown encouraging results. Increased Choline/Creatinin ratio was checked in lesions before a subsequent contrast enhancement [74]. Incorporation of spatial information from MRS guaranteed more accurate planning and prolonged survival in stereotactic radiosurgery for GBM [75].

PET with ^{18}F-fluorodeoxyglucose (FDG) has been widely used in diagnosis and treatment of systemic cancer. However, because there are some problematic obstacles as an imaging tool for brain [76], new PET tracers, such as ^{18}F-fluoro-L-thymidine (FLT) and ^{18}F-fluoromisonidazole (FMISO) , ^{11}C-methionine (MET) , and 3,4-dihydroxy-6-18F-fluoro-L-phenylalanine (FDOPA) have been developed and introduced to the clinics [33, 77]. FLT is the most extensively investigated tracer to image cell proliferation. FLT is a thymidine analogue and is correlated with expression of thymidine kinase-1 activity, an enzyme important in DNA synthesis. Thus, it can provide a measure of DNA synthesis and tumor cell proliferation [78]. With some limitations in correlation with Ki-67 labeling, FLT tracer uptake is essential for the in vivo assessment of tumor proliferation in high-grade gliomas [79, 80]. FLT-PET can be used as an imaging biomarker in assessing proliferation and serve as a predictive tool in overall survival for GBM, especially in the treatment with anti-angiogenic agents or with cytostatic therapy possibly leading to unreliable results on conventional MRI [81]. FMISO, as a tracer for determining tumor hypoxia, binds selectively to hypoxic cells [82]. In glioma patients, elevated FMISO uptake representing hypoxic area has been associated with cell proliferation and patient outcome after treatment [83, 84]. MET readily cross the intact blood-blood-barrier using specific amino acid transporters and incorporates into the active proliferative area. Elevated MET uptake correlates with grades, proliferation, accurate extension and biological aggressiveness in gliomas [85-87].

TREATMENT

In addition to the definitive antitumor therapy, the management of GBM patients involves providing effective supportive care. The most common problems include seizure, peritumoral edema, venous thromboembolism, gastrointestinal disturbance, osteoporosis, cognitive dysfunction, infection and mood disturbance [88].

It remains controversial to use prophylactic antiepileptic drugs (AEDs) in patients with malignant gliomas who have never had a seizure. However, given the potential for adverse effects and the lack of clear evidence that AEDs reduce the incidence of new-onset seizures, routine prophylactic AED therapy in brain tumor patients is probably unnecessary [89]. Patients with brain tumors who present with seizures should be treated with standard AED. Because some AEDs, such as phenytoin or carbamazepine, induce cytochrome P450 to increase the metabolism for chemotherapeutic agents, AED without induction of cytochrome P450, such as levetiracetam, are preferred [88].

To treat the peritumoral edema, the use of corticosteroid such as dexamethasone is indispensable. Glucose intolerance, Cushing's syndrome, steroid myopathy, and peptic ulceration may occur in prolonged treatment with high doses of corticosteroids. The use of moderate to high doses of corticosteroid can result in clinically significant suppression of the immune system and vulnerability to opportunistic infections. Among these infectious diseases, *Pneumocystis jiroveci (previously known as carinii)* can cause life-threatening pneumonitis. Although the clinical features of *Pneumocystis jiroveci* pneumonitis are usually those of an acute pneumonia, the presentation can be subtle and non-specific in immunocompromised state. Thus, physicians should maintain a high index of suspicion for this diagnosis in any patient developing respiratory symptoms. The use of prophylactic antibiotic therapy against this infection can be considered for brain tumor patients receiving prolonged corticosteroid treatment. However, its benefit is still controversial [88, 90]. As new treatment modalities improve survival rate of malignant glioma, long-term steroid complications previously unrecognized, including osteoporosis, compression fractures, and neuropsychiatric disturbance, are becoming more problematic. Vitamin D, calcium supplements, and bisphosphonates should be considered as the preventive measures [88].

Venous thromboembolism is the common cause of perioperative morbidity and mortality in malignant gliomas, with the incidence of 20 to 30% [91]. Old age (>60 years) , large sized tumor and paralytic leg can be regarded as risk factors [92]. Patients with malignant gliomas are often suppose to have increased risk of intracranial hemorrhage after anticoagulation therapy because of the increased vascularity of the tumors. According to a previous report, however, only 2% of intratumoral hemorrhage was complicated by anticoagulation therapy for venous thromboembolism. This complication rate was similar to that of the non-treated group [93]. Currently, it is generally accepted to use low-molecular weight heparin for venous thromboembolism, except in cases with intracerebral hemorrhage or other complications [94]. During and just after the surgery and chemoradiotherapy, patients with malignant gliomas frequently complain of profound fatigue. It is possibly associated with anemia, adverse effect of AED or steroid, and other various factors. Modafinil or methylphenidate may be useful in reducing the fatigue in this situation [95]. Donepezil may improve the decreased cognitive function including attention, mood and verbal memory after radiation treatment [96]. Neuropsychiatric problems can be overlooked in patients with malignant gliomas, and antidepressants and psychiatric support are often invaluable [97].

Although the mainstay of therapy for GBM consists of surgery, radiation and chemotherapy, several make GBM treatment notoriously difficult, including the intrinsic resistance of these lesions to conventional therapy, limited capacity of the brain to repair itself, infiltrative feature of the tumor cells into brain parenchyma, the variably disrupted blood–brain-barrier complicating drug delivery [98]. Current standard treatment is composed of maximal surgical resection and involved-field RT (60 Gy administered in 5 times weekly fractions over 6 weeks) with concurrent TMZ (75 $mg/m^2/d$) . After 4 weeks of rest, patients receive 6-12 cycles of adjuvant TMZ (150 $mg/m^2/d$ for 5 days at the beginning of the first 28-day cycle, followed by 200 $mg/m^2/d$ for 5 days at the beginning of the each subsequent 28-day cycle) [99, 100].

SURGERY

Surgical treatment for GBM remains critical for confirming the diagnosis, alleviating symptoms of mass effect and ICP, and reducing tumor volume [101].

There have been a lot of technical advances focusing on maximizing resection while minimizing injury to surrounding normal tissue. In addition, tissue obtained during the procedure can eventually be used for design of targeted therapies through the individualized analysis of the molecular signature [102]. The extent of surgical resection depends on location and eloquence of the brain areas involved.

However, surgery is always an incomplete debulking, since GBM is a highly infiltrating tumor and cannot be resected completely. Some advantages of radical resection include good relief of intracranial pressure, reversal of some neurologic deficits, lowering of seizure incidence, a definitive pathological diagnosis, and ultimately improved survival.

Although the value of radical microsurgical resection in GBM remains controversial, recent studies suggest that extent of resection is associated with better survival of the patients with GBM [103-106]. Especially, according to the most recent study, the extent of resection beyond critical threshold (eg, 78%) , may impact patient survival [105].

To resect the tumor to the greatest extent, several technical advances should be accompanied simultaneously. New techniques for preoperative radiological evaluations (DTI combined with functional MRI) , intraoperative MRI, three dimensional-image guidance or neuronavigation for tumor delineation, electrophysiological mapping for eloquent areas or 5-aminolevulinic acid (ALA) and, if needed, multimodal combined approach could be considered.

Neuronavigation, widely used for brain tumor surgery, has been assessed prospectively as to whether it improves resection or causes neurological deficits [107]. There was no benefit in terms of the extent of tumor resection and prognosis. This result may be closely related with brain shift and intraoperative distortion of anatomy, compared with that seen on preoperative imaging, mainly due to change of cerebrospinal fluid dynamics and tumor tissue volume [108-110].

Intraoperative collaboration with other techniques, however, has been attempted to overcome the limit of neuronavigation. In addition to integration with DTI, functional MRI, or PET [111-115], three dimensional ultrasonography [112, 114, 116, 117] and intraoperative neurophysiological monitoring [118-120] have been coupled with neuronavigation system.

Despite high cost, low quality of images, and limits of functional evaluation, intraoperative MRI also has been used in glioma surgery. It provides optimization of extent of resection in real time and can be coupled with other modalities, such as neuronavigation or electrophysiological studies [121-127].

The effects of a fluorescent tumor marker (5-ALA) on the degree of resection and survival in GBM surgery have also been recently analyzed [128-131]. The use of intraoperative 5-ALA and fluorescence-guided resection was shown to enhance the total resection rate and offer a survival benefit. Basically, the non-fluorescent prodrug is metabolized to fluorescent protoporphyrin IX in tumor tissue through the heme biosynthesis pathway. The accumulation of protoporphyrin IX in malignant gliomas may be explained by higher 5-ALA uptake in tumor tissue or increased enzyme activity for hemoglobin biosynthesis in tumor cells. Higher 5-ALA uptake may be related to disrupted BBB, increased neovascularization, and the overexpression of membrane transporters in glioma tissue.

Because the protoporphyrin IX level induced by 5-ALA in normal brain tissue is very low, macroscopic visualization of the tumor under the specialized microscope may allow more reliability to neurosurgeons than neuronavigation or standard microscope [102].

Radiation Therapy

External beam radiotherapy (RT) has been used to treat malignant gliomas for decades. It destructs tumor cells through the damage of ionizing radiation in the DNA helix by electrons and free radicals. Although the type of radiation has not been changed substantially, technical advancements have improved significantly to minimize the radiation dose for surrounding normal tissue. The rationale of RT in malignant gliomas is based on the landmark report that showed prolonged survival in treated group compared with the supportive group [132]. RT is usually started within 4 to 6 weeks after surgery and performed with a standard fractionated dose over 6 to 7 weeks [133-135]. Because of the infiltrative nature of malignant gliomas, wide margins are usually included to the treatment plan. The standard dose of external beam RT is 60 Gy in single daily fractions of 1.7-2 Gy, 5 times a week. The decision of margin generally follows the ECORTC and RTOG guidelines [136]. For initial treated volume, the margin expands 2 cm around abnormal area on FLAIR T_2 (46 grays [Gy] at 2 Gy/day) . It includes 2 cm around the enhancing tumor/tumor bed for the boost volume (14 Gy at 2 Gy/day, total 60 Gy) . Prior to therapy, the regions at risk are mapped and a conformal treatment plan is generated that encompasses target volume. Current processes render the significant sparing of surrounding normal tissues while maintaining high dose to the targeted area [137].

Although radiation has a major role in the standard therapy for newly diagnosed malignant gliomas, reirradiation is strongly restricted for recurrent cases because of significant risk for the development of necrosis [138]. However, considering factors such as the patient's performance status, the volume of recurrence tumor, the proximity of the recurrence to previous treated lesion, and the length of time since previous irradiation, reirradiation could be a useful modality with other salvage treatment [139, 140]. In a view of limiting treatment volume and dose reduction, single-fraction stereotactic radiosurgery (SRS) is used to a focal area of small (<3-4 cm) recurrence [141, 142]. SRS has not been associated with benefit for newly diagnosed GBMs as a boost to a standard RT [143]. In recurrence cases, however, it may lengthen the time to disease progression [144, 145]. Another option is the stereotactic brachytherapy, using stereotactic technique for implanting or infusing the radioactive isotope (eg, ^{125}I, ^{192}Ir, ^{252}Californium) within the confined tumor cavity [146, 147]. It delivers an additional 50-65 Gy of radiation during 4-7 days, bringing the total dose of radiation up to 110-120 Gy [138]. As a primary treatment, it is mainly adopted for well-defined, unilateral supratentorial tumors less than 5 cm in diameter without involvement of corpus callosum, brain stem, or ependymal surface. Although both SRS and brachytherapy are performed in a single treatment session, they can cause radiation necrosis of the residual tumor and sometimes the surrounding brain, which can necessitate surgery for relief of mass effect [148]. Recent studies, however, provide evidence that stereotactic RT has therapeutic effect in recurrent malignant gliomas both in terms of survival duration and morbidity, compared with other treatment strategies [149-152]. According to the most recent study, more favorable prognosis was found in younger patients, patients with less-extensive areas of disease progression or a short time interval between initial diagnosis and progression [149]. Reirradiation by means of hypofractionated delivery might have particular appeal for patients who have recurrent tumors that are too large to be considered for single-fraction SRS. Further investigations should be performed about the possibility of combining radiation with conventional chemotherapy, molecularly targeted therapy, or immunotherapy at the time of progression [153].

CHEMOTHERAPY

Among many chemotherapeutics tested for treatment of GBM, alkylating agents have frequently been used in clinical setting. Alkylating agents (including the nitrosoureas, procarbazine and TMZ) work by alkylating cellular DNA, leading to DNA cross-links and cell death. Alkylation at the O^6 site on guanine is particularly important [99, 154]. These agents can be classified into methylating drugs like TMZ and procarbazine, and chloroethylating drugs like carmustine (bis-(2-cholorethyl) -nitrosourea, BCNU) and lomustine (1-(2-chloroethyl) -3-cyclohexyl-1-nitrosourea, CCNU) , according to the alkyl group donated to O^6-guanine by O^6-alkylguanine DNA alkyltransferase (AGT) [154].

Nitrosourea compounds (BCNU and CCNU) act by forming O^6-chloroethylguanine lesions, converted to G-C interstrand crosslinks within 8-12 hours of formation [155], and these are very poorly repaired in mammalian cells. It is estimated that 2-5 crosslinks can kill a cell whereas over 5000 O^6-methylguanine lesions are required to do the same [156]. However, an aggressive regimen with these agents causes considerable side effects, leading to dose reductions and corresponding decreases in therapeutic efficacy [157]. Because of lipid solubility and ability to cross the blood-brain-barrier, nitrosoureas have been used for early randomized clinical trials as a adjuvant chemotherapy for malignant gliomas [158, 159]. In addition to the positive result from these studies, meta-analyses confirm that chemotherapy offers a modest survival benefit (a 6%–10% increase in 1-year survival) for patients with malignant glioma [160, 161]. Based on this data, the most commonly used regimens are BCNU or PCV (combination of procarbazine, CCNU, and vincristine) . However, prospective randomized trials using these regimens have failed to demonstrate a survival benefit [162].

TMZ, an oral alkylating agent, can reach maximum plasma concentration 30 to 90 minutes after intake with the plasma half-life of 2 hours [163]. Methylation of the O^6 site on guanine, the biologically most pertinent site of DNA methylation by TMZ, will trigger activation of the mismatch repair process [164] to result in G2 checkpoint activation leading to G2/M cell cycle arrest and eventually to induction of apoptosis [165-167]. Severe or life-threatening toxicity is rare. Common mild to moderate adverse effects are nausea and vomiting, constipation, and some fatigue. Noncumulative myelosuppression, particularly thrombocytopenia occurring 3 to 4 weeks after treatment start, is the most serious and dose-limiting toxicity, observed in less than 10% of patients [168-170].

A new standard of treatment for GBM emerged in 2005 [134]. A large, randomized, multicenter, phase III trial included 573 newly diagnosed GBM patients. The patients who were surgical candidates underwent maximal feasible resection. Then, all patients consecutively received standard RT (60 Gy over 6 weeks) and were randomly assigned to receive TMZ chemotherapy or no chemotherapy. In the chemotherapy arm, patients received radiotherapy with concurrent TMZ at a dose of 75 $mg/m^2/d$ for 6 weeks. After a 4-week break, patients received 6 cycles of adjuvant TMZ (150 to 200 $mg/m^2/d$ for 5 days during each 28-day cycle) . Median survival in chemotherapy group improved to 14.6 months (*vs* 12.1 mos in non-chemotherapy group) . More strikingly, the 2-year survival rate improved with TMZ therapy, from 10.4% to 26.5% ($P < 0.001$) . The trial tumor specimens were evaluated for O^6-methylguanine-DNA methyltransferase (MGMT) gene silencing [133]. Previous studies hypothesized that DNA methylation of the MGMT gene promoter region is an epigenetic modification that can reduce DNA repair activity and increase susceptibility to chemotherapy [171-173]. Among TMZ treated patients with MGMT promoter methylation, median survival was 21.7 months, and 2-year survival was a remarkable 46%. In contrast, temozolomide-treated patients without MGMT promoter methylation had a significantly shorter median survival of only 12.7 months, and a 2-year survival of 13.8%. This study provided evidence that MGMT promoter methylation was associated with better outcome in the RT and TMZ group, suggesting that it may be a predictive marker for sensitivity to alkylating chemotherapy. Several investigational approaches to suppress MGMT activity include dose intense TMZ regimens [174, 175] and combination therapy with O^6-benzylguanine or other MGMT inhibitors [176]. In addition to MGMT, the DNA repair enzyme poly(ADP-ribose) polymerase (PARP) may promote chemotherapy resistance in patients with malignant gliomas. PARP inhibitors such as BSI-201, ABT-888, and several others may be effective when combined with RT and TMZ [177, 178].

However, more than 50% of patients with GBM retain MGMT expression and demonstrate less sensitivity to TMZ, presumably because MGMT repairs the TMZ-induced DNA damage. These unmethylated patients who received TMZ had an approximate 10%–15% actuarial overall survival time at the 2-year survival point, compared with 0% in those who did not receive TMZ. Recent study showed that MGMT methylation is a predictive marker of radiation response, independently of TMZ treatment and may be a general surrogate marker of favorable prognosis in GBM [179]. This observation indicates that MGMT methylation status is not the sole predictor of GBM response to TMZ and this drug of choice, as the standard of care, should not be withheld from any GBM patient.

Gliadel wafer, an interstitial chemotherapy drug implanted within the tumor resection cavity, contains the BCNU and biodegradable polyanhydride copolymer. The advantages of this approach include achieving high concentrations of chemotherapeutic agent at the local resection site with minimal systemic toxicity and eliminating the problem of brain-blood-barrier penetration. Techniques that have been used include up to 8 Gliadel wafers that are placed in the resection cavity and designed to release BCNU slowly over a period of 2-3 weeks. Clinical trials results have shown that Gliadel prolonged survival in a statistically albeit modest manner in newly diagnosed patients [180]. The patients enrolled in this study received either conventional therapy (surgery followed by RT) with placement of a BCNU wafer or conventional therapy with placement of an identical placebo wafer. The median survival was increased for the BCNU wafer group (13.9 months) compared with the placebo wafer group (11.6 months) , with 1-year survival rates of 59.2% and 49.6%, respectively (P=0.03) , a 28% reduction in the risk of death and significant sustaining in neuroperformance status. This survival advantage was maintained at 2 and 3 years [181]. Although there have been reports that use of Gliadel wafer was not associated with an increase in perioperative morbidity after surgical treatment of malignant glioma, its use may have side-effects including seizure, brain edema, wound healing problems, intracranial infection, and delay in the administration of other drugs [180, 182]. Combination of both treatment strategies, local chemotherapy with Gliadel wafer and the standard concomitant radiochemotherapy, appears attractive in aggressive multimodal treatment schedules [183]. However, questionable survival benefit and possible increased toxicity warrant further evaluation [184, 185]. Although second line cytotoxic agents including carboplatin, etoposide, oxaliplatin, and irinotecan can be considered for the patients who do not respond to standard TMZ therapy, they produce low response rates and no significant survival benefit [101].

TARGET THERAPY

Various potential therapeutic targets have been developed based on the understanding of molecular mechanism and pathogenesis of glioma development and recognition of differences explaining various clinical courses among tumors with similar morphology. Molecular profiling of glioma has presented signaling pathways driving the malignant behavior of tumors and induction of cell migration and tumor invasiveness [186-188]. These pathways are activated by amplification of receptor tyrosine kinases such as the epidermal growth factor receptor (EGFR) , platelet-derived growth factor receptor (PDGFR) , insulin-like growth factor receptor (IGFR) , and others that lead to activation of downstream mediators if unopposed by tumor suppressors such as PTEN (phosphatase and tensin homolog on chromosome 10) . PTEN, frequently inactivated in malignant glioma, is a negative regulator of phosphatidylinositol-3 kinase (PI3K) , through several pathways linked with tumor-promoting function (eg, protein kinase C and the activated ras pathway) [99, 189]. Main targets have focused on receptor tyrosine kinases inhibitors such as EGFR and PDGFR, as well as on signal-transduction inhibitors targeting mTOR, farnesyltransferase, and PI3K [35, 190-193]. However, single agent therapies have been disappointing in malignant gliomas, with response rates of 10-15% or less and no prolongation of survival [100, 194, 195]. These results can be explained by some factors.

Malignant gliomas have coactivation of multiple tyrosine kinases [196], including redundant signaling pathway, and limit the activity of single agent. In addition, many of these agents have poor penetration ability through the blood-brain-barrier. Current developing strategies to increase the effectiveness of targeted molecular therapies include the use of a single agent targeted against several kinases, combinations of targeted agents, and targeted agents combined with radiotherapy and chemotherapy [194, 195, 197].

Vascular endothelial growth factor (VEGF) and its receptors (VEGFR) have emerged as other therapeutic targets. Because malignant gliomas are the most vascular among human tumors, VEGF is a critical stimulatory factor in tumor angiogenesis, as well as in the production of peritumoral edema [32, 198].

After bevacizumab (Avastin, humanized monoclonal antibody against VEGF) was approved by FDA for colon cancer, this agent had been introduced into neurooncological field for recurrent malignant gliomas often in combination with irinotecan.

According to the early clinical data, its response rate has been reported from 25% to 74%, with 6-month progression-free survival (PFS6) rate of 32% to 64% [199-205].

These results are superior to the 5-8% response rate and 21% PFS6 rate reported for TMZ [206]. The first trial randomly assigned 167 patients with recurrent GBM to bevacizumab therapy (10mg/kg IV every 2 weeks) with or without irinotecan (340 mg/m^2 IV with enzyme-inducing antiepileptic drug or 125 mg/m^2 without antiepileptic drug) [207]. Objective response rates were reported to be between 28% and 38%, and PFS6 rates ranged from 43% to 50%. In addition to hemorrhagic and thromboembolic complications, common toxicities observed in these studies included hypertension, proteinuria, fatigue, and wound-healing complications.

In another trial, bevacizumab monotherapy was tested in 48 heavily pretreated patients with recurrent GBM [208]. The radiological response rate was 35%, and the PFS6 rate was 29%. Phase III studies are ongoing for evaluation of the combination of bevacizumab with standard TMZ and RT. Preliminary results report that the addition of bevacizumab with standard TMZ and RT was found to be associated with minimal toxicity in patients newly diagnosed with GM [209].

Recently, a phase II trial for the combination of bevacizumab and irinotecan with standard TMZ and RT reported moderate toxicity and possible efficacy compared with the standard therapy [210].

Median overall survival was 21.2 months, and 65% of the patients were alive at 16 months. The median progression-free survival was 14.2 months. Combination of bevacizumab and other chemotherapeutics and targeted molecular drugs is also currently in clinical trial.

RECURRENT GBM

Recurrence is generally found as an increase in tumor size (≥25%) associated with increased edema and mass effect on MRI (or newly developed mass with a variable free interval, after complete removal documented on postoperative MRI) or unequivocal neurological deterioration. The Macdonald criteria, which rely on consecutive contrast-enhanced T1-weighted MRI or CT scans, use the enhancing tumor area as the primary parameter [211]. In addition to the difficulty of measuring the irregular-shaped glioma, however, recent observations have revealed the fundamental limitations to this approach [27, 212, 213]. These limitations include variable differences in different observers, the lack of assessment of non-enhancing component, the lack of the guidance for multifocal tumors, and the difficulty in measuring enhancing lesions in the wall of cystic or surgical cavities. Currently, it has been recommended to use the updated response assessment in Neuro-Oncology (RANO) criteria for radiological evaluation in malignant glioma treatment [214]. Although this criteria is also based on the maximal cross-sectional enhancing diameter to determine the size of the contrast-enhancing lesion (>5 mm increase in maximal diameter or ≥25% increase in sum of the products of perpendicular diameters of enhancing lesions) , it includes evaluation of non-enhancing MRI (T2-weighted or FLAIR images) for volume changes of tumor. The RANO criteria also modify the definition of measurable disease and introduce the clear definition for pseudoprogression. Tumor cyst, surgical cavity and nodular enhanced (< 10 mm) should not be measured in determining response. The neurological deterioration, based on the KPS, is defined as a decline to 70 or less from 90 or 100, a decline of at least 20 from 80 or less, or a decline to 50 or less without comorbid events or changes in steroid dose.

Pseudoprogression can be defined as radiological progression after adjuvant chemoradiotherapy, which stabilizes or improves with the same treatment or no further therapy [215]. Among the radiological aggravation after concurrent RT and TMZ, 20-50% of the cases were diagnosed with pseudoprogression [216-218]. According to the recent published data [219], median survival was significantly prolonged in pseudoprogression group compared with that of the patient with true progression (125 vs 36 weeks) . This survival prolongation can be explained by the possible correlation of pseudoprogression with the status of MGMT promoter methylation [220]. Considering the difficulty in differentiating pseudoprogression from true progression in the first 3 months after concurrent chemoradiotherapy, adjuvant TMZ should be continued for a minimum of 3 cycles with close observation unless new enhanced lesion develops clearly outside the RT field [214, 215]. Although various kinds of imaging modalities, such as MRS, diffusion or perfusion MR, and PET scan, have been introduced to help the diagnosis of pseudoprogression [27], repeated imaging studies may ultimately distinguish the true progression from pseudoprogression.

The treatment approach can be influenced by several factors including patient age, performance status, histology, extent initial resection, response to initial therapy, time since diagnosis, and recurrence feature (local vs diffuse) . Reoperation may be indicated in selected patients with a high KPS score and an easily accessible location [215]. Even though reirradiation or SRT has been shown to be beneficial, their usefulness remains controversial [138]. Medtromic TMZ, bevacizumab alone or in combination with irinotecan, nitrosourea-based regimens (BCNU, PCV) , and various investigational therapies have been used for recurrent GBM.

REFERENCES

[1] Kleihues P, Nakazato Y, Burger PC, Plate KH, Aldape KD, Giangaspero F, Brat DJ, von Deimling A, Biernat W, Ohgaki H *et al*: Glioblastoma. In: *WHO Classification of Tumours of the Central Nervous System.* Edited by Louis DN, Ohgaki H, Wiestler OD, Cavenee WK. Lyon: IARC Press; 2007: 33-49.

[2] Ohgaki H, Kleihues P: Population-based studies on incidence, survival rates, and genetic alterations in astrocytic and oligodendroglial gliomas. *Journal of neuropathology and experimental neurology* 2005, 64(6):479-489.

[3] Ohgaki H, Dessen P, Jourde B, Horstmann S, Nishikawa T, Di Patre PL, Burkhard C, Schuler D, Probst-Hensch NM, Maiorka PC et al: Genetic pathways to glioblastoma: a population-based study. Cancer research 2004, 64(19):6892-6899.

[4] Salcman M: Glioblastoma multiforme and anaplastic astrocytoma. In: *Brain tumors: an encyclopedic approach.* Edited by Kaye AH, Laws ER Jr. London: Churchill Livingstone; 2001: 494-523.

[5] Sanchez-Herrera F, Castro-Sierra E, Gordillo-Dominguez LF, Vaca-Ruiz MA, Santana-Montero B, Perezpena-Diazconti M, Gonzalez-Carranza V, Torres-Garcia S, Chico-Ponce de Leon F: Glioblastoma

multiforme in children: experience at Hospital Infantil de Mexico Federico Gomez. *Childs Nerv. Syst.* 2009, 25(5):551-557.
[6] Ohgaki H: Epidemiology of brain tumors. *Methods in molecular biology* 2009, 472:323-342.
[7] Fan KJ, Pezeshkpour GH: Ethnic distribution of primary central nervous system tumors in Washington, DC, 1971 to 1985. *Journal of the National Medical Association* 1992, 84(10):858-863.
[8] McLendon RE, Robinson JS, Jr., Chambers DB, Grufferman S, Burger PC: The glioblastoma multiforme in Georgia, 1977-1981. *Cancer* 1985, 56(4):894-897.
[9] Koch HJ, Klinkhammer-Schalke M, Hofstadter F, Bogdahn U, Hau P: Seasonal patterns of birth in patients with glioblastoma. *Chronobiology international* 2006, 23(5):1047-1052.
[10] Brenner AV, Linet MS, Shapiro WR, Selker RG, Fine HA, Black PM, Inskip PD: Season of birth and risk of brain tumors in adults. *Neurology* 2004, 63(2):276-281.
[11] Ohgaki H, Huang H, Haltia M, Vainio H, Kleihues P: More about: cell and molecular biology of simian virus 40: implications for human infections and disease. *Journal of the National Cancer Institute* 2000, 92(6):495-497.
[12] Vilchez RA, Kozinetz CA, Arrington AS, Madden CR, Butel JS: Simian virus 40 in human cancers. *The American journal of medicine* 2003, 114(8):675-684.
[13] Pandey JP: Genetic and Viral Etiology of Glioblastoma--a Unifying Hypothesis. *Cancer Epidemiol Biomarkers Prev* 2011, 20(6):1061-1063.
[14] Farrell CJ, Plotkin SR: Genetic causes of brain tumors: neurofibromatosis, tuberous sclerosis, von Hippel-Lindau, and other syndromes. *Neurologic clinics* 2007, 25(4):925-946, viii.
[15] Tamber MS, Rutka JT: Pediatric supratentorial high-grade gliomas. *Neurosurgical focus* 2003, 14(2):e1.
[16] Fisher JL, Schwartzbaum JA, Wrensch M, Wiemels JL: Epidemiology of brain tumors. *Neurologic clinics* 2007, 25(4):867-890, vii.
[17] Moss AR: Occupational exposure and brain tumors. *Journal of toxicology and environmental health* 1985, 16(5):703-711.
[18] Ron E, Modan B, Boice JD, Jr., Alfandary E, Stovall M, Chetrit A, Katz L: Tumors of the brain and nervous system after radiotherapy in childhood. *The New England journal of medicine* 1988, 319(16):1033-1039.

[19] Siemiatycki J, Richardson L, Straif K, Latreille B, Lakhani R, Campbell S, Rousseau MC, Boffetta P: Listing occupational carcinogens. *Environmental health perspectives* 2004, 112(15):1447-1459.

[20] Linos E, Raine T, Alonso A, Michaud D: Atopy and risk of brain tumors: a meta-analysis. *Journal of the National Cancer Institute* 2007, 99(20):1544-1550.

[21] Schoemaker MJ, Swerdlow AJ, Hepworth SJ, McKinney PA, van Tongeren M, Muir KR: History of allergies and risk of glioma in adults. *International journal of cancer* 2006, 119(9):2165-2172.

[22] Wiemels JL, Wiencke JK, Patoka J, Moghadassi M, Chew T, McMillan A, Miike R, Barger G, Wrensch M: Reduced immunoglobulin E and allergy among adults with glioma compared with controls. *Cancer research* 2004, 64(22):8468-8473.

[23] Wiemels JL, Wiencke JK, Kelsey KT, Moghadassi M, Rice T, Urayama KY, Miike R, Wrensch M: Allergy-related polymorphisms influence glioma status and serum IgE levels. *Cancer Epidemiol Biomarkers Prev* 2007, 16(6):1229-1235.

[24] Khurana VG, Teo C, Kundi M, Hardell L, Carlberg M: Cell phones and brain tumors: a review including the long-term epidemiologic data. *Surgical neurology* 2009, 72(3):205-214.

[25] Myung SK, Ju W, McDonnell DD, Lee YJ, Kazinets G, Cheng CT, Moskowitz JM: Mobile phone use and risk of tumors: a meta-analysis. *J. Clin. Oncol* 2009, 27(33):5565-5572.

[26] Baglietto L, Giles GG, English DR, Karahalios A, Hopper JL, Severi G: Alcohol consumption and risk of glioblastoma; evidence from the Melbourne Collaborative Cohort Study. *International journal of cancer*, 128(8):1929-1934.

[27] Sorensen AG, Batchelor TT, Wen PY, Zhang WT, Jain RK: Response criteria for glioma. *Nature clinical practice* 2008, 5(11):634-644.

[28] Jackson A, Kassner A, Annesley-Williams D, Reid H, Zhu XP, Li KL: Abnormalities in the recirculation phase of contrast agent bolus passage in cerebral gliomas: comparison with relative blood volume and tumor grade. *Ajnr.* 2002, 23(1):7-14.

[29] Law M, Oh S, Johnson G, Babb JS, Zagzag D, Golfinos J, Kelly PJ: Perfusion magnetic resonance imaging predicts patient outcome as an adjunct to histopathology: a second reference standard in the surgical and nonsurgical treatment of low-grade gliomas. *Neurosurgery* 2006, 58(6):1099-1107.

[30] Lev MH, Rosen BR: Clinical applications of intracranial perfusion MR imaging. *Neuroimaging clinics of North America* 1999, 9(2):309-331.

[31] Cha S: Update on brain tumor imaging: from anatomy to physiology. *Ajnr* 2006, 27(3):475-487.

[32] Jain RK, di Tomaso E, Duda DG, Loeffler JS, Sorensen AG, Batchelor TT: Angiogenesis in brain tumours. *Nature reviews* 2007, 8(8):610-622.

[33] Gerstner ER, Sorensen AG, Jain RK, Batchelor TT: Advances in neuroimaging techniques for the evaluation of tumor growth, vascular permeability, and angiogenesis in gliomas. *Current opinion in neurology* 2008, 21(6):728-735.

[34] Claes A, Wesseling P, Jeuken J, Maass C, Heerschap A, Leenders WP: Antiangiogenic compounds interfere with chemotherapy of brain tumors due to vessel normalization. *Molecular cancer therapeutics* 2008, 7(1):71-78.

[35] Batchelor TT, Sorensen AG, di Tomaso E, Zhang WT, Duda DG, Cohen KS, Kozak KR, Cahill DP, Chen PJ, Zhu M *et al*: AZD2171, a pan-VEGF receptor tyrosine kinase inhibitor, normalizes tumor vasculature and alleviates edema in glioblastoma patients. *Cancer cell* 2007, 11(1):83-95.

[36] Barajas RF, Jr., Chang JS, Segal MR, Parsa AT, McDermott MW, Berger MS, Cha S: Differentiation of recurrent glioblastoma multiforme from radiation necrosis after external beam radiation therapy with dynamic susceptibility-weighted contrast-enhanced perfusion MR imaging. *Radiology* 2009, 253(2):486-496.

[37] Henry RG, Vigneron DB, Fischbein NJ, Grant PE, Day MR, Noworolski SM, Star-Lack JM, Wald LL, Dillon WP, Chang SM *et al*: Comparison of relative cerebral blood volume and proton spectroscopy in patients with treated gliomas. *Ajnr.* 2000, 21(2):357-366.

[38] Lupo JM, Cha S, Chang SM, Nelson SJ: Dynamic susceptibility-weighted perfusion imaging of high-grade gliomas: characterization of spatial heterogeneity. *Ajnr.* 2005, 26(6):1446-1454.

[39] Maia AC, Jr., Malheiros SM, da Rocha AJ, da Silva CJ, Gabbai AA, Ferraz FA, Stavale JN: MR cerebral blood volume maps correlated with vascular endothelial growth factor expression and tumor grade in nonenhancing gliomas. *Ajnr.* 2005, 26(4):777-783.

[40] Sadeghi N, D'Haene N, Decaestecker C, Levivier M, Metens T, Maris C, Wikler D, Baleriaux D, Salmon I, Goldman S: Apparent diffusion coefficient and cerebral blood volume in brain gliomas: relation to tumor

cell density and tumor microvessel density based on stereotactic biopsies. *Ajnr.* 2008, 29(3):476-482.

[41] Sugahara T, Korogi Y, Kochi M, Ikushima I, Hirai T, Okuda T, Shigematsu Y, Liang L, Ge Y, Ushio Y *et al*: Correlation of MR imaging-determined cerebral blood volume maps with histologic and angiographic determination of vascularity of gliomas. *Ajnr.* 1998, 171(6):1479-1486.

[42] Le Bihan D, Breton E, Lallemand D, Grenier P, Cabanis E, Laval-Jeantet M: MR imaging of intravoxel incoherent motions: application to diffusion and perfusion in neurologic disorders. *Radiology* 1986, 161(2):401-407.

[43] Chenevert TL, Stegman LD, Taylor JM, Robertson PL, Greenberg HS, Rehemtulla A, Ross BD: Diffusion magnetic resonance imaging: an early surrogate marker of therapeutic efficacy in brain tumors. *Journal of the National Cancer Institute* 2000, 92(24):2029-2036.

[44] Higano S, Yun X, Kumabe T, Watanabe M, Mugikura S, Umetsu A, Sato A, Yamada T, Takahashi S: Malignant astrocytic tumors: clinical importance of apparent diffusion coefficient in prediction of grade and prognosis. *Radiology.* 2006, 241(3):839-846.

[45] Kitis O, Altay H, Calli C, Yunten N, Akalin T, Yurtseven T: Minimum apparent diffusion coefficients in the evaluation of brain tumors. *European journal of radiology.* 2005, 55(3):393-400.

[46] Sugahara T, Korogi Y, Kochi M, Ikushima I, Shigematu Y, Hirai T, Okuda T, Liang L, Ge Y, Komohara Y *et al*: Usefulness of diffusion-weighted MRI with echo-planar technique in the evaluation of cellularity in gliomas. *J Magn Reson Imaging* 1999, 9(1):53-60.

[47] Guo AC, Cummings TJ, Dash RC, Provenzale JM: Lymphomas and high-grade astrocytomas: comparison of water diffusibility and histologic characteristics. *Radiology.* 2002, 224(1):177-183.

[48] Stadnik TW, Chaskis C, Michotte A, Shabana WM, van Rompaey K, Luypaert R, Budinsky L, Jellus V, Osteaux M: Diffusion-weighted MR imaging of intracerebral masses: comparison with conventional MR imaging and histologic findings. *Ajnr.* 2001, 22(5):969-976.

[49] Gupta RK, Cloughesy TF, Sinha U, Garakian J, Lazareff J, Rubino G, Rubino L, Becker DP, Vinters HV, Alger JR: Relationships between choline magnetic resonance spectroscopy, apparent diffusion coefficient and quantitative histopathology in human glioma. *Journal of neuro-oncology.* 2000, 50(3):215-226.

[50] Mardor Y, Pfeffer R, Spiegelmann R, Roth Y, Maier SE, Nissim O, Berger R, Glicksman A, Baram J, Orenstein A *et al*: Early detection of response to radiation therapy in patients with brain malignancies using conventional and high b-value diffusion-weighted magnetic resonance imaging. *J. Clin. Oncol.* 2003, 21(6):1094-1100.

[51] Moffat BA, Chenevert TL, Lawrence TS, Meyer CR, Johnson TD, Dong Q, Tsien C, Mukherji S, Quint DJ, Gebarski SS *et al*: Functional diffusion map: a noninvasive MRI biomarker for early stratification of clinical brain tumor response. *Proceedings of the National Academy of Sciences of the United States of America.* 2005, 102(15):5524-5529.

[52] Hamstra DA, Galban CJ, Meyer CR, Johnson TD, Sundgren PC, Tsien C, Lawrence TS, Junck L, Ross DJ, Rehemtulla A *et al*: Functional diffusion map as an early imaging biomarker for high-grade glioma: correlation with conventional radiologic response and overall survival. *J. Clin. Oncol.* 2008, 26(20):3387-3394.

[53] Basser PJ, Pajevic S, Pierpaoli C, Duda J, Aldroubi A: In vivo fiber tractography using DT-MRI data. *Magn Reson Med* 2000, 44(4):625-632.

[54] Morita K, Matsuzawa H, Fujii Y, Tanaka R, Kwee IL, Nakada T: Diffusion tensor analysis of peritumoral edema using lambda chart analysis indicative of the heterogeneity of the microstructure within edema. *Journal of neurosurgery.* 2005, 102(2):336-341.

[55] Lu S, Ahn D, Johnson G, Law M, Zagzag D, Grossman RI: Diffusion-tensor MR imaging of intracranial neoplasia and associated peritumoral edema: introduction of the tumor infiltration index. *Radiology.* 2004, 232(1):221-228.

[56] Wu JS, Zhou LF, Tang WJ, Mao Y, Hu J, Song YY, Hong XN, Du GH: Clinical evaluation and follow-up outcome of diffusion tensor imaging-based functional neuronavigation: a prospective, controlled study in patients with gliomas involving pyramidal tracts. *Neurosurgery.* 2007, 61(5):935-948.

[57] Chaskis C, Stadnik T, Michotte A, Van Rompaey K, D'Haens J: Prognostic value of perfusion-weighted imaging in brain glioma: a prospective study. *Acta neurochirurgica.* 2006, 148(3):277-285.

[58] Pathak AP, Schmainda KM, Ward BD, Linderman JR, Rebro KJ, Greene AS: MR-derived cerebral blood volume maps: issues regarding histological validation and assessment of tumor angiogenesis. *Magn. Reson Med.* 2001, 46(4):735-747.

[59] Aronen HJ, Pardo FS, Kennedy DN, Belliveau JW, Packard SD, Hsu DW, Hochberg FH, Fischman AJ, Rosen BR: High microvascular blood volume is associated with high glucose uptake and tumor angiogenesis in human gliomas. *Clin. Cancer Res.* 2000, 6(6):2189-2200.

[60] Aronen HJ, Gazit IE, Louis DN, Buchbinder BR, Pardo FS, Weisskoff RM, Harsh GR, Cosgrove GR, Halpern EF, Hochberg FH *et al*: Cerebral blood volume maps of gliomas: comparison with tumor grade and histologic findings. *Radiology.* 1994, 191(1):41-51.

[61] Cha S, Johnson G, Wadghiri YZ, Jin O, Babb J, Zagzag D, Turnbull DH: Dynamic, contrast-enhanced perfusion MRI in mouse gliomas: correlation with histopathology. *Magn. Reson. Med.* 2003, 49(5):848-855.

[62] Sibtain NA, Howe FA, Saunders DE: The clinical value of proton magnetic resonance spectroscopy in adult brain tumours. *Clinical radiology.* 2007, 62(2):109-119.

[63] Young GS: Advanced MRI of adult brain tumors. *Neurologic clinics* 2007, 25(4):947-973, viii.

[64] Gajewicz W, Papierz W, Szymczak W, Goraj B: The use of proton MRS in the differential diagnosis of brain tumors and tumor-like processes. *Med. Sci. Monit.* 2003, 9(9):MT97-105.

[65] Del Sole A, Falini A, Ravasi L, Ottobrini L, De Marchis D, Bombardieri E, Lucignani G: Anatomical and biochemical investigation of primary brain tumours. *European journal of nuclear medicine.* 2001, 28(12):1851-1872.

[66] Delorme S, Weber MA: Applications of MRS in the evaluation of focal malignant brain lesions. *Cancer Imaging.* 2006, 6:95-99.

[67] Nelson SJ, McKnight TR, Henry RG: Characterization of untreated gliomas by magnetic resonance spectroscopic imaging. *Neuroimaging clinics of North America.* 2002, 12(4):599-613.

[68] Dowling C, Bollen AW, Noworolski SM, McDermott MW, Barbaro NM, Day MR, Henry RG, Chang SM, Dillon WP, Nelson SJ *et al*: Preoperative proton MR spectroscopic imaging of brain tumors: correlation with histopathologic analysis of resection specimens. *Ajnr.* 2001, 22(4):604-612.

[69] Nelson SJ: Multivoxel magnetic resonance spectroscopy of brain tumors. *Molecular cancer therapeutics.* 2003, 2(5):497-507.

[70] Pirzkall A, McKnight TR, Graves EE, Carol MP, Sneed PK, Wara WW, Nelson SJ, Verhey LJ, Larson DA: MR-spectroscopy guided target

delineation for high-grade gliomas. *International journal of radiation oncology, biology, physics.* 2001, 50(4):915-928.

[71] Rock JP, Scarpace L, Hearshen D, Gutierrez J, Fisher JL, Rosenblum M, Mikkelsen T: Associations among magnetic resonance spectroscopy, apparent diffusion coefficients, and image-guided histopathology with special attention to radiation necrosis. *Neurosurgery.* 2004, 54(5):1111-1117.

[72] Matsusue E, Fink JR, Rockhill JK, Ogawa T, Maravilla KR: Distinction between glioma progression and post-radiation change by combined physiologic MR imaging. *Neuroradiology*, 52(4):297-306.

[73] Zeng QS, Li CF, Liu H, Zhen JH, Feng DC: Distinction between recurrent glioma and radiation injury using magnetic resonance spectroscopy in combination with diffusion-weighted imaging. *International journal of radiation oncology, biology, physics.* 2007, 68(1):151-158.

[74] Graves EE, Nelson SJ, Vigneron DB, Verhey L, McDermott M, Larson D, Chang S, Prados MD, Dillon WP: Serial proton MR spectroscopic imaging of recurrent malignant gliomas after gamma knife radiosurgery. *Ajnr* 2001, 22(4):613-624.

[75] Chan AA, Lau A, Pirzkall A, Chang SM, Verhey LJ, Larson D, McDermott MW, Dillon WP, Nelson SJ: Proton magnetic resonance spectroscopy imaging in the evaluation of patients undergoing gamma knife surgery for Grade IV glioma. *Journal of neurosurgery.* 2004, 101(3):467-475.

[76] Vallabhajosula S: (18) F-labeled positron emission tomographic radiopharmaceuticals in oncology: an overview of radiochemistry and mechanisms of tumor localization. *Seminars in nuclear medicine.* 2007, 37(6):400-419.

[77] Chen W: Clinical applications of PET in brain tumors. *J. Nucl. Med.* 2007, 48(9):1468-1481.

[78] Barwick T, Bencherif B, Mountz JM, Avril N: Molecular PET and PET/CT imaging of tumour cell proliferation using F-18 fluoro-L-thymidine: a comprehensive evaluation. *Nuclear medicine communications.* 2009, 30(12):908-917.

[79] Ullrich R, Backes H, Li H, Kracht L, Miletic H, Kesper K, Neumaier B, Heiss WD, Wienhard K, Jacobs AH: Glioma proliferation as assessed by 3'-fluoro-3'-deoxy-L-thymidine positron emission tomography in patients with newly diagnosed high-grade glioma. *Clin. Cancer Res.* 2008, 14(7):2049-2055.

[80] Chen W, Cloughesy T, Kamdar N, Satyamurthy N, Bergsneider M, Liau L, Mischel P, Czernin J, Phelps ME, Silverman DH: Imaging proliferation in brain tumors with 18F-FLT PET: comparison with 18F-FDG. *J. Nucl. Med.*. 2005, 46(6):945-952.

[81] Chen W, Delaloye S, Silverman DH, Geist C, Czernin J, Sayre J, Satyamurthy N, Pope W, Lai A, Phelps ME *et al*: Predicting treatment response of malignant gliomas to bevacizumab and irinotecan by imaging proliferation with [18F] fluorothymidine positron emission tomography: a pilot study. *J. Clin. Oncol.* 2007, 25(30):4714-4721.

[82] Rasey JS, Grunbaum Z, Magee S, Nelson NJ, Olive PL, Durand RE, Krohn KA: Characterization of radiolabeled fluoromisonidazole as a probe for hypoxic cells. *Radiation research.* 1987, 111(2):292-304.

[83] Cher LM, Murone C, Lawrentschuk N, Ramdave S, Papenfuss A, Hannah A, O'Keefe GJ, Sachinidis JI, Berlangieri SU, Fabinyi G *et al*: Correlation of hypoxic cell fraction and angiogenesis with glucose metabolic rate in gliomas using 18F-fluoromisonidazole, 18F-FDG PET, and immunohistochemical studies. *J. Nucl. Med.* 2006, 47(3):410-418.

[84] Spence AM, Muzi M, Swanson KR, O'Sullivan F, Rockhill JK, Rajendran JG, Adamsen TC, Link JM, Swanson PE, Yagle KJ *et al*: Regional hypoxia in glioblastoma multiforme quantified with [18F]fluoromisonidazole positron emission tomography before radiotherapy: correlation with time to progression and survival. *Clin. Cancer Res.* 2008, 14(9):2623-2630.

[85] Kawai N, Maeda Y, Kudomi N, Miyake K, Okada M, Yamamoto Y, Nishiyama Y, Tamiya T: Correlation of biological aggressiveness assessed by 11C-methionine PET and hypoxic burden assessed by 18F-fluoromisonidazole PET in newly diagnosed glioblastoma. *European journal of nuclear medicine and molecular imaging*, 38(3):441-450.

[86] Hatakeyama T, Kawai N, Nishiyama Y, Yamamoto Y, Sasakawa Y, Ichikawa T, Tamiya T: 11C-methionine (MET) and 18F-fluorothymidine (FLT) PET in patients with newly diagnosed glioma. *European journal of nuclear medicine and molecular imaging.* 2008, 35(11):2009-2017.

[87] Miwa K, Shinoda J, Yano H, Okumura A, Iwama T, Nakashima T, Sakai N: Discrepancy between lesion distributions on methionine PET and MR images in patients with glioblastoma multiforme: insight from a PET and MR fusion image study. *Journal of neurology, neurosurgery, and psychiatry* 2004, 75(10):1457-1462.

[88] Wen PY, Schiff D, Kesari S, Drappatz J, Gigas DC, Doherty L: Medical management of patients with brain tumors. *Journal of neuro-oncology.* 2006, 80(3):313-332.
[89] Glantz MJ, Cole BF, Forsyth PA, Recht LD, Wen PY, Chamberlain MC, Grossman SA, Cairncross JG: Practice parameter: anticonvulsant prophylaxis in patients with newly diagnosed brain tumors. Report of the Quality Standards Subcommittee of the American Academy of Neurology. *Neurology.* 2000, 54(10):1886-1893.
[90] Green H, Paul M, Vidal L, Leibovici L: Prophylaxis of Pneumocystis pneumonia in immunocompromised non-HIV-infected patients: systematic review and meta-analysis of randomized controlled trials. *Mayo Clinic proceedings.* 2007, 82(9):1052-1059.
[91] Gerber DE, Grossman SA, Streiff MB: Management of venous thromboembolism in patients with primary and metastatic brain tumors. *J. Clin. Oncol.* 2006, 24(8):1310-1318.
[92] Pruitt AA: Medical management of patients with brain tumors. *Current treatment options in neurology*, 13(4):413-426.
[93] Ruff RL, Posner JB: Incidence and treatment of peripheral venous thrombosis in patients with glioma. *Annals. of neurology.* 1983, 13(3):334-336.
[94] Lee AY, Levine MN, Baker RI, Bowden C, Kakkar AK, Prins M, Rickles FR, Julian JA, Haley S, Kovacs MJ *et al*: Low-molecular-weight heparin versus a coumarin for the prevention of recurrent venous thromboembolism in patients with cancer. *The New England journal of medicine.* 2003, 349(2):146-153.
[95] Meyers CA, Weitzner MA, Valentine AD, Levin VA: Methylphenidate therapy improves cognition, mood, and function of brain tumor patients. *J. Clin. Oncol.* 1998, 16(7):2522-2527.
[96] Shaw EG, Rosdhal R, D'Agostino RB, Jr., Lovato J, Naughton MJ, Robbins ME, Rapp SR: Phase II study of donepezil in irradiated brain tumor patients: effect on cognitive function, mood, and quality of life. *J. Clin. Oncol.* 2006, 24(9):1415-1420.
[97] Litofsky NS, Farace E, Anderson F, Jr., Meyers CA, Huang W, Laws ER, Jr.: Depression in patients with high-grade glioma: results of the Glioma Outcomes Project. *Neurosurgery.* 2004, 54(2):358-366.
[98] Chamberlain MC: Treatment options for glioblastoma. *Neurosurgical focus* 2006, 20(4):E19.
[99] Norden AD, Wen PY: Glioma therapy in adults. *The neurologist.* 2006, 12(6):279-292.

[100] Wen PY, Kesari S: Malignant gliomas in adults. *The New England journal of medicine.* 2008, 359(5):492-507.

[101] Grossman SA, Batara JF: Current management of glioblastoma multiforme. *Seminars in oncology.* 2004, 31(5):635-644.

[102] Van Meir EG, Hadjipanayis CG, Norden AD, Shu HK, Wen PY, Olson JJ: Exciting new advances in neuro-oncology: the avenue to a cure for malignant glioma. *CA: a cancer journal for clinicians*, 60(3):166-193.

[103] Lacroix M, Abi-Said D, Fourney DR, Gokaslan ZL, Shi W, DeMonte F, Lang FF, McCutcheon IE, Hassenbusch SJ, Holland E *et al*: A multivariate analysis of 416 patients with glioblastoma multiforme: prognosis, extent of resection, and survival. *Journal of neurosurgery.* 2001, 95(2):190-198.

[104] Sanai N, Berger MS: Glioma extent of resection and its impact on patient outcome. *Neurosurgery* 2008, 62(4):753-764.

[105] Sanai N, Polley MY, McDermott MW, Parsa AT, Berger MS: An extent of resection threshold for newly diagnosed glioblastomas. *Journal of neurosurgery.* 2011, 115(1):3-8.

[106] Vuorinen V, Hinkka S, Farkkila M, Jaaskelainen J: Debulking or biopsy of malignant glioma in elderly people - a randomised study. *Acta neurochirurgica.* 2003, 145(1):5-10.

[107] Willems PW, Taphoorn MJ, Burger H, Berkelbach van der Sprenkel JW, Tulleken CA: Effectiveness of neuronavigation in resecting solitary intracerebral contrast-enhancing tumors: a randomized controlled trial. *Journal of neurosurgery.* 2006, 104(3):360-368.

[108] Letteboer MM, Willems PW, Viergever MA, Niessen WJ: Brain shift estimation in image-guided neurosurgery using 3-D ultrasound. *IEEE transactions on bio-medical engineering.* 2005, 52(2):268-276.

[109] Trantakis C, Tittgemeyer M, Schneider JP, Lindner D, Winkler D, Strauss G, Meixensberger J: Investigation of time-dependency of intracranial brain shift and its relation to the extent of tumor removal using intra-operative MRI. *Neurological research.* 2003, 25(1):9-12.

[110] Nimsky C, Grummich P, Sorensen AG, Fahlbusch R, Ganslandt O: Visualization of the pyramidal tract in glioma surgery by integrating diffusion tensor imaging in functional neuronavigation. *Zentralblatt fur Neurochirurgie.* 2005, 66(3):133-141.

[111] Braun V, Dempf S, Tomczak R, Wunderlich A, Weller R, Richter HP: Multimodal cranial neuronavigation: direct integration of functional magnetic resonance imaging and positron emission tomography data: technical note. *Neurosurgery.* 2001, 48(5):1178-1181.

[112] Rasmussen IA, Jr., Lindseth F, Rygh OM, Berntsen EM, Selbekk T, Xu J, Nagelhus Hernes TA, Harg E, Haberg A, Unsgaard G: Functional neuronavigation combined with intra-operative 3D ultrasound: initial experiences during surgical resections close to eloquent brain areas and future directions in automatic brain shift compensation of preoperative data. *Acta neurochirurgica.* 2007, 149(4):365-378.

[113] Coenen VA, Krings T, Weidemann J, Hans FJ, Reinacher P, Gilsbach JM, Rohde V: Sequential visualization of brain and fiber tract deformation during intracranial surgery with three-dimensional ultrasound: an approach to evaluate the effect of brain shift. *Neurosurgery.* 2005, 56(1 Suppl):133-141.

[114] Berntsen EM, Gulati S, Solheim O, Kvistad KA, Torp SH, Selbekk T, Unsgard G, Haberg AK: Functional magnetic resonance imaging and diffusion tensor tractography incorporated into an intraoperative 3-dimensional ultrasound-based neuronavigation system: impact on therapeutic strategies, extent of resection, and clinical outcome. *Neurosurgery*, 67(2):251-264.

[115] Pirotte B, Goldman S, Dewitte O, Massager N, Wikler D, Lefranc F, Ben Taib NO, Rorive S, David P, Brotchi J *et al*: Integrated positron emission tomography and magnetic resonance imaging-guided resection of brain tumors: a report of 103 consecutive procedures. *Journal of neurosurgery.* 2006, 104(2):238-253.

[116] Muns A, Meixensberger J, Arnold S, Schmitgen A, Arlt F, Chalopin C, Lindner D: Integration of a 3D ultrasound probe into neuronavigation. *Acta neurochirurgica*, 153(7):1529-1533.

[117] Schlaier JR, Warnat J, Dorenbeck U, Proescholdt M, Schebesch KM, Brawanski A: Image fusion of MR images and real-time ultrasonography: evaluation of fusion accuracy combining two commercial instruments, a neuronavigation system and a ultrasound system. *Acta neurochirurgica.* 2004, 146(3):271-276.

[118] Nossek E, Korn A, Shahar T, Kanner AA, Yaffe H, Marcovici D, Ben-Harosh C, Ben Ami H, Weinstein M, Shapira-Lichter I *et al*: Intraoperative mapping and monitoring of the corticospinal tracts with neurophysiological assessment and 3-dimensional ultrasonography-based navigation. Clinical article. *Journal of neurosurgery*, 114(3):738-746.

[119] Gonzalez-Darder JM, Gonzalez-Lopez P, Talamantes F, Quilis V, Cortes V, Garcia-March G, Roldan P: Multimodal navigation in the functional

microsurgical resection of intrinsic brain tumors located in eloquent motor areas: role of tractography. *Neurosurgical focus*, 28(2):E5.

[120] Shamov T, Spiriev T, Tzvetanov P, Petkov A: The combination of neuronavigation with transcranial magnetic stimulation for treatment of opercular gliomas of the dominant brain hemisphere. *Clinical neurology and neurosurgery*, 112(8):672-677.

[121] Senft C, Franz K, Ulrich CT, Bink A, Szelenyi A, Gasser T, Seifert V: Low field intraoperative MRI-guided surgery of gliomas: a single center experience. *Clinical neurology and neurosurgery*, 112(3):237-243.

[122] Muragaki Y, Iseki H, Maruyama T, Kawamata T, Yamane F, Nakamura R, Kubo O, Takakura K, Hori T: Usefulness of intraoperative magnetic resonance imaging for glioma surgery. *Acta. Neurochir. Suppl.* 2006, 98:67-75.

[123] Hatiboglu MA, Weinberg JS, Suki D, Rao G, Prabhu SS, Shah K, Jackson E, Sawaya R: Impact of intraoperative high-field magnetic resonance imaging guidance on glioma surgery: a prospective volumetric analysis. *Neurosurgery.* 2009, 64(6):1073-1081.

[124] Jankovski A, Francotte F, Vaz G, Fomekong E, Duprez T, Van Boven M, Docquier MA, Hermoye L, Cosnard G, Raftopoulos C: Intraoperative magnetic resonance imaging at 3-T using a dual independent operating room-magnetic resonance imaging suite: development, feasibility, safety, and preliminary experience. *Neurosurgery.* 2008, 63(3):412-424.

[125] Sun GC, Chen XL, Zhao Y, Wang F, Hou BK, Wang YB, Song ZJ, Wang D, Xu BN: Intraoperative High-Field Magnetic Resonance Imaging Combined With Fiber Tract Neuronavigation Guided Resection Of Cerebral Lesions Involving Optic Radiation. *Neurosurgery.* 2011, *Jun. 7.*

[126] Parney IF, Goerss SJ, McGee K, Huston J, 3rd, Perkins WJ, Meyer FB: Awake craniotomy, electrophysiologic mapping, and tumor resection with high-field intraoperative MRI. *World neurosurgery*, 73(5):547-551.

[127] Kuhnt D, Ganslandt O, Schlaffer SM, Buchfelder M, Nimsky C: Quantification of glioma removal by intraoperative high-field magnetic resonance imaging - an update. *Neurosurgery.* 2011, *May 26.*

[128] Pichlmeier U, Bink A, Schackert G, Stummer W: Resection and survival in glioblastoma multiforme: an RTOG recursive partitioning analysis of ALA study patients. *Neuro-oncology.* 2008, 10(6):1025-1034.

[129] Stummer W, Pichlmeier U, Meinel T, Wiestler OD, Zanella F, Reulen HJ: Fluorescence-guided surgery with 5-aminolevulinic acid for

resection of malignant glioma: a randomised controlled multicentre phase III trial. *The lancet oncology.* 2006, 7(5):392-401.

[130] Stummer W, Reulen HJ, Meinel T, Pichlmeier U, Schumacher W, Tonn JC, Rohde V, Oppel F, Turowski B, Woiciechowsky C *et al*: Extent of resection and survival in glioblastoma multiforme: identification of and adjustment for bias. *Neurosurgery.* 2008, 62(3):564-576.

[131] Tonn JC, Stummer W: Fluorescence-guided resection of malignant gliomas using 5-aminolevulinic acid: practical use, risks, and pitfalls. *Clinical neurosurgery.* 2008, 55:20-26.

[132] Walker MD, Strike TA, Sheline GE: An analysis of dose-effect relationship in the radiotherapy of malignant gliomas. *International journal of radiation oncology, biology, physics.* 1979, 5(10):1725-1731.

[133] Hegi ME, Diserens AC, Gorlia T, Hamou MF, de Tribolet N, Weller M, Kros JM, Hainfellner JA, Mason W, Mariani L *et al*: MGMT gene silencing and benefit from temozolomide in glioblastoma. *The New England journal of medicine.* 2005, 352(10):997-1003.

[134] Stupp R, Mason WP, van den Bent MJ, Weller M, Fisher B, Taphoorn MJ, Belanger K, Brandes AA, Marosi C, Bogdahn U *et al*: Radiotherapy plus concomitant and adjuvant temozolomide for glioblastoma. *The New England journal of medicine.* 2005, 352(10):987-996.

[135] Stupp R, van den Bent MJ, Hegi ME: Optimal role of temozolomide in the treatment of malignant gliomas. *Current neurology and neuroscience reports.* 2005, 5(3):198-206.

[136] Ataman F, Poortmans P, Stupp R, Fisher B, Mirimanoff RO: Quality assurance of the EORTC 26981/22981; NCIC CE3 intergroup trial on radiotherapy with or without temozolomide for newly-diagnosed glioblastoma multiforme: the individual case review. *Eur. J. Cancer* 2004, 40(11):1724-1730.

[137] Chan MF, Schupak K, Burman C, Chui CS, Ling CC: Comparison of intensity-modulated radiotherapy with three-dimensional conformal radiation therapy planning for glioblastoma multiforme. *Med. Dosim.* 2003, 28(4):261-265.

[138] Butowski NA, Sneed PK, Chang SM: Diagnosis and treatment of recurrent high-grade astrocytoma. *J. Clin. Oncol.* 2006, 24(8):1273-1280.

[139] Nieder C, Astner ST, Mehta MP, Grosu AL, Molls M: Improvement, clinical course, and quality of life after palliative radiotherapy for recurrent glioblastoma. *American journal of clinical oncology.* 2008, 31(3):300-305.

[140] Mayer R, Sminia P: Reirradiation tolerance of the human brain. *International journal of radiation oncology, biology, physics.* 2008, 70(5):1350-1360.

[141] Larson DA, Gutin PH, McDermott M, Lamborn K, Sneed PK, Wara WM, Flickinger JC, Kondziolka D, Lunsford LD, Hudgins WR *et al*: Gamma knife for glioma: selection factors and survival. *International journal of radiation oncology, biology, physics.* 1996, 36(5):1045-1053.

[142] Kondziolka D, Flickinger JC, Bissonette DJ, Bozik M, Lunsford LD: Survival benefit of stereotactic radiosurgery for patients with malignant glial neoplasms. *Neurosurgery.* 1997, 41(4):776-783.

[143] Souhami L, Seiferheld W, Brachman D, Podgorsak EB, Werner-Wasik M, Lustig R, Schultz CJ, Sause W, Okunieff P, Buckner J *et al*: Randomized comparison of stereotactic radiosurgery followed by conventional radiotherapy with carmustine to conventional radiotherapy with carmustine for patients with glioblastoma multiforme: report of Radiation Therapy Oncology Group 93-05 protocol. *International journal of radiation oncology, biology, physics.* 2004, 60(3):853-860.

[144] Larson DA, Prados M, Lamborn KR, Smith V, Sneed PK, Chang S, Nicholas KM, Wara WM, Devriendt D, Kunwar S *et al*: Phase II study of high central dose Gamma Knife radiosurgery and marimastat in patients with recurrent malignant glioma. *International journal of radiation oncology, biology, physics.* 2002, 54(5):1397-1404.

[145] Combs SE, Widmer V, Thilmann C, Hof H, Debus J, Schulz-Ertner D: Stereotactic radiosurgery (SRS): treatment option for recurrent glioblastoma multiforme (GBM) . *Cancer* 2005, 104(10):2168-2173.

[146] Bernstein M, Laperriere N, Glen J, Leung P, Thomason C, Landon AE: Brachytherapy for recurrent malignant astrocytoma. *International journal of radiation oncology, biology, physics.* 1994, 30(5):1213-1217.

[147] Gabayan AJ, Green SB, Sanan A, Jenrette J, Schultz C, Papagikos M, Tatter SP, Patel A, Amin P, Lustig R *et al*: GliaSite brachytherapy for treatment of recurrent malignant gliomas: a retrospective multi-institutional analysis. *Neurosurgery.* 2006, 58(4):701-709.

[148] Quant EC, Drappatz J, Wen PY, Norden AD: Recurrent high-grade glioma. *Current treatment options in neurology*, 12(4):321-333.

[149] Fogh SE, Andrews DW, Glass J, Curran W, Glass C, Champ C, Evans JJ, Hyslop T, Pequignot E, Downes B *et al*: Hypofractionated stereotactic radiation therapy: an effective therapy for recurrent high-grade gliomas. *J. Clin. Oncol*, 28(18):3048-3053.

[150] Fokas E, Wacker U, Gross MW, Henzel M, Encheva E, Engenhart-Cabillic R: Hypofractionated stereotactic reirradiation of recurrent glioblastomas: a beneficial treatment option after high-dose radiotherapy? *Strahlenther Onkol.* 2009, 185(4):235-240.
[151] Combs SE, Thilmann C, Edler L, Debus J, Schulz-Ertner D: Efficacy of fractionated stereotactic reirradiation in recurrent gliomas: long-term results in 172 patients treated in a single institution. *J. Clin. Oncol.* 2005, 23(34):8863-8869.
[152] Grosu AL, Weber WA, Franz M, Stark S, Piert M, Thamm R, Gumprecht H, Schwaiger M, Molls M, Nieder C: Reirradiation of recurrent high-grade gliomas using amino acid PET (SPECT) /CT/MRI image fusion to determine gross tumor volume for stereotactic fractionated radiotherapy. *International journal of radiation oncology, biology, physics.* 2005, 63(2):511-519.
[153] Pollack IF: Neuro-oncology: Therapeutic benefits of reirradiation for recurrent brain tumors. *Nat. Rev. Neurol*, 6(10):533-535.
[154] Gerson SL: MGMT: its role in cancer aetiology and cancer therapeutics. *Nat. Rev. Cancer* 2004, 4(4):296-307.
[155] Gonzaga PE, Brent TP: Affinity purification and characterization of human O6-alkylguanine-DNA alkyltransferase complexed with BCNU-treated, synthetic oligonucleotide. *Nucleic. acids research* 1989, 17(16):6581-6590.
[156] Day RS, 3rd, Ziolkowski CH, Scudiero DA, Meyer SA, Lubiniecki AS, Girardi AJ, Galloway SM, Bynum GD: Defective repair of alkylated DNA by human tumour and SV40-transformed human cell strains. *Nature.* 1980, 288(5792):724-727.
[157] Lonardi S, Tosoni A, Brandes AA: Adjuvant chemotherapy in the treatment of high grade gliomas. *Cancer treatment reviews.* 2005, 31(2):79-89.
[158] Hildebrand J, Sahmoud T, Mignolet F, Brucher JM, Afra D: Adjuvant therapy with dibromodulcitol and BCNU increases survival of adults with malignant gliomas. EORTC Brain Tumor Group. *Neurology.* 1994, 44(8):1479-1483.
[159] Walker MD, Green SB, Byar DP, Alexander E, Jr., Batzdorf U, Brooks WH, Hunt WE, MacCarty CS, Mahaley MS, Jr., Mealey J, Jr. *et al*: Randomized comparisons of radiotherapy and nitrosoureas for the treatment of malignant glioma after surgery. *The New England journal of medicine.* 1980, 303(23):1323-1329.

[160] Fine HA, Dear KB, Loeffler JS, Black PM, Canellos GP: Meta-analysis of radiation therapy with and without adjuvant chemotherapy for malignant gliomas in adults. *Cancer.* 1993, 71(8):2585-2597.

[161] Stewart LA: Chemotherapy in adult high-grade glioma: a systematic review and meta-analysis of individual patient data from 12 randomised trials. *Lancet.* 2002, 359(9311):1011-1018.

[162] Randomized trial of procarbazine, lomustine, and vincristine in the adjuvant treatment of high-grade astrocytoma: a Medical Research Council trial. *J. Clin. Oncol.* 2001, 19(2):509-518.

[163] Brada M, Judson I, Beale P, Moore S, Reidenberg P, Statkevich P, Dugan M, Batra V, Cutler D: Phase I dose-escalation and pharmacokinetic study of temozolomide (SCH 52365) for refractory or relapsing malignancies. *British journal of cancer.* 1999, 81(6):1022-1030.

[164] Kaina B, Ziouta A, Ochs K, Coquerelle T: Chromosomal instability, reproductive cell death and apoptosis induced by O6-methylguanine in Mex-, Mex+ and methylation-tolerant mismatch repair compromised cells: facts and models. *Mutation research.* 1997, 381(2):227-241.

[165] Hirose Y, Berger MS, Pieper RO: p53 effects both the duration of G2/M arrest and the fate of temozolomide-treated human glioblastoma cells. *Cancer research.* 2001, 61(5):1957-1963.

[166] Hirose Y, Berger MS, Pieper RO: Abrogation of the Chk1-mediated G(2) checkpoint pathway potentiates temozolomide-induced toxicity in a p53-independent manner in human glioblastoma cells. *Cancer research.* 2001, 61(15):5843-5849.

[167] Hirose Y, Kreklau EL, Erickson LC, Berger MS, Pieper RO: Delayed repletion of O6-methylguanine-DNA methyltransferase resulting in failure to protect the human glioblastoma cell line SF767 from temozolomide-induced cytotoxicity. *Journal of neurosurgery.* 2003, 98(3):591-598.

[168] Newlands ES, Stevens MF, Wedge SR, Wheelhouse RT, Brock C: Temozolomide: a review of its discovery, chemical properties, pre-clinical development and clinical trials. *Cancer treatment reviews.* 1997, 23(1):35-61.

[169] Friedman HS, Kerby T, Calvert H: Temozolomide and treatment of malignant glioma. *Clin. Cancer. Res* 2000, 6(7):2585-2597.

[170] Mutter N, Stupp R: Temozolomide: a milestone in neuro-oncology and beyond? *Expert review of anticancer therapy.* 2006, 6(8):1187-1204.

[171] Hegi ME, Diserens AC, Godard S, Dietrich PY, Regli L, Ostermann S, Otten P, Van Melle G, de Tribolet N, Stupp R: Clinical trial substantiates the predictive value of O-6-methylguanine-DNA methyltransferase promoter methylation in glioblastoma patients treated with temozolomide. *Clin. Cancer Res.* 2004, 10(6):1871-1874.
[172] Esteller M, Garcia-Foncillas J, Andion E, Goodman SN, Hidalgo OF, Vanaclocha V, Baylin SB, Herman JG: Inactivation of the DNA-repair gene MGMT and the clinical response of gliomas to alkylating agents. *The New England journal of medicine.* 2000, 343(19):1350-1354.
[173] Paz MF, Yaya-Tur R, Rojas-Marcos I, Reynes G, Pollan M, Aguirre-Cruz L, Garcia-Lopez JL, Piquer J, Safont MJ, Balana C *et al*: CpG island hypermethylation of the DNA repair enzyme methyltransferase predicts response to temozolomide in primary gliomas. *Clin. Cancer Res.* 2004, 10(15):4933-4938.
[174] Robinson CG, Palomo JM, Rahmathulla G, McGraw M, Donze J, Liu L, Vogelbaum MA: Effect of alternative temozolomide schedules on glioblastoma O(6) -methylguanine-DNA methyltransferase activity and survival. *British journal of cancer*, 103(4):498-504.
[175] Tolcher AW, Gerson SL, Denis L, Geyer C, Hammond LA, Patnaik A, Goetz AD, Schwartz G, Edwards T, Reyderman L *et al*: Marked inactivation of O6-alkylguanine-DNA alkyltransferase activity with protracted temozolomide schedules. *British journal of cancer.* 2003, 88(7):1004-1011.
[176] Broniscer A, Gururangan S, MacDonald TJ, Goldman S, Packer RJ, Stewart CF, Wallace D, Danks MK, Friedman HS, Poussaint TY *et al*: Phase I trial of single-dose temozolomide and continuous administration of o6-benzylguanine in children with brain tumors: a pediatric brain tumor consortium report. *Clin. Cancer Res.* 2007, 13(22 Pt 1):6712-6718.
[177] Donawho CK, Luo Y, Luo Y, Penning TD, Bauch JL, Bouska JJ, Bontcheva-Diaz VD, Cox BF, DeWeese TL, Dillehay LE *et al*: ABT-888, an orally active poly(ADP-ribose) polymerase inhibitor that potentiates DNA-damaging agents in preclinical tumor models. *Clin. Cancer Res.* 2007, 13(9):2728-2737.
[178] Clarke MJ, Mulligan EA, Grogan PT, Mladek AC, Carlson BL, Schroeder MA, Curtin NJ, Lou Z, Decker PA, Wu W *et al*: Effective sensitization of temozolomide by ABT-888 is lost with development of temozolomide resistance in glioblastoma xenograft lines. *Molecular cancer therapeutics.* 2009, 8(2):407-414.

[179] Rivera AL, Pelloski CE, Gilbert MR, Colman H, De La Cruz C, Sulman EP, Bekele BN, Aldape KD: MGMT promoter methylation is predictive of response to radiotherapy and prognostic in the absence of adjuvant alkylating chemotherapy for glioblastoma. *Neuro-oncology*, 12(2):116-121.

[180] Westphal M, Hilt DC, Bortey E, Delavault P, Olivares R, Warnke PC, Whittle IR, Jaaskelainen J, Ram Z: A phase 3 trial of local chemotherapy with biodegradable carmustine (BCNU) wafers (Gliadel wafers) in patients with primary malignant glioma. *Neuro-oncology*. 2003, 5(2):79-88.

[181] Westphal M, Ram Z, Riddle V, Hilt D, Bortey E: Gliadel wafer in initial surgery for malignant glioma: long-term follow-up of a multicenter controlled trial. *Acta neurochirurgica*. 2006, 148(3):269-275.

[182] Attenello FJ, Mukherjee D, Datoo G, McGirt MJ, Bohan E, Weingart JD, Olivi A, Quinones-Hinojosa A, Brem H: Use of Gliadel (BCNU) wafer in the surgical treatment of malignant glioma: a 10-year institutional experience. *Annals of surgical oncology*. 2008, 15(10):2887-2893.

[183] McGirt MJ, Than KD, Weingart JD, Chaichana KL, Attenello FJ, Olivi A, Laterra J, Kleinberg LR, Grossman SA, Brem H *et al*: Gliadel (BCNU) wafer plus concomitant temozolomide therapy after primary resection of glioblastoma multiforme. *Journal of neurosurgery*. 2009, 110(3):583-588.

[184] Bock HC, Puchner MJ, Lohmann F, Schutze M, Koll S, Ketter R, Buchalla R, Rainov N, Kantelhardt SR, Rohde V *et al*: First-line treatment of malignant glioma with carmustine implants followed by concomitant radiochemotherapy: a multicenter experience. *Neurosurgical review*. 2010, 33(4):441-449.

[185] Noel G, Schott R, Froelich S, Gaub MP, Boyer P, Fischer-Lokou D, Dufour P, Kehrli P, Maitrot D: Retrospective Comparison of Chemoradiotherapy Followed by Adjuvant Chemotherapy, With or Without Prior Gliadel Implantation (Carmustine) After Initial Surgery in Patients With Newly Diagnosed High-Grade Gliomas. *International journal of radiation oncology, biology, physics*. 2011, Feb 5.

[186] Tysnes BB, Mahesparan R: Biological mechanisms of glioma invasion and potential therapeutic targets. *Journal of neuro-oncology*. 2001, 53(2):129-147.

[187] Louis DN: Molecular pathology of malignant gliomas. *Annual review of pathology*. 2006, 1:97-117.

[188] Comprehensive genomic characterization defines human glioblastoma genes and core pathways. *Nature.* 2008, 455(7216):1061-1068.
[189] Stupp R, Hegi ME, Gilbert MR, Chakravarti A: Chemoradiotherapy in malignant glioma: standard of care and future directions. *J. Clin. Oncol.* 2007, 25(26):4127-4136.
[190] Rich JN, Reardon DA, Peery T, Dowell JM, Quinn JA, Penne KL, Wikstrand CJ, Van Duyn LB, Dancey JE, McLendon RE *et al*: Phase II trial of gefitinib in recurrent glioblastoma. *J. Clin. Oncol.* 2004, 22(1):133-142.
[191] Galanis E, Buckner JC, Maurer MJ, Kreisberg JI, Ballman K, Boni J, Peralba JM, Jenkins RB, Dakhil SR, Morton RF *et al*: Phase II trial of temsirolimus (CCI-779) in recurrent glioblastoma multiforme: a North Central Cancer Treatment Group Study. *J. Clin. Oncol.* 2005, 23(23):5294-5304.
[192] Chang SM, Wen P, Cloughesy T, Greenberg H, Schiff D, Conrad C, Fink K, Robins HI, De Angelis L, Raizer J *et al*: Phase II study of CCI-779 in patients with recurrent glioblastoma multiforme. *Investigational new drugs.* 2005, 23(4):357-361.
[193] Cloughesy TF, Wen PY, Robins HI, Chang SM, Groves MD, Fink KL, Junck L, Schiff D, Abrey L, Gilbert MR *et al*: Phase II trial of tipifarnib in patients with recurrent malignant glioma either receiving or not receiving enzyme-inducing antiepileptic drugs: a North American Brain Tumor Consortium Study. *J. Clin. Oncol.* 2006, 24(22):3651-3656.
[194] Chi AS, Wen PY: Inhibiting kinases in malignant gliomas. *Expert opinion on therapeutic targets.* 2007, 11(4):473-496.
[195] Sathornsumetee S, Reardon DA, Desjardins A, Quinn JA, Vredenburgh JJ, Rich JN: Molecularly targeted therapy for malignant glioma. *Cancer.* 2007, 110(1):13-24.
[196] Stommel JM, Kimmelman AC, Ying H, Nabioullin R, Ponugoti AH, Wiedemeyer R, Stegh AH, Bradner JE, Ligon KL, Brennan C *et al*: Coactivation of receptor tyrosine kinases affects the response of tumor cells to targeted therapies. *Science.* 2007, 318(5848):287-290.
[197] Furnari FB, Fenton T, Bachoo RM, Mukasa A, Stommel JM, Stegh A, Hahn WC, Ligon KL, Louis DN, Brennan C *et al*: Malignant astrocytic glioma: genetics, biology, and paths to treatment. *Genes and development.* 2007, 21(21):2683-2710.
[198] Schmidt NO, Westphal M, Hagel C, Ergun S, Stavrou D, Rosen EM, Lamszus K: Levels of vascular endothelial growth factor, hepatocyte growth factor/scatter factor and basic fibroblast growth factor in human

gliomas and their relation to angiogenesis. *International journal of cancer.* 1999, 84(1):10-18.

[199] Norden AD, Young GS, Setayesh K, Muzikansky A, Klufas R, Ross GL, Ciampa AS, Ebbeling LG, Levy B, Drappatz J *et al*: Bevacizumab for recurrent malignant gliomas: efficacy, toxicity, and patterns of recurrence. *Neurology.* 2008, 70(10):779-787.

[200] Narayana A, Kelly P, Golfinos J, Parker E, Johnson G, Knopp E, Zagzag D, Fischer I, Raza S, Medabalmi P *et al*: Antiangiogenic therapy using bevacizumab in recurrent high-grade glioma: impact on local control and patient survival. *Journal of neurosurgery.* 2009, 110(1):173-180.

[201] Nghiemphu PL, Liu W, Lee Y, Than T, Graham C, Lai A, Green RM, Pope WB, Liau LM, Mischel PS *et al*: Bevacizumab and chemotherapy for recurrent glioblastoma: a single-institution experience. *Neurology.* 2009, 72(14):1217-1222.

[202] Poulsen HS, Grunnet K, Sorensen M, Olsen P, Hasselbalch B, Nelausen K, Kosteljanetz M, Lassen U: Bevacizumab plus irinotecan in the treatment patients with progressive recurrent malignant brain tumours. *Acta oncologica.* 2009, 48(1):52-58.

[203] Zuniga RM, Torcuator R, Jain R, Anderson J, Doyle T, Ellika S, Schultz L, Mikkelsen T: Efficacy, safety and patterns of response and recurrence in patients with recurrent high-grade gliomas treated with bevacizumab plus irinotecan. *Journal of neuro-oncology.* 2009, 91(3):329-336.

[204] Pope WB, Lai A, Nghiemphu P, Mischel P, Cloughesy TF: MRI in patients with high-grade gliomas treated with bevacizumab and chemotherapy. *Neurology.* 2006, 66(8):1258-1260.

[205] Vredenburgh JJ, Desjardins A, Herndon JE, 2nd, Marcello J, Reardon DA, Quinn JA, Rich JN, Sathornsumetee S, Gururangan S, Sampson J *et al*: Bevacizumab plus irinotecan in recurrent glioblastoma multiforme. *J. Clin. Oncol.* 2007, 25(30):4722-4729.

[206] Yung WK, Albright RE, Olson J, Fredericks R, Fink K, Prados MD, Brada M, Spence A, Hohl RJ, Shapiro W *et al*: A phase II study of temozolomide vs. procarbazine in patients with glioblastoma multiforme at first relapse. *British journal of cancer.* 2000, 83(5):588-593.

[207] Friedman HS, Prados MD, Wen PY, Mikkelsen T, Schiff D, Abrey LE, Yung WK, Paleologos N, Nicholas MK, Jensen R *et al*: Bevacizumab alone and in combination with irinotecan in recurrent glioblastoma. *J. Clin. Oncol.* 2009, 27(28):4733-4740.

[208] Kreisl TN, Kim L, Moore K, Duic P, Royce C, Stroud I, Garren N, Mackey M, Butman JA, Camphausen K *et al*: Phase II trial of single-

agent bevacizumab followed by bevacizumab plus irinotecan at tumor progression in recurrent glioblastoma. *J. Clin. Oncol.* 2009, 27(5):740-745.

[209] Vredenburgh JJ, Desjardins A, Kirkpatrick JP, Reardon DA, Peters KB, Herndon JE, 2nd, Marcello J, Bailey L, Threatt S, Sampson J *et al*: Addition of Bevacizumab to Standard Radiation Therapy and Daily Temozolomide Is Associated with Minimal Toxicity in Newly Diagnosed Glioblastoma Multiforme. *International journal of radiation oncology, biology, physics.* 2010, Oct 30.

[210] Vredenburgh JJ, Desjardins A, Reardon DA, Peters KB, Herndon JE, 2nd, Marcello J, Kirkpatrick JP, Sampson JH, Bailey L, Threatt S *et al*: The addition of bevacizumab to standard radiation therapy and temozolomide followed by bevacizumab, temozolomide, and irinotecan for newly diagnosed glioblastoma. *Clin. Cancer. Res*, 17(12):4119-4124.

[211] Macdonald DR, Cascino TL, Schold SC, Jr., Cairncross JG: Response criteria for phase II studies of supratentorial malignant glioma. *J. Clin. Oncol.* 1990, 8(7):1277-1280.

[212] Henson JW, Ulmer S, Harris GJ: Brain tumor imaging in clinical trials. *Ajnr.* 2008, 29(3):419-424.

[213] van den Bent MJ, Vogelbaum MA, Wen PY, Macdonald DR, Chang SM: End point assessment in gliomas: novel treatments limit usefulness of classical Macdonald's Criteria. *J. Clin. Oncol.* 2009, 27(18):2905-2908.

[214] Wen PY, Macdonald DR, Reardon DA, Cloughesy TF, Sorensen AG, Galanis E, Degroot J, Wick W, Gilbert MR, Lassman AB *et al*: Updated response assessment criteria for high-grade gliomas: response assessment in neuro-oncology working group. *J. Clin. Oncol.* 2010, 28(11):1963-1972.

[215] Easaw JC, Mason WP, Perry J, Laperriere N, Eisenstat DD, Del Maestro R, Belanger K, Fulton D, Macdonald D: Canadian recommendations for the treatment of recurrent or progressive glioblastoma multiforme. *Current oncology.* 2011, 18(3):e126-e136.

[216] Roldan GB, Scott JN, McIntyre JB, Dharmawardene M, de Robles PA, Magliocco AM, Yan ES, Parney IF, Forsyth PA, Cairncross JG *et al*: Population-based study of pseudoprogression after chemoradiotherapy in GBM. *The Canadian journal of neurological sciences.* 2009, 36(5):617-622.

[217] Taal W, Brandsma D, de Bruin HG, Bromberg JE, Swaak-Kragten AT, Smitt PA, van Es CA, van den Bent MJ: Incidence of early pseudo-

progression in a cohort of malignant glioma patients treated with chemoirradiation with temozolomide. *Cancer.* 2008, 113(2):405-410.

[218] Chamberlain MC, Glantz MJ, Chalmers L, Van Horn A, Sloan AE: Early necrosis following concurrent Temodar and radiotherapy in patients with glioblastoma. *Journal of neuro-oncology.* 2007, 82(1):81-83.

[219] Sanghera P, Perry J, Sahgal A, Symons S, Aviv R, Morrison M, Lam K, Davey P, Tsao MN: Pseudoprogression following chemoradiotherapy for glioblastoma multiforme. *The Canadian journal of neurological sciences.* 2010, 37(1):36-42.

[220] Brandes AA, Franceschi E, Tosoni A, Blatt V, Pession A, Tallini G, Bertorelle R, Bartolini S, Calbucci F, Andreoli A *et al*: MGMT promoter methylation status can predict the incidence and outcome of pseudoprogression after concomitant radiochemotherapy in newly diagnosed glioblastoma patients. *J. Clin. Oncol.* 2008, 26(13):2192-2197.

In: Glioblastoma
Editors: M. F. Bezerra et.al, pp. 43-75

ISBN: 978-1-62100-858-3

Chapter 2

THERAPEUTIC POTENTIAL OF SCORPION TOXINS AGAINST GLIOBLASTOMA

Ilhem Rjeibi, Mohamed ElAyeb and Najet Srairi-Abid*

Laboratoire des Venins et Toxines, Institut Pasteur de Tunis, 13, place pasteur, BP 74, 1002, Belvédère, Tunis, Tunisia

ABSTRACT

Despite advances in standard therapy, including surgical resection, radiotherapy and chemotherapy, the prognosis for patients with glioblastoma remains poor. A unique feature contributing to the disease aggressiveness is the ability of malignant glioma cells to actively migrate along brain vasculature instead of passive metastasis through vascular circulation.

During the last decade, different ion channel types have been found to be overexpressed in a variety of tumors, thus emerging as possible tumoral markers. Ion channels may be considered as a suitable pharmacological target for glioblastoma therapy.

Because scorpion toxins have well defined structures, constrained by disulfide bridges, and interact with ionic channels (their targets) through multiple contacts, they bind with much higher affinity and specificity than most other ionic channel blockers available to date.

* Correspondence to: Najet Srairi-Abid, Laboratoire des Venins et Toxines, Institut Pasteur de Tunis, 13, Place Pasteur. 1002, Tunis - Belvédère, Tunisie, Tel.: (216) 71 783 022, Fax: (216) 71 791 833, E-mail: najet.abid@pasteur.rns.tn

Scorpion toxins represent thus promising agents for treatment and early detection of malignant glioma brain tumors. In this review we present the main results of years of research involving glioma ionic channels and scorpion toxins that have anti-glioblastoma activity on the basis of recent publications and our experience.

Keywords: Glioblastoma, scorpion toxins, ionic channels, brain cancer.

I. INTRODUCTION

Evidence tracing back to the seventies indicates that ion channel blockers, especially for K^+ and Cl^- channels, impair neoplastic cell proliferation. These observations were subsequently extended, thus opening a wide field of research on the functional implications of ion channels in cancer cells biology (Pardo et al., 2004; Kunzelmann et al., 2005) . A rapidly increasing number of ion-channel types are now known to be expressed in various cancers, and some of them are selectively expressed in aggressive cancers (Diss *et al.*, 2004; Fiske *et al.*, 2006; Roger *et al.*, 2006; Schönherr, 2005; Villalonga *et al.*, 2007) . In agreement with the many observations carried out *in vitro*, recent studies indicate that blocking the activity of certain voltage-gated channels impairs the growth of some tumors *in vivo* (Fiske, et al., 2006; Gomez-Varela et al., 2007; Pillozzi et al., 2011) . Scorpion toxins have proven to be among the most potent and selective antagonists available for voltage-gated channels permeable to K^+, Na^+, Ca^{2+} and Cl^-, (Possani et al., 2000; Possani et al., 1999; Srinivasan et al., 2001; DeBin et al., 1993; Olamendi-Portugal et al., 2002) . Due to their small size, compact and rigid structure, high potency and selectivity, scorpion toxins have emerged as highly valuable tools for research and drug development for numerous indications. Some of these toxins are currently under evaluation for a number of pathologies.

II. BRAIN TUMORS AND IONIC CHANNELS

Brain tumor is a mass of abnormal cells in the brain that have grown and multiplied in an uncontrolled fashion. They belong to a group of diverse tumors that affect the brain and spinal cord known as *central nervous system (CNS) neoplasm* (Amberger et al., 1997; Noble et al., 1997) . Brain tumors that develop from various types of cells making up the brain are called *primary brain tumors.* These types of brain tumors are usually localized to the brain itself and only rarely spread to other parts of the body. *Metastatic brain tumors*, also known as *secondary brain tumors*, originate from cancer cells in another part of the body and spread to the brain through the bloodstream. The distinction between primary and secondary brain tumors is important for a clinical perspective because they are usually treated differently.

Approximately 50% of all primary brain tumors originate from specialized nerve cells, the *glial cells* and are called *gliomas* (Berninger et al., 2007) . Among the many different types of gliomas, the most common, *astrocytomas,* develop from astrocytes. The World Health Organization (WHO) classifies astrocytomas into four distinct grades designated as Grade I, II, III, and IV on the basis of how quickly the cells grow and spread and how the cells appear under a microscope (Louis et al., 2007) . Glioblastoma, technically known as glioblastoma multiforme (GBM) , is the fastest growing type of astrocytoma (Grade IV astrocytoma) that quickly spreads and invades nearby normal brain tissue and contains areas of dead cells (necrosis) in the center of the tumor. Glioblastoma multiforme is the most common type of primary malignant brain tumor in adults and accounts for about 60-70% of cases. Although standard treatment with surgery, irradiation, and temozolomide postpones progression and extends survival to some extent, these tumors universally recur and unrelentingly result in death (Stupp et al., 2009) . Therefore, improvement of treatment options for patients with glioblastoma is imperative. Great effort is thus being devoted to develop new drugs, targeted on specific cancer-related molecules, to improve response and avoid systemic toxicity. Since ion channel's expression is often altered in human cancers and their blockade often impairs important aspects of neoplastic progression, they appear to be very promising diagnostic and therapeutic targets. A major advantage of ion channels is their accessibility from the extracellular side, which facilitates many aspects of the physiological, pharmacological and clinical approaches.

Ion channels in glia types have been shown by many laboratories to be functionally involved in proliferation (Bringmann et al., 2000; Chin et al., 1997; DeCoursey et al., 1984; Schlichter et al., 1996) . Human glioma cells express a variety of ion channels (Werner and Southeimer 2009) . These include voltage-gated K^+ (Chin et al., 1997) , voltage gated Na^+ (Brismar and Collins 1989; Schrey et al., 2002) , Ca^{2+}-activated K^+ (Brismar and Collins, 1989; Pallotta et al., 1987) , voltage-gated Cl^- (Ullrich and Sontheimer, 1996) , and volume-regulated Cl^- channels (Bakhramov et al., 1995; Brismar, 1995) . Furthermore it has been shown that glioma migration/invasion requires complex and well-arranged interactions of molecular motors with the cytoskeleton and adhesion sites of cells interacting with other cells or the extracellular matrix surrounding them (Giese et al., 1995; Gladson, 1999; Demuth and Berens, 2004; Zamecnik, 2005) . It also involves the production and release of matrix-degrading enzymes (Ohnishi et al., 1993; Maidment et al., 1996; Gladson, 1999; Nakada et al., 2003) and chemotactic interactions with neighboring cells (Merzak et al., 1994; Giese et al., 1995; Maidment et al., 1997; Ritch et al., 2003; Farin et al., 2006) . Many of these features are shared with other cancers. However, in stark contrast to other cancers, glioma cells spread by active cell migration rather than spreading passively via hematogenous routes. As a result, gliomas rarely ever metastasize outside the central nervous system (CNS); they readily invade and metastasize within the brain and spinal cord. This is surprising since the extracellular space in the mature brain is very small. Cells that navigate the narrow and tortuous extracellular space will need to be able to adjust their shape and volume to fit through these narrow spaces. Indeed, glioma cells that penetrate through the extracellular space are elongated, wedge-shaped with slender cell processes (Soroceanu et al., 1999) . This morphology is consistent with an overall shrinkage of the cell body and an elongation of invadopodia, the leading processes of cells actively engaged in invasion. Cell shrinkage requires the secretion of cytoplasm, principally KCl and water from the cell. This is accomplished by the coordinated activity of defined K^+ and Cl^- channels, which are the principal diffusional release pathways for these ions (Soroceanu et al., 1999) . K^+ and Cl^- channels represent thus an interesting pharmacological target for new drugs (Ulrich and Sontheimer, 1997) .

II.1. Potassium Channels in Glial and Glioma Cells

In the field of cell biology, potassium channels are the most widely distributed type of ion channel and are found in virtually all living organisms (Littleton and Ganetzky, 2000) . Furthermore, potassium channels are found in most cell types and control a wide variety of cell functions (Hille and Bertil, 2001; Jessell, et al., 2000) . They form potassium-selective pores that span cell membranes. There are four major classes of potassium channels:

- Calcium-activated potassium channels - open in response to the presence of calcium ions or other signalling molecules.
- Inwardly rectifying potassium channels - passe current (positive charge) more easily in the inward direction (into the cell) .

- Tandem pore domain potassium channels - are constitutively open or possess high basal activation, such as the "resting potassium channels" or "leak channels" that set the negative membrane potential of neurons. When open, they allow potassium ions to cross the membrane at a rate which is nearly as fast as their diffusion through bulk water.
- Voltage-gated potassium channels - are voltage-gated ion channels that open or close in response to changes in the transmembrane voltage.

The architectural structure of the ion channel families consists of four variations built on a common pore-forming structural theme (Yu and Catterall 2004, Ashcroft 2006) . Voltage-gated K^+ channels exemplify the first basic structure consists of six regions that form membrane-spanning helices (termed segments S1 to S6) and a membrane-spanning loop between the S5 and S6 segments. Their principal subunits are composed of four homologous Kv domains (I to IV) that form the common structural motif for this family (Yu and Catterall 2004; Shieh et al., 2000) . Experimental analysis of ion channel structures shows that the four homologous domains surround a central pore. The inward rectifying K^+ channels are complexes of four subunits that each has only two transmembrane segments, termed M1 and M2, which are analogous in structure and function to the S5 and S6 segments of voltage-gated K^+ channels. Two of these pore motifs are linked together to generate the structural theme of the two-pore K^+ channels.

In the last decade, this field has advanced due to the resolution of the three-dimensional structure of a number of K^+-channels, including KcsA, KvAP and Kv1.2 by Roderick MacKinnon's group, for which he was awarded the 2003 Nobel Prize in chemistry (Doyle et al., 1998, Lee et al., 2005, Long et al., 2005) .

K^+channels are well-characterized as having key regulatory roles in the cell cycle progression of both normally proliferating (e.g. lymphocytes, Schwann cells and glia) and abnormally proliferating (cancerous) cell types (Chandy et al., 2004; Pardo, 2004; Vautier et al., 2004; Wilson and Chiu, 1993) . It is well established that healthy glial cells express an abundance of voltage-gated K^+ channels (Kv) including the Shaker (Kv1) subfamily (Verkhratsky, 2000) . It was reported that particular members of this channel family are closely related to cell growth and cell cycle progression. In rat oligodendrocyte precursor cells, for instance, the transition of quiescent cells into the G1 phase is accompanied by a selective increase of Kv1.3 and Kv1.5

protein expression (Chittajallu et al., 2002) . Specific blocking of Kv1.3-containing channels alone was sufficient to elicit G1 arrest (Attali et al., 1997) . In contrast, Kv1.5 antisense treatment in astrocytes inhibited cell growth (MacFarlane et al., 2000) . This channel was preferably expressed in low-grade astrocytomas and had a low level of expression or was lacking in most oligodendrogliomas and glioblastomas (PreuBat et al., 2003) .

Large-conductance Ca^{2+}-activated K^+ (BK) channels are ubiquitously expressed in cells derived from the most common human brain tumors, namely meningiomas and gliomas (Kraft et al., 2000; Ransom and Sontheimer, 2001; Weydt et al, 1997) . The activation of BK channels is triggered by membrane depolarization and enhanced by an increase in Ca^{2+} (Toro et al, 1998) . Prior studies have implicated BK channels in the proliferation and migration of glioblastoma cells (Basrai et al, 2002; Weaver et al, 2004; Weaver et al, 2006) . Furthermore, it has been shown in malignant glioma biopsy samples that BK channel expression correlates with glioma malignancy (Liu et al., 2002) . The use of selective pharmacological inhibitors shows prominent expression of currents that are inhibited by the BK channel specific inhibitors. However, despite the presence of transcripts for intermediate conductance Ca^{2+}-activated K^+ channels (IK) and small conductance Ca^{2+}-activated K^+ channels (SK) , neither clotrimazole, an inhibitor of IK channels, nor apamin, known to block most SK channels inhibited any current. The exclusive expression of functional BK channels was further demonstrated by short hairpin RNA knockdown experiments. Western blotting of patient biopsies with antibodies specific for all three KCa channel types further substantiated the exclusive expression of BK type KCa channels *in vivo*. This finding is in contrast to other cancers that express primarily IK channels (Weaver et al., 2006) .

BK has also been associated with growth control in cervical, ovarian, prostate, and breast cancer derived cell lines (Coiret and al, 2007; Bloch et al., 2007) . However, a number of other studies contradict these findings and suggest that BK channels are not required for proliferation or even have anti-tumorogenic properties, including in glioma cells (Chin et al., 1997; Cambien et al. 2008) . In addition to BK, IK1 channels have also been investigated to regulate growth rate in numerous types of malignant and non-malignant mammalian cells (Parihar et al., 2003; Jager et al., 2004; Grgic et al., 2005; Wang et al., 2007; Tao et al., 2008) . Recent studies show that the pharmacological inhibitors of both BK and IK1 strongly suppress glioma cell growth in an additive fashion. However, low concentration of the same blockers that were sufficient to inhibit channel activity had no effect on cell proliferation suggestting that Ca^{2+}-activated K^+ channels do not play a critical role in proliferation of glioma cells and that the effects of pharmacological inhibitors occur through their off-target actions (Abdullaev et al., 2010) .

II.2. Chloride Channels Are Signature of GBM

Chloride channels reside both in the plasma membrane and in intracellular organelles. They display a variety of important physiological and cellular roles that include regulation of pH, volume homeostasis, organic solute transport, cell migration, cell proliferation and differentiation (Wilson and Chiu, 1993; Pappas and Ritchie, 1998; Shen et al., 2000) . They are also essential for salt and fluid movements across epithelia (Venglarik et al., 1990; O'Grady et al., 2000) , volume regulation (Jackson and Madsen, 1997; Valverde, 1999) .

Chloride channels allow the passive flux of anions across biological membranes. Although they generally also transport other anionic species, sometimes even more efficiently than they transport Cl^-, they are often called Cl^- channels because Cl^- is the physiologically most important anion. In common with other channels, Cl^- channels are able to regulate ion flow by switching on or off in response to stimuli such as ligand binding, changes in intracellular Ca^{2+}, or changes in voltage (a process called gating) . Several classes of Cl^- channels have not yet been identified at the molecular level. Three molecularly distinct Cl^- channel families are well established (Jentsch et al., 2002):

- The cystic fibrosis transmembrane conductance regulator (CFTR) channel. It was the first anion channel to be identified by positional cloning. Its gene emerged from the search for the cystic fibrosis locus in 1989 and yielded a rather unexpected sequence, that of an ABC transport protein, with a tandem repeat of a transmembrane domain of six putative transmembrane helices and a nucleotide binding fold, linked by a regulator domain containing numerous phosphorylation sites (Riordan et al., 1989) . On the basis of this structure, the protein was rather cautiously named "conductance regulator." CFTR channel is now known to be a voltage-independent anion channel, which requires the presence of hydrolyzable nucleoside triphosphate for efficient activity.
- Ligand-gated GABA and glycine receptors. The neurotransmitters GABA and glycine mediate fast inhibitory neurotransmission in the mammalian CNS. Glycine is predominantly used in the spinal cord

and the brain stem, whereas GABA is more commonly used in the brain. Their binding to their receptors opens intrinsic anion channels. In the adult CNS, this mostly leads to a Cl^- influx, which hyperpolarizes the neuron and thereby inhibits neuronal activity. Early in development, GABA and glycine induce a strong depolarizing response that can cause Ca^{2+} influx via voltage-gated Ca^{2+} channels and thus triggers neurotransmitter release (Owens et al., 1996, Reichling et al., 1994) . This excitatory action results from a more positive Cl^- equilibrium potential in undifferentiated neurons. During further development, the intracellular Cl^- concentration is decreased, in part as a consequence of the upregulation of the cation cotransporter KCC2 (Hubner et al., 2001.; Rivera et al., 1999) . This inverts the GABA- and glycine-mediated current from excitatory to inhibitory (Wang et al., 1994.) .

- CLC channels (Jentsch et al., 2002) . Measurements of Cl^- currents have revealed that these channels are gated by cell volume, membrane potential, extracellular ligands, intracellular ions (H^+ and Ca^{2+}) and protein kinases. Mammals have nine different CLC genes. Using homology, they can be grouped into three branches. Members of the first branch (ClC-1, ClC-2, ClC-Ka and ClC-Kb) exert their function in the plasma membrane, whereas members of the two other branches (ClC-3, ClC-4 and ClC-5 in one branch, and ClC-6 and ClC-7 in the other) function primarily in intracellular membranes. Many, but possibly not all, CLC chloride channels are gated in a voltage-dependent manner (Jentsch et al., 2002) . Because of the diversity of factors regulating the activity on these channels, it is not surprising that they are involved in many physiological functions. The importance of one such group, the CLC family of chloride channels, is highlighted by diseases that develop when these channels does not function normally (Ishiguro, et al. 2010; Xu et al., 2010) . All members of the ClC family share a conserved structural organization consisting of a complex transmembrane transport domain and a soluble regulatory domain. To date, representative structures for the two parts are available, the transmembrane domain from the structure of a bacterial homologue (EcClC) (Dutzler et al., 2002; 2003) , the soluble domain from a eukaryotic family member (Meyer and Dutzler 2006) . EcClC is a homodimeric protein with two structurally identical subunits, each containing an independent ion translocation pore. The subunits exhibit a complex topology with two structurally related halves spanning the membrane with opposite orientations to form an 'antiparallel architecture' (Dutzler et al., 2002) . The chloride translocation path is located at the interface between the two halves and contains a Cl^- selectivity filter in the neck of an hourglass-like shaped pore. The cytoplasmic domain consists of two well defined and tightly interacting cystathionine beta-synthetase subdomains (CBS) , which constitute about two-thirds of the protein. The remaining third, which is of low sequence complexity, is disordered (Meyer and Dutzler 2006) . CBS domains are strategically positioned to regulate the ion-transport pathway, and many disease-causing mutations in human CLCs reside on the CBS-transmembrane interface. (Feng et al., 2010) .

The Sounthener's group shows that voltage-gated chloride channels are expressed in human gliomas (Ullrich et al., 1998) . They made a concerted effort to identify and characterize the underlying Cl^- channels in glioma cells and showed that three members of the ClC family are consistently present in patient biopsies (Olsen et al., 2003) . These include ClC-2, ClC-3 and ClC-5. ClC-2 and ClC-3 are upregulated in glioma membranes, and may play an important role in cell migration and invasion by means of the excretion of chloride ions and the associated obligatory movement of water (Sanchez-Olea et al., 1993; Olsen et al., 2003; Hermoso et al., 2002; Parkerson et al., 2004) . The treatment of glioma cells with ClC-2 antisense causes the selective loss of inwardly rectifying Ca^{2+} sensitive Cl^- currents with biophysical features characteristic of ClC-2 channels (Olsen et al., 2003) . Glioma cells show an unusual resting conductance for ClC3 which can be attributed to channels that are sensitive to NPPB, DIDS and tamoxifen (Sontheimer, 2008, Soroceanu et al., 1999; Ransom et al., 2001) . These data suggest that ClC-2 and ClC-3 channels are excellent candidates mediating the resting Cl^- conductance and hence may be involved in Cl^- efflux that mediates cell shrinkage of invading cells.

Interestingly, Sontheimer's group remarked that low grade tumors (e.g., pilocytic astrocytomas) , containing more differentiated, astrocyte-like cells showed expression of glioma chloride currents in concert with voltage-activated sodium and potassium currents also seen in normal astrocytes. By contrast, high grade tumors (e.g., glioblastoma multiforme) expressed almost exclusively chloride currents, suggesting a gradual loss of Na^+ currents and gain of Cl^- currents with increasing pathological tumor grade. They demonstrate that these chloride currents are a glioma-specific feature (Ullrich et al., 1998) .

All these suggest that ClC channels are signature of GBM and that future therapy for glioblastoma should aim at pharmacologic blockade by targeting multiple ClCs activities (Cuddapah and Sontheimer, 2010) .

III. Potassium and Chloride Channels Modulators

III.1. Small Ions

K^+ Blockers

Several compounds were found in the early 1980s to block K^+ channels at micromolar to millimolar concentrations (Chandy et al., 2006) , including the classical Kv channel inhibitors 4-aminopyridine (4AP) and tetraethylammonium (TEA) .

- 4AP is an organic compound with the chemical formula $H_2NC_5H_4N$. The molecule is one of the three isomeric amines of pyridine. In the laboratory, it is a useful pharmacological tool in studying various potassium conductances in physiology and biophysics. It is a relatively selective blocker of members of voltage activated Kv1 (Shaker, KCNA) family channels. It selectively and reversibly inhibits Shaker channels at concentration of 1 mM.
- TEA is a quaternary ammonium cation consisting of four ethyl groups attached to a central nitrogen atom. It is used in neurophysiology experiments to block the voltage activated potassium channels involved in the trailing part of the transmission of an action potential along a neuron. TEA is also known to reverse the action of drugs such as tubocurarine, a non-depolarizing blocker.

Since the mid-1990s efforts by scientists at pharmaceutical companies and in academia have yielded more potent and more drug-like small molecule potassium channels blockers (Chandy et al., 2006) . These compounds fall roughly into two groups (DeCoursey et al., 1984): typical combinatorial library compounds, like CP-339818 (Fukushima, et al., 1984) , UK-78280 (Cahalan, et al., 1985) and phenyl-stilbene A (Hess, et al., 1993) that have a relatively simple structure and low molecular weight, and are rich in nitrogen and halogen atoms.

Cl^- Blockers

Voltage dependent chloride channels appear to be quite unresponsive to blockade by the classical anion channel blockers. ClC-2 requires millimolar concentrations of DIDS, 9-AC, and DPC for efficient block (Clark et al., 1998; Thiemann et al., 1992.) and ClC-5 is not significantly blocked by DIDS, DPC, NPPB, 9-AC, and niflumic acid (Schmieder et al., 1998; Steinmeyer et al., 1995.) . However, ClC-1 can be inhibited by 9-AC, DPC, and niflumic acid in the micromolar range (Astill et al.,1996., Steinmeyer et al.,1991.) , and a high-affinity block by derivatives of clofibric acid has been described (Aromataris et al.,1999., Pusch et al., 2000.) . Both ClC-1 and ClC-2 are sensitive to extracellular Zn^{2+} in the micromolar range (Clark et al., 1998; Kür et al., 1997; 1999.) , but it is currently not known if this applies to all ClC channels. Cd^{2+} was also often used to inhibit native ClC-2-like currents (Schwiebert et al., 1998; Blaisdell et al., 2000; Chesnoy-Marchais and Fritsch, 1994; Clark et al., 1998) . However, none of these inhibitors is specific.

With few exceptions, K^+ or Cl^- channels blockers are rather unspecific and have a low potency, with effective concentrations in the range of micromolar to even millimolar. It has been shown that they interact with these channels by only a simple binding with only one amino acids of the channel (Kavanaugh et al., 1991) .

The low specificity for individual ion channels is compounded by side effects of these substances, mainly on ion transporters and components of intracellular signalling pathways. It is therefore highly desirable to have specific blockers for each channel type available.

Peptide- and protein-based drugs have long been recognized as having distinct advantages over their small molecule chemical counterparts. Endogenous peptides are often more potent and specific to their in vivo receptor subtype targets, potentially resulting in fewer adverse effects.

III.2. Scorpion Toxins: High Affinity Ligands for Ionic Channels

The understanding of the biophysical and pharmacological properties of channels has been greatly improved by the use of scorpion toxins, particularly in differentiation of specific channel activity. The electrical currents generated by different channels can be modulated by the use of toxins. Although numerous toxins have been discovered, they represent only a minute fraction of the toxin repertoire present in venoms (Escoubas et al., 2006; Terlau and Olivera, 2004) . Scorpion toxins are variously used as a defensive biotoxin to ward off predation, or as both defensive and predatory venom acting on a vast array of targets. They are small proteins with a potent pharmacological action towards ion channels and are useful pharmacological probes to investigate ion-specific channel proteins and their functions (Kaczorowski and Garcia, 1999) . Most scorpion toxins share a common structural fold consisting of an alpha-helix connected by a network of disulfide bridges to three β strands (Bontems et al., 1991) . This Csαβ motif is a versatile scaffold with which evolution has played to generate a huge diversity of sequences and their associated biological activities (Zhu et al., 2004) , leading to a combinatorial library of pharmacologically active peptides (Sollod et al., 2005)

Scorpion toxins have been classified into several classes, based on the channel they target. Toxins binding to Na^+ channels are 60-70 amino acid-long proteins stabilized by 4 disulfide bridges, they are called long-chain scorpion toxins. Toxins active on K^+ channels are 30-40 residues-long with three or four disulfide bonds. There are also a few short-type, scorpion toxins that bind to Ca^{2+} channels (Valdivia et al., 1992; Kuniyasu et al., 1999; Shahbazzedeh et al., 2007; Fajloun et al., 2000) and to Cl^- channels (Debin et al., 1993; Fu et al., 2007; Fuller et al., 2007) . Lastly, another structural group of toxins with 58 amino acids and only three disulfide bridges called birtoxin-like peptides have been characterized (Inceglu et al., 2001) . This structural group contains peptides showing similar sequences but differences in activity. Some of them are active on Na^+ channels (Inceglu et al., 2001; Martin-Eauclair et al., 2005; Abbas et al., 2011) , whereas others are active on K^+ channels (Srairi-Abid et al., 2005; Soli et al., 2009) .

Due to their high affinity and specificity, scorpion toxins provide powerful tools to study the structure and function of ionic channels. Scorpion toxins strongly alter channel function by binding to several different receptor sites. The mode of action of scorpion toxins can be roughly divided into two major groups: the "pore-plungers" and the "voltage-sensor modulators" or "gating-modifiers". The most studied toxins in pharmacological point of view are potassium channel toxins. The majority of these toxins are "pore-plungers": i.e. they bind to the pore region and physically block the ion transport through the pore. These toxins are characterized by the presence of a dyad or triad, having a Lys in structural proximity to either one or two hydrophobic residues (Phe, Tyr, Trp) (Dauplais et al., 1997, Mouhat et al., 2005; Srairi-Abid 2005) . The Lys residue is "plunged" into the pore and interacts with the channel's

Asp residues inside the pore, while the hydrophobic residues of the toxin interact with hydrophobic residues on the pore outer-surface (Dauplais et al., 1997) . Toxin selectivity is achieved by additional protein-protein interactions, thus discriminating between closely related channels (Lebrun et al.,1997; Srairi-Abid, 2008) . "Gating-modifier" toxins bind to the voltage sensor moiety (S4 helix) , which is partially exposed to the intracellular space, modulate its movement, and thus modulate the mechanism of pore gating (Philips et al., 2005)

IV. Anti-Gliomas Effect of Scorpion Venoms and Their Toxins

IV.1. Scorpion Venoms Effect on Malignant Glioma

Scorpion and its venom have been used as traditional and folk therapy in various pathophysiological conditions in India, China, Africa and Cuba. Moreover, very efficient medicines, including anticancer agents, are being to be developed on the basis of toxins isolated from scorpion venom (Gomes et al., 2010) .

Several studies have demonstrated the cancer preventive and therapeutic efficacy of scorpion venom in different animal tumor models and cell culture systems including prostate, breast, colon and skin cancers (Jia et al., 2001; Yang et al., 2002; Zhang et al., 2006) . *Buthus martenzii Karsch* (BmK) scorpion venom, a rich source of various ion channels blockers/modulators, induces cell death (apoptosis) of cultured malignant glioma U251-MG cells (Wang and Ji, 2005) . Furthermore, using U251-MG tumor xenografts on severe combined immunodeficiency mice, BmK venom could significantly inhibit the tumor growth. Recently, Zargan and his collaborators report the apoptotic and antiproliferative effects of *Odontobuthus doriae* scorpion venom in human neuroblastoma cells (Zargan et al., 2011) .

IV.2. Potassium Channel Scorpion Toxins Affecting Glioma Cells

Scorpion toxins charybdotoxin (ChTX) and iberiotoxin (IbTX) , specific BK-channel inhibitors, inhibited glioma cell migration in a dose-dependent fashion (Weaver et al., 2006; McFerrin and Sontheimer, 2006) . In cerebellar granule cells, migration is accompanied by oscillatory changes in intracellular Ca^{2+} (Rakic and Komuro, 1995; Komuro and Rakic, 1996) and these changes are mediated by activation of NMDA receptors. In migratory glioma cells, similar Ca^{2+} oscillations were reported in response to activation of ACh-R (Bordey et al., 2000) , which activate charybdotoxin-sensitive BK K^{+} channels. Moreover, glioma cells express Ca^{2+}-permeable AMPA receptors, and Ca^{2+} influx through these receptors is required for cell migration (Ishiuchi et al., 2002) .

Cell proliferation could be also inhibited by IbTX or ChTX *via* their inhibition of the ATP-stimulated DNA synthesis in Müller cells (Moll et al., 2002) . Similarly carbachol, known to activate glioma BK channels (Chavis et al., 1998) , stimulates DNA synthesis in glioma cells (Ashkenazi et al., 1989) . BK channel inhibition by IbTXcaused a dose- and time-dependent decrease in cell number discernible as early as 72 hr after exposure and maximal after 4-5 days. Flowcytometry analysis showed that IbTX treatment arrests glioma cells in S phase of the cell cycle, whereupon cells undergo cell death.

IV.3. Chloride Channel Scorpion Toxins as Specific Anti-Glioblastomas

Chlorotoxin (ClTX) , a 36 amino acid peptide from the venom of the giant yellow Israeli scorpion *Leiurus quinquestriatus,* was described to block small-conductance Cl^{-} channels, derived from epithelial cells, when applied to the cytoplasmic surface (DeBin et al., 1993) .

This peptide binds to essentially all glioma cells *in vivo*, as illustrated by an example staining using an Oregon Green conjugated peptide (Sontheimer 2008) . Using native and recombinant ^{125}I-labeled chlorotoxin, Soroceanu and his collaborators showed that in radioreceptor assays, ^{125}I-labeled chlorotoxin binds to presumably glioma-specific chloride channels (GCC) or a receptor that modulates GCC activity. Moreover, ^{131}I-labeled chlorotoxin distribution, visualized through *in vivo* imaging by gamma ray camera scans, demonstrated specific and persistent intratumoral localization of the radioactive ligand. Immunohistochemical studies using biotinylated and fluorescently tagged chlorotoxin showed highly selective staining of glioma cells *in vitro*, *in situ*, and in sections of patient biopsies. Tissues comparison including normal human brain, kidney, and colon were consistently negative for chlorotoxin immunostaining. Deshane et al, showed that chlorotoxin inhibit the migration and invasion of glioma cells possibly *via* the modulation of ion channels (Deshane et al., 2003) . Subsequent studies suggested that chlorotoxin modulates the chloride ion channel in glioma cells by facilitating the internalization and hence, the down-regulation of the cell surface levels of the CLC-3 chloride channel (McFerrin and Sontheimer, 2006) . Surprisingly, further studies on the interaction of chlorotoxin with Cl^- channels suggested that these effects were indirect.

Chlorotoxin was shown to bind a macromolecular complex containing MMP-2, MT1-MMP, TIMP-2 (Deshane et al., 2003) and CLC-3 at the surface of glioma cells and mediate the internalization and down-regulation of both MMP-2 and CLC-3 (McFerrin and Sontheimer, 2006; Deshane et al., 2003) . Chlorotoxin was also able to inhibit the MMP-2 activity *in vitro*, and the cell surface gelatinolytic activity in D54-MG cells, supporting an interaction between MMP-2 and chlorotoxin in glioma cells (Deshane et al., 2003; Sontheimer, 2008) . This is a surprising action for a scorpion peptide, but could explain the irreversible action of this peptide and its relatively slow time course of Cl^- channel block (Ullrich and Sontheimer, 1996) . Even preceding the identification of this mechanism of action, the relative glioma specificity of this peptide spurred research toward a clinical application of chlorotoxin as a drug to target gliomas clinically. This work demonstrated that chlorotoxin binds exclusively to glial derived tumors and some cancers that are embryologically related like melanoma (Lyons et al., 2002) . No binding was observed to normal human tissues in numerous autopsies and biopsies evaluated.

A synthetic version of chlorotoxin, TM-601, showed equal biological activity and tumor specificity to the native toxin and was submitted to the FDA for clinical evaluation. Beginning in 2004, a phase 1 clinical study began administering chlorotoxin labeled with 10 mCi ^{131}I to patients with late stage, high-grade malignant glioma. These patients had received labeled peptide prior radiation and chemotherapy and have shown recurrence. As predicted from prior animal studies, chlorotoxin showed remarkable tumor specificity and did not show any non-specific labeling. Results from the completed phase 1 study have been published (Mamelak et al., 2006) . Overall the drug was deemed safe and tumor specific and FDA approved the use of this compound in a multi-center phase II efficacy study in which multiple doses of chlorotoxin are administered.

Using mouse tumor model, a bio-conjugate of chlorotoxin with the near-infrared dye Cy5.5 (chlorotoxin:Cy5.5) , was shown to efficiently detect and monitor multiple tumor types, including glioma and medulloblastoma (Veiseh et al., 2007) . Chlorotoxin, conjugated with iron oxide nanoparticles through a polyethylene glycol linker, could successfully attach to both drug and targeting ligands. The target nanoparticle demonstrated preferential accumulation and increased cytotoxicity in tumor cells (Sun et al., 2008) . I*n vivo*, these nanoparticles were retained within tumors. It was suggested that this multifunctional nanoparticle system may find potential applications in cancer diagnosis and treatment (Sun et al., 2008; Jiaqi et al., 2010) . Recent results suggested that chlorotoxin could be exploited as a special glioma-targeting ligand, and a potential delivery system for gene therapy of glioma *via* intravenous administration (Huang et al., 2011) .

These data suggest that chlorotoxin and chlorotoxin-conjugated molecules may serve as glioma-specific markers with diagnostic and therapeutic potential.

Nevertheless, the lack of selective inhibitors for Cl^- channels doses not permit an unequivocal identification of the carrying Cl^- channels in glioma cells by pharmacological means nor the molecular basis of the specific interaction of chlorotoxin to glioma cells.

Chlorotoxin Analogs and Structure- Function Relationship Study

A recombinant chlorotoxin-like peptide from *Buthus martenzii Karsch,* namedrBmKCta, was shown to have activity toward chloride channels and inhibit the growth of glioma cells. It exhibited specific toxicity against glioma cells, but not towards normal astrocytes (Fu et all., 2007) as well as chlorotoxin. The primary sequence of rBmKCTa consists of 35 amino acids, with four disulfide bridges and shows 68 % sequence similarity with chlorotoxin. ^{131}I-labeled or Cy5.5-conjugated BmKCTa prevented the metastasis of glioma (Fan et al., 2010) .

Recently, our team identified and isolated a chlorotoxin-like peptide, AaCtx, from *Androctonus australis* scorpionvenom (Rjeibi et al., 2011) . Its amino acid sequence shares 70% similarity (60% identity) with chlorotoxin from which it differs by twelve amino acids (Rjeibi et al., 2011) . sAaCtx, a synthetic version of AaCtx, has been shown to inhibit invasion and migration of U87 glioma cells with IC50 values of 125 μM and 10 μM respectively. It was reported that the inhibitory effect observed with chlorotoxin on the invasion and migration of U251MG, D54MG and U87 glioma cell lines is of 600 nM (Soroceanu et al., 1999) . These results showed that AaCtx displays lower efficacies than chlorotoxin on glioma cells. However, the activity of chlorotoxin-like peptides could be ameliorated with a suitable structure-function relationship study.

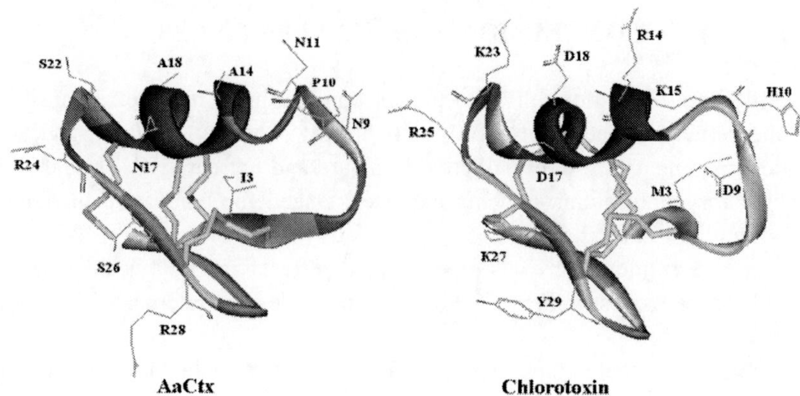

Figure 1. Homology model of AaCtx:Backbone ribbon representation of the model of AaCtx compared with the structure of chlorotoxin (PDB code1CHL [Lippens et al., 1995]) , which, besides I5A (PDB code1SIS (Lomize et al., 1991)) , is one of the two structures used as template for molecular modeling. Disulfide bridges are in yellow stick representation. Amino acids different between AaCtx and chlorotoxin are represented.

We started by inspecting unrelated classes of compounds used to block chloride channels. Our inspection reveals that these compounds bear, with few exceptions, a negative charge at physiological pH (Jentsch et al. 2002) . This suggests that the negative charge or the acidic character of some structural motifs of chlorotoxin-like peptides is expected to favor inhibition of glioma cells migration and invasion.

From the different 12 amino acids, the three aspartic acid residues in positions 9, 17 and 18 of chlorotoxin are replaced by neutral amino acids N9, N17 and A18 respectively, on AaCtx. As shown in figure 1, these amino acid residues are well exposed on the AaCtx 3D surface. N9 is localised on its *N*-terminal loop whereas N17 and A18 are localized on its α-helix. These results showed, in one hand, that N9, N17 and/or A18 are probably responsible of the weak activity of AaCtx and in another hand, that *N*-terminal loop and/or α-helix are the main structural elements of chlorotoxin-like peptides interacting with glioblastoma cells. Work is in progress in our laboratory to synthesize AaCtx analogs by targeting amino acids of its N-terminal loop and α-helix to improve the efficacy of the molecule then to design a more potent peptide than chlorotoxin.

Conclusion and Perspectives

Infiltration of tumor cells into the surrounding brain may be responsible for the refractory nature of GBM to treatment (Lassman, 2004) . Indeed, surgical treatments are only palliative in nature and not curative. The limited survival for glioblastoma patients indicates a need for innovative therapies targeting glioblastomas.

Because chemotherapy has unwanted side-effects and kills healthy tissue around the tumor, researchers have been trying to develop alternative forms of therapy.

The aim of targeted therapies, as their name implies, is to target cancerous cells while leaving surrounding cells unaffected.

Here, we review that ion channels should be included among the novel targets for glioblastoma therapy, which may open an entire pharmaceutical and clinical field.

First, their expression is often grossly altered in human cancers. Second, channel dysfunction can have a strong impact on cell physiology and signalling, with ensuing effects on cancer progression. Third, ion channels represent one of the few pharmaceutically tractable molecular classes. A major advantage is their accessibility from the extracellular side, which makes ion channel modulators particularly effective.

Purposes for therapeutic applications consist of many organic compounds which are not highly selective for these channels. One type of targeted therapy, which looks promising, is based on the use of scorpion toxins, which specifically target conductance glioma-chloride channels. Short chain scorpion toxins have various pharmacological advantages including high specificity, high activity no accumulation in organs, low toxicity and low immunogenicity. Furthermore, their compact structures lead to enhance chemical and thermal stability and relative low sensitivity to proteases.

The study of scorpion venom components, clinical toxin manifestation in human being and potential development of new drugs is just beginning. Characterization of AaCtx, even if it is less active than chlorotoxin, brought useful information on amino acids responsible for the activity of chlorotoxin-like peptides, and may serve as starting point for structure–function relationship studies which may lead to design highly active anti-glioblastoma drugs. The coming years are promising and many novel anti-glioblastoma potent toxins will probably be synthesised or isolated from scorpion venoms.

ACKNOWLEDGEMENTS

We thank Pr. José Luis (INSERM UMR 911-CRO2, Aix-Marseille Université, France) and Dr. Khadija Essafi-Benkhadir K (Unité de Biochimie et Pathologie Expérimentale Institut Pasteur de Tunis, Tunisie) for helpful discussion and critical comments on the manuscript.

REFERENCES

Abbas, N, Rosso; JP, Céard, B; Belghazi, M; Lebrun, R; Bougis, PE; Martin-Eauclaire, MF. Characterization of three "Birtoxin-like" toxins from the Androctonus amoreuxi scorpion venom. *Peptides*. 2011; 32(5):911-9.

Abdullaev, IF; Rudkouskaya, A; Mongin, AA; Kuo, YH. Calcium-activated potassium channels BK and IK1 are functionally expressed in human gliomas but do not regulate cell proliferation. *PLoS One*. 2010;5(8):e12304.

Amberger, VR; Avellana-Adalid V; Hensel T; Baron-Van Evercooren A; Schwab ME. Oligodendrocyte-type 2 astrocyte progenitors use a metalloendoprotease to spread and migrate on CNS myelin. *Eur. J. Neurosci.* 1997; 9;:151–162.

Arcangeli, A;; Crociani, O; Lastraioli, E; Masi, A; Pillozzi, S; Becchetti, A. Targeting ionchannels in cancer: a novel frontier in antineoplastic therapy. *Curr. Med. Chem*. 2009; 16: 66–93.

Aromataris, EC; Astill, DS; Rychkov, GY; Bryant, SH; Bretag, AH; Roberts, ML. Modulation of the gating of CIC-1 by S-() -2-(4-chlorophenoxy) propionic acid. *Br. J. Pharmacol.* 1999;126: 1375–1382.

Ashcroft, FM. K(ATP) channels and insulin secretion: a key role in health and disease. *Biochem. Soc. Trans*. 2006; 34:243-246. Review.

Ashkenazi, A; Ramachandran, J; Capon, DJ.Acetylcholine analogue stimulates DNA synthesis in brain-derived cells via specific muscarinic receptor subtypes. *Nature.* 1989; 340:146-50.

Astill, DS; Rychkov, G; Clarke, JD; Hughes, BP; Roberts, ML; Bretag, AH. Characteristics of skeletal muscle chloride channel ClC-1 and point mutant R304E expressed in Sf-9 insect cells. *Biochim. Biophys. Acta* 1996; 1280: 178–186.

Attali, B; Wang, N; Kolot, A; Sobko, A; Cherepanov, V; Soliven, B. Characterization of delayed rectifier Kv channels in oligodendrocytes and progenitor cells, *J. Neurosci.* 1997;17: 8234–8245.

Bakhramov, A; Fenech, C; Bolton, TB. Chloride current activated by hypotonicity in cultured human astrocytoma cells. *Exp. Physiol.* 1995; 80: 379–389.

Basrai, D; Kraft, R; Bollensdorff, C; Liebmann, L; Benndorf, K; Patt, S. BK channel blockers inhibit potassium-induced proliferation of human astrocytoma cells. *Neuroreport* 2002; 13: 403–407.

Berninger, B; Costa, MR; Koch, U; Schroeder, T; Sutor, B; Grothe, B; Götz, M. Functional Properties of Neurons Derived from In Vitro Reprogrammed Postnatal Astroglia - *Journal of Neuroscience* 2007; 27: 8654-8664.

Blaisdell, CJ; Edmonds, RD; Wang, XT; Guggino, S; Zeitlin, PL. pH-regulated chloride secretion in fetal lung epithelia. *Am. J. Physiol. Lung Cell Mol. Physiol.* 2000; 278:1248–1255.

Bloch, M; Ousingsawat, J; Simon, R; Schraml, P; Gasser, TC; Mihatsch, MJ; Kunzelmann, K; Bubendorf, L. KCNMA1 gene amplification promotes tumor cell proliferation in human prostate cancer. *Oncogene* 2007; 26: 2525–2534.

Bontems, F; Roumestand, C; Boyot, P; Gilquin, B; Doljansky, Y; Menez, A; Toma, F. Three-dimensional structure of natural charybdotoxin in aqueous solution by 1H-NMR. Charybdotoxin possesses a structural motif found in other scorpion toxins. *Eur. J. Biochem.* 1991; 196(1):19-28.

Bordey, A; Sontheimer, H; Trouslard, J. Muscarinic activation of BK channels induces membrane oscillations in glioma cells and leads to inhibition of cell migration. *J. Membr. Biol.* 2000; 176:31-40.

Brandes, AA. State-of-the-art treatment of high-grade brain tumors. *Semin. Oncol.* 2003; 30:4-9.

Bringmann, A; Francke, M; Pannicke, T; Biedermann, B; Kodal, H; Faude, F; Reichelt, W; Reichenbach, A. Role of glial K1 channels in ontogeny and gliosis: a hypothesis based upon studies on Muller cells. *Glia 2000;* 29: 35–44.

Brismar, T. Physiology of transformed glial cells. *Glia* 1995; 15:231–243.

Brismar, T; Collins VP. Potassium and sodium channels in human malignant glioma cells. *Brain Res. 1989;* 480: 259–267.

Cahalan, MD; Chandy, KG; DeCoursey, TE; Gupta, S. A voltage-gated potassium channel in human T lymphocytes. *J. Physiol.* (Lond.) 1985, 358:197–237.

Cambien, B; Rezzonico, R; Vitale, S; Rouzaire-Dubois, B; Dubois, JM; Barthel, R; Karimdjee, BS; Mograbi, B; Schmid-Alliana, A; Schmid-Antomarchi, H. Silencing of hSlo potassium channels in human osteosarcoma cells promotes tumorigenesis. *Int. J. Cancer* 2008; 123: 365–371.

Carpentier, A. Neuro-oncology: The growing role of chemotherapy in glioma. *Lancet Neurol.* 2005; 4:4–5.

Chandy, KG; Wulff, H; Beeton, C; Pennington, M; Gutman, GA; Cahalan, MD. K+ channels as targets for specific immunomodulation. *Trends Pharmacol. Sci.* 2004; 25:280-289. Review.

Chandy, G; Wulff, H; Beeton, C; Galabresi P; Gutman, G; Pennington, M. Voltage-gated ion channels as drug targets, Chapter Kv1.3 potassium channel: physiology, pharmacology and therapeutic indications. In: Editor Triggle DJ, Editor Gopalakrishnan M, Editor Rampe D, Editor Zheng W. Title: Voltage-gated ion channels as drug targets. Weinheim: John Wiley; 2006; 214-274.

Chavis, P; Ango, F; Michel, JM; Bockaert, J; Fagni, L. Modulation of big K+ channel activity by ryanodine receptors and L-type Ca2+ channels in neurons. *Eur. J. Neurosci.* 1998; 10:2322-2327.

Chesnoy-Marchais, D; and Fritsh, J. Activation of hyperpolarization and atypical osmosensitivity of a Cl- current in rat osteoblastic cells. *J. Membr. Biol.* 1994; 140: 173–188.

Chin, LS; Park, CC; Zitnay, KM; Sinha, M; DiPatri, AJ; Perillan, P; Simard, JM, 4-Aminopyridine causes apoptosis and blocks an outward rectifier K+ channel in malignant astrocytoma cell lines. *J. Neurosci. Res.*, 1997. 48:122-127.

Chittajallu, R; Chen, Y; Wang, H; Yan, X; Ghiani, CA; Heckman, T; McBain, CJ; Gallo, V. Regulation of Kv1 subunit expression in oligodendrocyte progenitor cells and their role in G1/S phase progression of the cell cycle, *Proc. Natl. Acad. Sci. USA*; 2002, 99:2350–2355.

Clark, S; Jordt, SE; Jentsch, TJ; Mathie, A. Characterization of the hyperpolarization-activated chloride current in dissociated rat sympathetic neurons. *J. Physiol.* (Lond) 1998; 506: 665–678.

Coiret, G; Borowiec, AS; Mariot, P; Ouadid-Ahidouch, H; Matifat, F. The antiestrogen tamoxifen activates BK channels and stimulates proliferation of MCF-7 breast cancer cells. *Mol. Pharmacol.* 2007; 71:843–851.

Cuddapah, VA; and Sontheimer, H. Molecular interaction and functional regulation of ClC-3 by Ca2+/calmodulin-dependent protein kinase II

(CaMKII) in human malignant glioma. *J. Biol. Chem.* 2010; 285: 11188-11196.

Dauplais, M; Lecoq, A; Song, J; Cotton, J; Jamin, N; Gilquin, B; Roumestand, C; Vita, C; De Medeiros, CL; Rowan, EG; Harvey, AL; Ménez, A. On the convergent evolution of animal toxins. Conservation of a diad of functional residues in potassium channel-blocking toxins with unrelated structures. *J. Biol. Chem.* 1997; 272, 4302–4309.

DeBin, JA; Maggio, JE; Strichartz, GR. Purification and characterization of chlorotoxin, a chloride channel ligand from the venom of the scorpion. *Am J. Physiol.* 1993; 264:361-369.

DeCoursey, TE; Chandy, KG; Gupta, S; Cahalan, MD; Voltage-gated K+ channels in human T lymphocytes: a role in mitogenesis *Nature,* 1984; 307:465–468.

Demuth, T; Berens, ME. Molecular mechanisms of glioma cell migration and invasion. *J. Neurooncol.* 2004; 70(2):217-228.

Deshane, J; Garner, CC; Sontheimer, H. Chlorotoxin inhibits glioma cell invasion via matrix metalloproteinase-2. *J. Biol. Chem.* 2003; 278:4135-44.

Doyle, D.A; Morais Cabral, J; Pfuetzner, RA; Kuo, A; Gulbis, JM; Cohen, SL; Chait, BT; MacKinnon, R. The structure of the potassium channel: molecular basis of K+ conduction and selectivity. *Science.* 1998; 280:69-77.

Dutzler, R; Campbell, EB; Cadene, M; Chait, BT; MacKinnon, R. X-ray structure of a ClC chloride channel at 3.0 Å reveals the molecular basis of anion selectivity. *Nature* 2002; 415:287-294.

Dutzler, R; Campbell, EB; MacKinnon, R. Gating the selectivity filter in ClC chloride channels. *Science* 2003; 300:108-112.

Ernest, NJ; Weaver, AK; Van Duyn, LB; Sontheimer; HW; Relative contribution of chloride channels and transporters to regulatory volume decrease in human glioma cells. *Am J. Physiol. Cell Physiol.* 2005; 288:1451-1460.

Escoubas, P; Sollod, B; King, GF. Venom landscapes: mining the complexity of spider venoms via a combined cDNA and mass spectrometric approach. *Toxicon.* 2006; 47:650-63.

Fajloun, Z; Kharrat, R; Chen, L; Lecomte, C; Di Luccio, E; Bichet, D; El Ayeb, M; Rochat, H; Allen, PD; Pessah, IN; De Waard, M; Sabatier, JM.Chemical synthesis and characterization of maurocalcine, a scorpion toxin that activates Ca(2+) release channel/ryanodine receptors. *FEBS Lett.* 2000;469(2-3):179-85.

Fan, S; Sun, Z; Jiang, D; Dai, C; Ma, Y; Zhao, Z; Liu, H; Wu, Y; Cao, Z; Li, W. BmKCT toxin inhibits glioma proliferation and tumor metastasis. *Cancer Lett.* 2010 291:158-66.

Farin, A; Suzuki, SO; Weiker, M; Goldman, JE; Bruce, JN; Canoll, P. Transplanted glioma cells migrate and proliferate on host brain vasculature: a dynamic analysis. *Glia.* 2006; 53(8):799-808.

Feng L, Campbell EB, Hsiung Y, MacKinnon R. Structure of a eukaryotic CLC transporter defines an intermediate state in the transport cycle. *Science.* 2010;330:635-641.

Fine, HA; Dear, KB; Loeffler, JS;Black, PM; Canellos, GP. Meta-analysis of radiation therapy with and without adjuvant chemotherapy for malignant gliomas in adults. *Cancer* 1993; 71:2585–2597.

Fiske, JL; Fomin, VP; Brown, ML; Duncan, RL; Sikes, RA. Voltage-sensitive ion channels in cancer. *Cancer Metastasis Rev.* 2006, 25: 439–500.

Fu, YJ; Yin, LT; Liang, AH; Zhang, CF; Wang, W; Chai, BF; Yang, JY; Fan, XJ. Therapeutic potential of chlorotoxin-like neurotoxin from the Chinese scorpion for human gliomas. *Neurosci. Lett.* 2007; 412:62–67.

Fukushima, Y; Hagiwara, S; Henkart, M. Potassium current in clonal cytotoxic T lymphocytes from the mouse. *J. Physiol.* 1984; 351:645–656.

Fuller, MD; Thompson, CH; Zhang, ZR; Freeman, CS; Schay, E; Szakacs, G; Bakos, E; Sarkadi, B; McMaster, D; French, RJ; Pohl, J; Kubanek, J; McCarty, NA. State dependent inhibition of cystic fibrosis transmembrane conductance regulator chloride channels by a novel peptide toxin. *J. Biol. Chem.* 2007; 282:37545–37555.

Giese, A; Loo, MA; Rief, MD; Tran, N; Berens, ME. Substrates for astrocytoma invasion. *Neurosurgery* 1995; 37(2):294-301.

Gladson CL. The extracellular matrix of gliomas: modulation of cell function. *J. Neuropathol. Exp. Neurol.* 1999. 58(10):1029-1040.

G□mez-Varela, D; Zwick-Wallasch, ER; Knötgen, H; Sanchez, A; Hettmann, T; Ossipov, O; Weseloh, R; Contreras-Jurado, C; Rothe, M; Stühmer, W; Pardo, LA. Monoclonal antibody blockade of the human Eag1 potassium channel function exerts antitumor activity. *Cancer Res.* 2007; 67:7343–7349.

Gomes, A; Bhattacharjee, P; Mishra, R; Biswas, AK; Dasgupta, SC; Giri, B. Anticancer potential of animal venoms and toxins. *Indian Journal of Experimental Biology* 2010; 48:93-103.

Grgic, I; Eichler, I; Heinau, P; Si, H; Brakemeier, S; Hoyer, J; Köhler, R. Selective blockade of the intermediate-conductance Ca2+-activated K+ channel suppresses proliferation of microvascular and macrovascular endothelial cells and angiogenesis in vivo. *Arterioscler Thromb Vasc Biol* 2005; 25:704–709.

Hermoso, M; Satterwhite, CM; Andrade, YN; Hidalgo, J; Wilson, SM; Horowitz, B. ClC-3 is a fundamental molecular component of volume-sensitive outwardly rectifying Cl channelsand volume regulation in HeLa cells and Xenopus laevis oocytes. *J. Biol. Chem.* 2002; 277: 40066-40074.

Hess, SD; Oortgiesen, M; Cahalan, MD. Calcium oscillations in human T and natural killer cells depend upon membrane potential and calcium influx. *J. Immunol.* 1993; 150:2620–2633.

Hille, B. "Chapter 5: Potassium Channels and Chloride Channels". Ion channels of excitable membranes. 3rd edition. Sunderland: Mass: Sinauer Associates; 2001; 131-168.

Huang, R; Ke, W; Han, L; Li, J; Liu, S; Jiang, C. Targeted delivery of chlorotoxin-modified DNA-loaded nanoparticles to glioma via intravenous administration. *Biomaterials.* 2011; 32(9):2399-406.

Hubner, C; Stein, V; Hermanns-Borgmeyer, I; Meyer, T; Ballanyi, K; Jentsch, TJ. Disruption of KCC2 reveals an essential role of K-Cl-cotransport already in early synaptic inhibition. *Neuron* 2001; 30: 515–524.

Inceoglu, B; Lango, J; Jennifer, W; Hawkins, P; Southern, J; Hammock, BD. Isolation and characterization of a novel type of neurotoxic peptide from the venom of the South African scorpion Parabuthus transvaalicus. *Eur. J. Biochem.* 2001; 268:5407–5413.

Ishiguro, T; Avila, H; Lin, SY; Nakamura, T; Yamamoto, M. Boyd, DD. Gene trapping identifies chloride channel 4 as a novel inducer of colon cancer cell migration, invasion and metastases. *British Journal of Cancer*; 2010; 102:774–782.

Ishiuchi S, Tsuzuki K, Yoshida Y, Yamada N, Hagimura N, Okado H, Miwa A, Kurihara H, Nakazato Y, Tamura M, Sasaki T, Ozawa S. Blockage of Ca(2+) -permeable AMPA receptors suppresses migration and induces apoptosis in human glioblastoma cells. *Nat. Med.* 2002; 8:971-978.

Jackson, PS; Madsen, JR. Cerebral edema, cell volume regulation, and the role of organic osmolyte transport. *Pediatr Neurosurg.* 1997; 27:279-285.

Jager, H; Dreker, T; Buck, A; Giehl, K; Gress, T; Grissmer, S. Blockage of intermediate-conductance Ca2+-activated K+ channels inhibit human pancreatic cancer cell growth in vitro. *Mol. Pharmacol.* 2004; 65:630–638.

Jentsch, TJ; Stein, V; Weinreich, F; Zdebik, AA. Molecular structure and physiological function of chloride channels. *Physiol. Rev.* 2002; 82:503-568.

Jessell, TM; Schwartz, JH.. "Chapter 6: Ion Channels". Principles of Neural *Science* 2000; 105–124.

Jia L, Patwari Y, Srinivasula SM, Newland AC, Fernandes-Alnemri T, Alnemri ES, Kelsey SM. Bax translocation is crucial for the sensitivity of leukaemic cells to etoposide-induced apoptosis. *Oncogene*. 2001; 20:4817-26.

Jiaqi, W; X, M; Enzhong, Liu; Kezheng, Chen. Incorporation of magnetite nanoparticle clusters in fluorescent silica nanoparticles for high-performance brain tumor delineation. *Nanotechnology* 2010; 23:235104,

Kaczorowski, GJ; Garcia, ML. Pharmacology of voltage-gated and calcium-activated potassium channels. *Curr. Opin. Chem. Biol.* 1999; 4:448-58.

Kavanaugh, MP; Osborne, PO; Varnum, M; Bush, AE; Adelma, JP; North, RA. Interaction between tetraethylammonium and amino acid residues in the pore of rat cloned voltage-dependent potassium channels. *J. Biol. Chem.* 1991; 266: 7583-7587.

Komuro, H; Rakic, P. Intracellular Ca2+ fluctuations modulate the rate of neuronal migration. *Neuron*. 1996;17:275-85.

Kraft, R; Benndorf, K; Patt, S. Large conductance Ca2+activated K+ channels in human meningioma cells. *J. Membr. Biol.*; 2000; 175:25–33.

Kürz, LL; Klink, H; Jakob, I; Kuchenbecker, M; Benz, S; Lehmann-horn, F; Rüdel, R. Identification of three cysteines as targets for the Zn2+ blockade of the human skeletal muscle chloride channel. *J. Biol. Chem.* 1999; 274:11687–11692.

Kürz, LL; Wagner, S; George, JR; Rüdel, R. Probing the major skeletal muscle chloride channel with Zn2+ and other sulfhydryl reactive compounds. *Pflu¨ gers. Arch.* 1997; 433:357–363.

Kuniyasu, A; Kawano, S; Hirayama, Y; Ji, YH; Xu, K; Ohkura, M; Furukawa, K; Ohizumi, Y; Hiraoka, M; Nakayama, H. A new scorpion toxin (BmK-PL) stimulates Ca2+-release channel activity of the skeletal-muscle ryanodine receptor by an indirect mechanism. *Biochem. J.* 1999; 339:343-50.

Kunzelmann, K. Ion channels and cancer. J. Memb. Biol. 2005; 205:159–173.

Lassman, AB. Molecular biology of gliomas. *Curr. Neurol. Neurosci. Rep.* 2004; 4:228–233.

Lebrun, B; Romi-Lebrun, R; Martin-Eauclaie, MF; Yasuda, A; Ishiguro, M; Oyamoe, Y; Pongs, O; Nakajima, T. A four-disulphide-bridged toxin, with high affinity towards voltage-gated K+ channels, isolated from Heterometrus spinnifer (Scorpionidae) venom. *Biochem. J.* 1997; 328, 321±327.

Lee, SY;Lee, A; Chen, J; MacKinnon, R. Structure of the KvAP voltage-dependent K+ channel and its dependence on the lipid membrane. *Proc. Natl Acad Sci USA*. 2005; 102: 15441-15446.

Lippens, G; Najib, J; Wodak, SJ; Tartar, A. NMR sequential assignments and solution structure of chlorotoxin, a small scorpion toxin that blocks chloride channels. *Biochemistry* 1995; 34:13–21.

Littleton, JT; Ganetzky, B. "Ion channels and synaptic organization: analysis of the Drosophila genome". *Neuron* 2000; 26:35–43.

Liu, X; Chang, Y; Reinhart, PH; Sontheimer, H; Chang, Y. Cloning and characterization of glioma BK, a novel BK channel isoform highly expressed in human glioma cells. *J. Neurosci.* 2002; 22: 1840–1849.

Liu, YF; Hu, J; Zhang, JH; Wang, SL; Wu, CF. Isolation, purification and N-terminal partial sequence of an antitumor peptide from the venom of the Chinese scorpion *Buthus martenzii KarschPrep, Biochem. Biotechnol.* 2002; 32:317-327.

Lomize, AL; Maiorov, VN; Arsen'ev, AS. Determination of the spatial structure of insectotoxin 15A from Buthus erpeus by (1) H-NMR spectroscopy data. *Bioorg. Khim.* 1991; 17:1613–32.

Long, SB; Campbell, EB; Mackinnon, R. Crystal structure of a mammalian voltage-dependent Shaker family K+ channel. *Science*, 2005;309:897-903.

Louis, DN; Ohgaki, H; Wiestler, OD; Cavenee, WK; Burger, PC; Jouvet, A; Scheithauer, BW; Kleihues, P. The 2007 WHO classification of tumours of the central nervous system. *Acta Neuropathol.* 2007; 114: 97-109.

Lyons, SA; O'Neal, J; Sontheimer, H. Chlorotoxin, a scorpion-derived peptide, specifically binds to gliomas and tumors of neuroectodermal origin. *Glia* 2002; 39:162-73.

Lyons, SA; O'Neal, J; Sontheimer, H. Chlorotoxin, a scorpion-derived peptide, specifically binds to gliomas and tumors of neuroectodermal origin. *Glia.* 2002; 39:162-73.

Lyons, SA; Chung, WJ; Weaver, AK; Ogunrinu, T; Sontheimer, H. Autocrine glutamate signaling promotes glioma cell invasion. *Cancer Res.* 2007; 67, 9463-9471.

MacFarlane, SN; Sontheimer, H. Modulation of Kv1.5 currents by scr tyrosine phosphorylation: potential role in the differentiation of astrocytes, *J. Neurosci.* 2000; 20:5245–5253.

Maidment, SL; Merzak, A; Koochekpour, S; Rooprai, HK; Rucklidge, GJ; Pilkington, GJ. The effect of exogenous gangliosides on matrix metalloproteinase secretion by human glioma cells in vitro. *Eur. J. Cancer*. 1996; 32:868-871.

Maidment, SL; Rucklidge, GJ; Rooprai, HK; Pilkington, GJ. An inverse correlation between expression of NCAM-A and the matrix-metalloproteinases gelatinase-A and gelatinase-B in human glioma cells in vitro. *Cancer Lett.* 1997; 116:71-77.

Mamelak, AN; Rosenfeld, S; Bucholz, R; Raubitschek, A; Nabors, LB; Fiveash, JB. Phase I single-dose study of intracavitary administered iodine-131-TM-601 in adults with recurrent highgrade glioma. *J. Clin. Oncol.* 2006; 24:3644-3650.

Martin-Eauclaire, MF; Ceard, B; Bosmans, F; Rosso, JP; Tytgat, J; Bougis, PE. New "Birtoxin analogs" from Androctonus australis venom. *Biochem Biophys Res Commun.* 2005; 333(2):524-30.

McFerrin, MB; Sontheimer, H: A role for ion channels in glioma cell invasion. Neuron *Glia Biol*; 2006;2:39-49.

Merzak, A; McCrea, S; Koocheckpour, S; Pilkington, GJ. Control of human glioma cell growth, migration and invasion in vitro by transforming growth factor beta 1. *Br. J. Cancer*. 1994; 70:199-203.

Meyer, S; Dutzler, R: Crystal structure of the cytoplasmic domain of the chloride channel ClC-0. *Structure* 2006; 14:299-307.

Moll, V; Weick, M; Milenkovic, I; Kodal, H; Reichenbach, A; Bringmann, A. P2Y receptor-mediated stimulation of Müller. glial DNA synthesis. *Invest Ophthalmol. Vis. Sci.* 2002; 43:766-73.

Mouhat, S; De Waard, M; Sabatier, JM. Contribution of the functional dyad of animal toxins acting on voltage-gated Kv1-type channels. *J. Pept. Sci.* 2005; 11(2):65-8. Review.

Nakada, M; Okada, Y; Yamashita, J. The role of matrix metalloproteinases in glioma invasion. *Front Biosci.* 2003, 8:261:269. Review.

Noble, M; Mayer-Proschel, M. Growth factors, glia and gliomas. *J Neurooncol.* 1997; 35:193–209.

O'Grady, SM; Jiang, X; Ingbar, DH. Cl^- channel activation is necessary for stimulation of Na transport in adult alveolar epithelial cells. *Am. J. Physiol.*; 2000; 278:239–244.

Ohnishi, T; Arita, N; Hayakawa, T; Kawahara, K; Kato, K; Kakinuma, A. Purification of motility factor (GMF) from human malignant glioma cells and its biological significance in tumor invasion. *Biochem. Biophys. Res. Commun.* 1993; 193(2):518-25.

Olamendi-Portugal, T; Ines-Garcia, B; Lopez-Gonzalez, I; Van-Der-Walt, J; Dyason, K; Ulens, C; Tytgat, J; Felix, R; Darszon, A; Possani, LD. Two new scorpion toxins that target voltage-gated Ca2+ and Na+ channels. *Biochem. Biophys. Res. Commun.* 2002; 299:562-568.

Olsen, ML; Schade, S; Lyons, SA; Amaral, MD; Sontheimer, H. Expression of voltage-gated chloride channels in human glioma cells. *J. Neurosci.* 2003; 23: 5572-5582.

Owens, DF; Boyce, LH; Davis, MB; Kriegstein, AR. Excitatory GABA responses in embryonic and neonatal cortical slices demonstrated by gramicidin perforated-patch recordings and calcium imaging. *J. Neurosci.* 1996; 16:6414–6423.

Pallotta, B; Hepler, J; Oglesby, S; Harden, TA. comparison of calcium-activated potassium channel currents in cell-attached and excised patches. *J. Gen. Physiol.* 1987; 89:985–997.

Pappas, CA; Ritchie, JM. Effect of specific ion channel blockers on cultured Schwann cell proliferation. *Glia* 1998; 22:113–120.

Pardo, LA. Voltage-gated potassium channels in cell proliferation. *Physiology* (Bethesda) . 2004; 19:285-292.

Pardo, LA; Contreras-Jurado, C; Zientkowska, M; Alves, F; Stuhmer, W. Role of voltage-gated potassium channels in cancer. *J. Membr. Biol.* 2005; 205:115-124.

Parihar, AS; Coghlan, MJ; Gopalakrishnan, M; Shieh, CC. Effects of intermediate-conductance Ca2+-activated K+ channel modulators on human prostate cancer cell proliferation. *Eur. J. Pharmacol.* 2003; 471: 157–164.

Parkerson, KA; and Sontheimer, H. Biophysical and pharmacological characterization of hypotonically activated chloride currents in cortical astrocytes. *Glia* 2004; 46:419-436.

Phillips, LR; Milescu, M; Li-Smerin, Y; Mindell, JA; Kim, JI; Swartz, KJ. Voltage-sensor activation with a tarantula toxin as cargo. *Nature* 2005; 436:857-860.

Pillozzi, S; Masselli, M; De Lorenzo, E; Cilia, E; Crociani, O; Amedei, A; Accordi, B; Veltroni, M; Basso, G; Campana, D; Becchetti, A; Arcangeli, A. Overcoming chemotherapy resistance in childhood acute lymphoblastic leukemia by targeting ion channels. *Blood* 2011; 117:902-914.

Possani, LD; Becerril, B; Delepierre, M; Tytgat, J. Scorpion toxins specific for Na+-channels. *Eur. J. Biochem.* 1999; 264:287–300.

Possani, LD; Merino, E; Corona, M; Bolivar, F; Becerril, B. Peptides and genes coding for scorpion toxins that affect ion-channels. *Biochimie* 2000; 82:861–868.

PreuBat, K; Beetz, C; Michael, S; Kraft, R; Wolfl, S; Kalff, R; Patt, S. Expression of voltage-gated potassium channels Kv1.3 and Kv1.5 in human gliomas, *Neurosci. Lett.* 2003; 346:33–36.

Pusch, M; Liantonio, A; Bertorello, L; Accardi, A; De Luca, A; Pierno, S; Tortorella, V; Camerino, DC. Pharmacological characterization of chloride channels belonging to the ClC family by the use of chiral clofibric acid derivatives. *Mol. Pharmacol* 2000; 58:498–507.

Rakic, P; Komuro, H. The role of receptor/channel activity in neuronal cell migration. *J. Neurobiol.* 1995; 26(3):299-315. Review.

Ransom, CB; O'Neal, JT; Sontheimer, H. Volume-activated chloride currents contribute to the resting conductance and invasive migration of human glioma cells. *J. Neurosci.* 2001; 21:7674–7683.

Ransom, CB; and Sontheimer, H. BK channels in human glioma cells. *J. Neurophysiol.* 2001; 85:790–803.

Reichling, DB; Kyrozis, A; Wang, J; Macdermott, AB. Mechanisms of GABA and glycine depolarization-induced calcium transients in rat dorsal horn neurons. *J. Physiol.* (Lond) 1994; 476: 411–421,

Riordan, JR; Rommens, JM; Kerem, B; Alon, N; Rozmahel, R; Grzelczak, Z; Zielenski, J; Lok, S; Plavsic, N; Chou, JL. Identification of the cystic fibrosis gene: cloning and characterization of complementary DNA. *Science.* 1989; 245:1066–1073.

Ritch PA, Carroll SL, Sontheimer H. Neuregulin-1 enhances motility and migration of human astrocytic glioma cells. *J. Biol. Chem.*. 2003 Jun 6;278(23):20971-8.

Rivera, C; Voipio, J; Payne, JA; Ruusuvuori, E; Lahtinen, H; Lamsa, K; Pirvola, U; Saarma, M; Kaila, K. The K+/Cl- co-transporter KCC2 renders GABA hyperpolarizing during neuronal maturation. *Nature* 1999; 397: 251–255,.

Rjeibi, I; Mabrouk, K; Mosrati, H; Berenguer, C; Mejdoub, H; Villard, C; Laffitte, D; Bertin, D; Ouafik, L; Luis, J; Elayeb, M; Srairi-Abid, N. Purification, synthesis and characterisation of AaCtx, the first chlorotoxin-like peptide from Androctonus australis scorpion venom. *Peptides* 2011; 32:656-663.

Sanchez-Olea, R; Pena, C; Moran, J; Pasantes-Morales, H. Inhibition of volume regulation and efflux of osmoregulatory amino acids by blockers of Cl– transport in cultured astrocytes. *Neurosci. Lett.* 1993; 156:141-144.

Schlichter, L; Sakellaropoulos Ballyk; Pennefather, P; Phipps, D. Properties of K1 and Cl2 channels and their involvement in proliferation of rat microglial cells. *Glia.* 1996; 17:225–236.

Scmieder, S; Lindenthal, S; Banderall, U; Ehrebfeld, J. Characterization of the putative chloride channel xClC-5 expressed in Xenopus laevis oocytes and comparison with endogenous chloride currents. *J. Physiol.* (Lond) , 1998, 511:379–393.

Schwiebert, EM; Cid-Soto, LP; Stafford, D; Carter, M; Blaisdell, CJ; Zeitlin, PL; Guggino, WB; Cutting, GR. Analysis of ClC-2 channels as an alternative pathway for chloride conduction in cystic fibrosis airway cells. *Proc Natl Acad Sci* USA 1998; 95:3879–3884.

Schrey, M; Codina, C; Kraft, R; Beetz, C; Kalff, R; Wölfl, S; Patt, S. Molecular characterization of voltage-gated sodium channels in human gliomas. *Neuroreport,* 2002; 13:2493-2498.

Shahbazzadeh, D; Srairi-Abid, N; Feng, W; Ram, N; Borchani, L; Ronjat, M; Akbari, A; Pessah, IN; De Waard, M; El Ayeb, M. Hemicalcin, a new toxin from the Iranian scorpion Hemiscorpius lepturus which is active on ryanodine-sensitive Ca2+ channels. *Biochem. J.* 2007; 404:89-96.

Shen, MR; Droogmans, G; Eggermont, J; Voets, T; Ellory, JC; Nilius, B. Differential expression of volume-regulated anion channels during cell cycle progression of human cervical cancer cells. *J. Physiol. (Lond)* 2000; 529:385–394.

Soli, R; Kaabi, B; Barhoumi, M; El-Ayeb, M; Srairi-Abid, Najet. Bioinformatics' Characterizations and Prediction of K^+ and Na^+ Ion Channels Gating-modifier Toxins. *BMC Pharmacology.* 2009; 9:4-15.

Sollod, BL; Wilson, D; Zhaxybayeva, O; Gogarten, JP; Drinkwater, R; King, GF. Were arachnids the first to use combinatorial peptide libraries? *Peptides.* 2005; 26:131-9. Review.

Sontheimer, H. An unexpected role for ion channels in brain tumor metastasis. *Exp. Biol. Med.* 2008; 233:779-791.

Soroceanu, L; Manning, J; Sontheimer, H. Modulation of glioma cell migration and invasion using Cl(−) and K(+) ion channel blockers. *J. Neurosci.* 1999; 19:5942–5954.

Srairi-Abid, N; Guijarro, JI; Benkhalifa, R; Mantegazza, M; Cheikh, A; Ben Aissa, M; Haumont, PY; Delepierre, M; El Ayeb, M. A new type of scorpion Na+-channel-toxin-like polypeptide active on K+ channels. *Biochem. J.* 2005; 388:455-64.

Srairi-Abid, N; Shahbazzadeh, D; Chatti, I; Mlayah-Bellalouna, S; Mejdoub, H; Borchani, L; Benkhalifa, R; Akbari, A; El Ayeb, M. Hemitoxin, the first potassium channel toxin from the venom of the Iranian scorpion Hemiscorpius lepturus *FEBS J.* 2008, 275:4641-4650.

Srinivasan, KN; Gopalakrishnakone, P; Tan, PT; Chew, KC; Cheng, B; Kini, RM; Koh, JL; Seah, SH; Brusic, V. Sorpion, a molecular database of scorpion toxins. *Toxicon* 2001; 40:23–31.

Steinmeyer, K; Ortland, C; Jentsch, TJ. Primary structure and functional expression of a developmentally regulated skeletal muscle chloride channel. *Nature* 1991; 354:301–304.

Steinmeyer, K; Scwappach, B; Bens, M; Vandewalle, A; Jentsch, TJ. Cloning and functional expression of rat CLC-5, a chloride channel related to kidney disease. *J. Biol. Chem.*. 1995; 270:31172–31177.

Stupp, R; Hegi, ME; Mason, WP; et al. Effects of radiotherapy with concomitant and adjuvant temozolomide versus radiotherapy alone on survival in glioblastoma in a randomised phase III study. *Lancet Oncol.* 2009; 10:459–466.

Sun, C; Veiseh, O; Gunn, J; Fang, C; Hansen, S; Lee, D; Sze, R; Ellenbogen, RG; Olson, J; Zhang, M. In vivo MRI detection of gliomas by chlorotoxin-conjugated superparamagnetic nanoprobes. *Small* 2008; 4:372-379.

Tao, R; Lau, CP; Tse, HF; Li, GR. Regulation of cell proliferation by intermediate-conductance Ca2+-activated potassium and volume-sensitive chloride channels in mouse mesenchymal stem cells. *Am. J. Physiol. Cell Physiol.* 2008; 295:1409–1416.

Terlau, H; and Olivera, BM. Conus venoms: a rich source of novel ion channel-targeted peptides. 2004; *Phsiol. Rev.* 84:41-68.

Thiemann, A; Gru¨ nder, S; Push, M; Jentsch, TJ. A chloride channel widely expressed in epithelial and non-epithelial cells. *Nature.* 1992; 356:57–60.

Toro, L; Wallner, M; Meera, P; Tanaka, Y. Maxi-KCa, a unique member of the voltage gated K channel superfamily. *News Physiol. Sci.*1998; 13:112–117.

Ullrich, N; and Sontheimer, H. Biophysical and pharmacological characterization of chloride currents in human astrocytoma cells. *Am. J. Physiol. Cell Physiol.* 1996; 270: 1511–1521.

Ullrich, N; Sontheimer, H. Cell cycle-dependent expression of a glioma-specific chloride current: proposed link to cytoskeletal changes. *Am. J. Physiol.*. 1997; 273:1290-1297.

Ullrich, N; Bordey, A; Gillespie, GY; Sontheimer, H. Expression of voltage-activated chloride currents in acute slices of human gliomas. *Neuroscience*. 1998; 83:1161-1173.

Valdivia, HH; Kirby, MS; Lederer, WJ; Coronado, R. Scorpion toxins targeted against the sarcoplasmic reticulum Ca(2+) -release channel of skeletal and cardiac muscle. *Proc. Natl. Acad. Sci. USA*. 1992; 89:12185-12189.

Valverde, MA. CLC channels: leaving the dark ages on the verge of a new millenium. *Curr Opin Cell Biol.*1999; 11:509–516.

Vautier, F; Belachew, S; Chittajallu, R; Gallo, V. Shaker-type potassium channel subunits differentially control oligodendrocyte progenitor proliferation. *Glia.* 2004; 48, 337-345.

Veiseh, M; Gabikian, P; Bahrami, SB; Veiseh, O; Zhang, M; Hackman, R. C; Ravanpay, AC; Stroud, MR; Kusuma, Y; Hansen, SJ; Kwok, D; Munoz, NM; Sze, RW; Grady, WM; Greenberg, NM; Ellenbogen, RG; Olson, JM. Tumor paint: a chlorotoxin:Cy5.5 bioconjugate for intraoperative visualization of cancer foci. *Cancer Res.* 2007; 67, 6882-6888 11.

Venglarik, CJ; Bridges, RJ; Frizzell, RA. A simple assay for agonist-regulated Cl and K conductances in salt-secreting epithelial cells. *Am. J. Physiol.*. 1990; 259:358–364.

Verkhratsky, A; Steinhauser, C. Ion channels in glial cells. *Brain Res. Rev.* 2000; 32:380–412.

Wang, J; Reichling, DB; Kyrozis, A; Macdermott, AB. Developmental loss of GABA- and glycine-induced depolarization and Ca2_ transients in embryonic rat dorsal horn neurons in culture. *Eur. J. Neurosci.* 1994; 6:1275–1280.

Wang, WX; and Ji, YH. Scorpion venom induces glioma cell apoptosis in vivo and inhibits glioma tumor growth in vitro, *J. Neurooncol.* 2005; 73:1-7.

Wang, ZH; Shen, B; Yao, HL; Jia, YC; Ren, J;Feng, YJ; Wang, YZ. Blockage of intermediate-conductance-Ca(2+) -activated K(+) channels inhibits progression of human endometrial cancer. *Oncogene.* 2007; 26:5107–5114.

Weaver, AK; Bomben, VC; Sontheimer, H. Expression and function of calcium-activated potassium channels in human glioma cells. *Glia* 2006; 54:223–233.

Weaver, AK; Liu, X; Sontheimer, H. Role for calcium-activated potassium channels (BK) in growth control of human malignant glioma cells. *J. Neurosci. Res.* 2004; 78:224–234.

Weydt, P; Moller, T; Labrakakis, C; Patt, S; Kettenmann, H. Neuroligand-triggered calcium signalling in cultured human glioma cells. *Neurosci. Lett.* 1997; 228:91–94.

Xu, B; Mao, J; Wang, L; Zhu, L; Li, H; Wang, W; Jin, X; Zhu, J; Chen, L. ClC-3 chloride channels are essential for cell proliferation and cell cycle progression in nasopharyngeal carcinoma cells. *Acta Biochim. Biophys.* 2010; 42:370-380.

Yu, FH; Catterall, WA. The VGL-chanome: a protein superfamily specialized for electrical signaling and ionic homeostasis. *Sci. STKE.* 2004; 253:15.

Yang D, Zhang J. Pay great attention to early diagnosis and treatment of breast cancer*Zhonghua Yi Xue Za Zhi.* 2002; 82:1227-1228.

Zamecnik, J. The extracellular space and matrix of gliomas. *Acta Neuropathol.* 2005; 110:435-42.

Zargan, J; Sajad, M; Umar, S; Naime, M; Ali, S; Khan, HA. Scorpion (Odontobuthus doriae) venom induces apoptosis and inhibits DNA synthesis in human neuroblastoma cells. *Mol. Cell Biochem.* 2011; 348:173-181.

Zhang, QY; Zhao, WH; Kang, XM. Relation between c-erbB1, c-erbB2, MAPK expression and resistance to tamoxifen in breast cancer cells in vitro. *Zhonghua Zhong Liu Za Zhi*. 2006 28:826-830. Chinese.

Zhu, S; Huys, I; Dyason, K; Verdonck, F; Tytgat, J. Evolutionary trace analysis of scorpion toxins specific for K-channels. *Proteins.* 2004; 54:361-70.

In: Glioblastoma
Editors: M. F. Bezerra et.al, pp. 77-99
ISBN: 978-1-62100-858-3

Chapter 3

GLIOBLASTOMA: EPIDEMIOLOGY, RISK FACTORS, DIAGNOSIS, AND TREATMENT OPTIONS

Nicholas Butowski*

Department of Neuro-Oncology. Brain Tumor Research Center.
University of California, San Francisco. San Francisco, California
400 Parnassus Avenue,
A808San Francisco, California

ABSTRACT

Glioblastomamultiforme (GBM) is the most common central nervous system malignancy. Why patients develop GBM is still unknown. These aggressive tumors may present in a number of ways, depending on such factors as growth rate and anatomic location. While standard histopathology and epidemiology studies have helped us categorize patients with GBM into risk groups, treatment results for most patients remain unsatisfactory. An improved epidemiological understanding in conjunction with continued advances in the use of molecular markers will hopefully lead to better treatment and prevention strategies. This chapter serves as an introduction into the epidemiology of GBM and its associated risk factors. Also presented are the neurological signs and

* Associate Professor.94143-0350. Phone: 415-353-7500. Fax: 415-353-2187. Email: butowski@neurosurg.ucsf.edu

symptoms that a GBM may cause, and the prognostic factors used for estimating survival. Lastly, there is a brief review of standard and experimental treatment options.

Keywords:glioblastoma, brain tumor, glioma, epidemiology

1. Introduction

This manuscript reviews epidemiologic data and risk factors for glioblastomamultiforme (GBM) . Also reviewed are the neurological signs and symptoms that a GBM may cause and associated prognostic factors. Lastly, a brief review of treatment options for GBM is given.

2. Epidemiology

Approximately 51,000 primary brain tumors are diagnosed in the United States each year; approximately half are GBM, the most aggressive form of glioma.[1-3]GBM continues to be among the top ten causes of cancer-related death despite a relatively low incidence when compared to other cancers. The incidence rate of primary malignant brain tumor is 4-9 cases per 100,000 person-years. This rate is higher in males (7.6 per 100,000 person-years) than females (5.4 per 100,000 person-years) .[1] The global incidence rate of primary malignant brain tumor is 4 per 100,000 person-years in males and 2.5 per 100,000 person-years in females. The incidence rates are higher in more developed countries. The prevalence rate for primary malignant brain tumors is 29.5 per 100,000 persons.[1]

Recently, some have questioned whether brain tumor incidence is increasing. Review and comparison across time periods or across studies is difficult due to diagnostic discrepancies and ascertainment bias in registry data. Nonetheless, after extensive review, this apparent increase is thought to be due to many factors including better diagnostic ability, better access to medical care, and better care for the elderly, all leading to greater detection rather than an increased incidence.[2, 3] Nevertheless, more uniform and unbiased diagnosis and registration methods must be employed before this issue is resolved.

2.1. Age, Gender, Ethnicity, Geography

While a GBM can occur at any age, the average age of onset is early sixties. In general, GBMs affect males 40% more frequently than females.[4] According to a recent study, this greater incidence of GBM in males becomes evident around the age of menarche, is greatest around the age of menopause, then decreases, suggesting a possible protective effect provided by female hormones, though this is merely speculation.[5]

GBM incidence data is subject to variations in diagnostic and reporting techniques amongst different ethnicities or geographic regions. Brain tumor incidence is higher in countries with more developed medical care; however, this is not always the case. For example, the incidence rate for brain tumors in Japan is less than half that in Northern Europe.[3]In the United States, GBMs are more common in Caucasians than in African Americans, non-white Hispanics, Chinese, Japanese, and Filipinos. These dissimilarities are hard to attribute wholly to differences in access to health care or diagnostic practices. Plausibly, genetic predisposition influences incidence in a manner that is not understood. Such discoveries warrant further research into the possible implications of differences in genetics amongst races playing a significant role in tumorigenesis.

2.2. Risk Factors

Research into the etiology of GBM continues, but is mired by many factors including the rarity of disease and the relatively short survival after diagnosis. Studies reveal little with regard to specific causal factors. High-dose therapeutic ionizing radiation to the head, administered for benign conditions or for cancer treatment, does increase the risk of GBM as well as meningioma [6].

Other established risk factors include the hereditary genetic syndromes listed in Table 1. These syndromes explain <5% of brain tumor cases and outside of them, information on familial aggregation is poorly understood. There appears to be an increased incidence of brain tumor in first-degree relatives, and gender predominance with brain tumors being more common in males;

However, an exact mode of inheritance is not evident. Several "glioma families" have been followed over time, but the pattern of inheritance is unclear as tumors skip generations, have variable times of onset and, in parent-child pairs, the child is often diagnosed before the parent.[7] Various segregation analyses of familial GBM favor an autosomal recessive mode of inheritance while others favor a polygenic model. [8]

Armed with this information, investigators have initiated studies of genetic polymorphisms that when coupled with certain environmental exposures, may lead to brain tumors. Unfortunately, several studies of genetic alterations involved in oxidative metabolism, DNA stability and repair, and immune response have led to conflicting reports.[3]

Numerous non-inherited risk factors were examined with several studies suggesting a possible role of the immune system in tumorogenesis. For instance, people who received polio vaccines contaminated with the SV40 virus were shown to be at increased risk of developing a brain tumor, though other studies failed to support this claim.[3] Viral antigens from JC virus and human herpes virus 6 were detected in brain tumor subtypes, but their possible etiologic role is unclear.[9, 10]

Nucleic acids and proteins from human cytomegalovirus were also found in GBM.[9] Intriguingly, other studies indicate that prior infection with varicella zoster may decrease glioma risk. Likewise, there is an inverse association of allergic diseases (asthma, eczema, general allergy) with glioma, further suggesting an immunologic role in the formation of brain tumors.[3]

Table 1. Heritable Genetic Syndromes

SYNDROME	GENE AFFECTED	CNS LESION	CHROMOSOME
Li-Fraumeni syndrome	p53	malignant glioma	17q
Neurofibromatosis 1	NF1	glioma of optic pathway/brainstem	17q11
Neurofibromatosis 2	NF2	acoustic neuroma, meningioma	22q12
Tuberous sclerosis	TSC1, TSC 2	subependymal giant cell astrocytoma, cortical tuber	9q34, 16p13.3
Von-Hippel-Lindau	VHL	hemangioblastoma of cerebellum/spine	3p25
Turcot's syndrome	APC	GBM, medulloblastoma	5q21
Retinoblastoma	RB1	pineoblastoma	13q14
Gorlin's Syndrome	PTCH	medulloblastoma	9q22.3
Lhermitte-Duclos/ Cowden	PTEN	gangliocytoma of cerebellum	10q23.2

Another area, discussed in the media, is that of a possible risk from exposure to electromagnetic fields. The overwhelming amount of evidence does not support any such relationship.[11, 12] Nonetheless, there continues to be anecdotal concern over such matters fueled by increased exposure to radio frequency involved in the increased use of handheld phones and wireless radio devices. Again, numerous studies fail to indicate a causal relationship.[13, 14] In fact, a recent case-control study found no relationship between brain cancer mortality and radiofrequency exposure.[15] Of course, the effects of long-term exposure remain to be determined. Another area of popular concern is the possible association between head trauma and brain tumor risk. To date, no correlation between head trauma and GBM has been supported. In fact, a study that compared adult patients with glioma and a history of head injury requiring medical attention to control patients failed to support an association during an average of 8 years of follow up;[16] however, there was a slight increased risk in the first year following the injury that the authors attributed to increased detection.

Studies of diet, vitamins, alcohol, tobacco, and environmental exposures reveal little about the cause of glioma. Nitrate exposure from cured meats does not influence brain-tumor development;[3] however, reliable assessment of true exposure to nitrates is difficult, due to widespread exposure through tobacco smoke and cosmetics, not to mention the endogenous digestive exposure. Although tobacco is a ubiquitous environmental source of carcinogens, studies have not supported a role in developing a brain tumor. Alcohol consumption does not increase one's risk of developing a GBM, and may actually decrease risk.[17]Lastly, no significant association with increased brain-tumor risk has been found with exposure to pesticides, synthetic rubber, or agents known to be carcinogens, including vinyl chloride and petrochemicals.[3]

2.3. Stem Cells

Several genetic abnormalities in genes governing growth factor-signaling pathways or cell-cycle control are evident in GBM. Discovering how and why these genetic mutations occur may lead to an improved understanding of the disease and to better treatments. The undifferentiated character of brain tumors and recentinvestigation into cancer stem cellshave fueled debate as to whether or not neural stem cells give rise to brain tumors via acquisition of oncogenic mutations. Until recently, the adult brain was thought to be a static environment. It is now known that several regions of the brain contain cells capable of proliferation. Such cells are either stem cells (multi-potent and self-renewing) or progenitor cells (self-renewing precursors capable of producing astrocytes or oligodendrocytes) . Thus, either stem cells or progenitor cells, in addition to differentiated glia, could be the substrate for neoplastic transformation into brain tumors.[18]

As stem cells already possess the machinery for self-renewal, and their longevity targets them for accumulation of genetic mutations, it is easy to see why the stem cell theory is appealing. Regions of the brain with stem cell populations are more sensitive to viral or chemical oncogenesis, [19]and it has been shown that differentiated cells in the brain can give rise to tumors when infectedwith activated *Ras*and*Akt*and *c-Myc* gene transfer. Additionally, the concept of cancer stem cell clonal population implies that with tumor recurrence, mutations found in the first tumor should be found in the second. However, this is not always the case.[20] It also seems that neural stem cells are recruited by brain tumors, leading to the possibility of heterogeneous and or polyclonal cell population with one tumor. Thus, the appearance of stem cells in a brain tumor may be a consequence of dedifferentiating mutations and not the cause of the tumor. Whether the transforming event(s) causing a brain tumor occurs in a stem cell or a more differentiated cell that has reacquired stem cell characteristics remains to be proven. Certainly, the role of stem cells in the ontogeny of brain tumors is complex.

3. ClinicalPresentation

Symptoms or signs of brain tumors are produced by tumor mass, adjacent edema, or infiltration and destruction of normal tissue. Symptoms and signs are best appreciated by considering tumor location and growth rate. For example, rapidly growing tumors located in eloquent cortex or along the ventricular system may manifest themselves after only a small amount of growth. Those in less eloquent areas of the brain may manifest themselves only after substantial growth. No specific sign or symptom is pathognomonic for a brain tumor.

Brain tumors can cause either ‘generalized’ or ‘focal’ neurological dysfunction. Included within the ‘generalized’ grouping are those signs and symptoms related to increased intracranial pressure (ICP) and seizures. Increases in ICP may be due to cerebral edema, vasogenic edema (produced by leakage of the blood-brain barrier) , obstruction of cerebrospinal fluid

(CSF) flow, or obstruction of venous flow. Under these conditions, the patient may develop headache, nausea, vomiting, lethargy, and visual abnormalities like papilledema or diplopia. An acute rise in ICP may cause a sudden onset of these symptoms accompanied by a significant change in level of alertness.

Headache occurs in approximately fifty percent of patients with brain tumors. The headaches usually are not severe and are classically more noticeable in the morning, tend to improve later in the day, and worsen with coughing, straining, or another activity that may increase ICP. Headaches can occur in brain-tumor patients without an increase in ICP, and are subsequently thought to be due to traction on pain-sensitive structures such as the meninges or blood vessels. Of course, headache is a nonspecific symptom occurring in most people as the result of many causes other than a brain tumor. As such, one should always consider other possible reasons why a patient may experience a headache. Furthermore, remember that the most distinguishing feature of a brain-tumor headache is its association with other neurological signs such as personality changes, motor deficits, or seizures.

The incidence of seizures at presentation of a brain tumor varies with histological subtype, ranging from 90% in patients with low-grade gliomas to 35% of patients with GBM.[21] Seizures may occur during the clinical course in approximately 30% of patients with any sort of brain tumor, which is why many patients are prophylactically treated with anti-seizure medicine. However, randomized controlled studies have demonstrated that prophylactic anticonvulsants are unlikely to be useful in brain-tumor patients who have not had a seizure.[22] Whether a tumor will produce a seizure and what type of seizure depend on the location and growth rate of the tumor. Seizures are more frequent when the tumor is cortical and slow growing.[23] Several commonly used anticonvulsants, including Dilantin, Tegretol, and phenobarbital, induce hepatic enzymes and thus may lower the blood levels of a variety of medicines used as palliative or chemotherapeutic agents. This point must be considered when designing and evaluating the efficacy and toxicity of treatment regimens. As with headaches, other etiologies need to be considered in the evaluation of a patient with new-onset seizures; nevertheless, timely imaging should be performed to rule out a focal lesion like a tumor.

Within the 'focal' group of signs and symptoms are those neurological deficits due to the anatomic location of the tumor. These focal findings are generally gradual in onset and progressive, in contrast to acute occurrences like those seen with vascular events. A site-specific discussion of signs and symptoms follows, but a few general principles can be easily recalled: supratentorial tumors may produce motor or sensory deficits, visual field deficits, dysphasia, or a combination of these; cognitive or personality changes of considerable variety can be seen in patients with frontal lobe involvement, gliomatosis, or meningeal dissemination; and infratentorial tumors or posterior fossa tumors generally produce multiple cranial nerve deficits, cerebellar dysfunction, or long tract signs. Tumors within the frontal lobe often cause progressive cognitive decline, emotional liability, and contralateral grasp reflexes. If the left anterior frontal gyrus is involved, the patient may experience productive aphasia. Focal motor seizures or contralateral motor weakness may result from involvement of the precentralgyrus.

In the temporal lobes, left-sided involvement may lead to receptive aphasia while right-sided lesions may disturb the perception of musical notes or quality of speech. More generalized involvement may lead to emotional changes, behavioral difficulties, and auditory hallucinations. Lastly, involvement of the temporal optic radiations may result in crossed upper quadrantonopia.

Tumors of the parietal region may cause contralateral dysfunction of sensation or sensory seizures. Involvement of the optic radiations passing through this region can cause contralateral lower quadrantonopia. If the left supramarginalgyrus is affected, the patient may experience ideational apraxia. Tumor infiltration into the left angular gyrus can result in alexia, agraphia, right-left confusion, and finger agnosia, or a combination thereof. Nondominant (usually right-sided) involvement often manifests itself with anoagnosia (neglect or denial of an affected limb) or constructional apraxia.

Tumors of the occipital lobe generally produce crossed homonymous hemianopia or visual hallucinations. Involvement of the left occipital lobe can result in visual agnosia for objects and/or colors. Bilateral damage results in cortical blindness. In the case of cerebellar lesions, if the vermis is affected, the patient will experience truncal ataxia. If the hemispheres are affected the patient will experience appendicular ataxia (incoordination of the limbs usually accompanied by hypotonia) . Vertical nystagmus can also be observed with cerebellar involvement. Tumors affecting the brainstem generally manifest themselves with cranial nerve palsies, nystagmus, and long tract signs (pyramidal or sensory) .

4. Radiological Assessment

Magnetic resonance (MR) imaging with intravenous contrast is the standard technique used to diagnose and monitor GBMs before, during, and after therapy. When a brain tumor is suspected, the initial step in evaluation is brain imaging with CT or MRI, with gadolinium administration. These studies will assist in determining the location and size of the lesion in addition to the extent of mass effect and degree of cerebral edema. MRI is generally the preferred study, as it is superior to CT in a number of ways:1) MRI resolution and sensitivity are higher, 2) there is less chance of artifact in the posterior fossa or pituitary fossa, and 3) MRI provides a more accurate three-dimensional reconstruction of the tumor, which can better guide surgical resection or biopsy. CT does remain superior for demonstrating acute hemorrhage.

Recent advances in MR imaging methods such as diffusion-weighted imaging, perfusion imaging, and spectroscopic imaging can provide quantitative cellular, hemodynamic, and metabolic information that may enhance our understanding of brain tumor biology. Such imaging advances may improve assessment of treatment response, more accurately determine tumor activity during therapy, and differentiate between recurrent tumor and treatment-related complications. [24-28] These imaging techniques render the greatest amount of information when used together. Research continues to be performed in this area and validation studies that correlate image-guided acquisition of tissue with histopathology are needed.

5. Prognostic Factors

The overall survival for patients with GBM has not improved much in the past 30 years with an average survival of less than one year and less than 3% of patients with GBM surviving 5 years.[23]Increased mitotic activity and or increased MIB-1 labeling correlate with reduced survival in GBM patients.[29, 30]

Rather than rely on the phenomenological pathological classification currently in use, a gene-expression based classification is gaining favor and may assist in determining prognosis and guiding treatment. As GBM appears to be a polygenic disease, further study is ongoing into the prognostic value of molecular signatures to understand how they may guide effective therapy. For example, a recent study demonstrated that gene-expression profiling, when coupled with class prediction methodology, classified diagnostically challenging malignant glioma in a manner that better correlated with clinical outcome compared to histopathologic identification.[31]Nevertheless, further studies and reproducible results are needed before this technique is widely utilized, especially considering the increasing evidence that a sequential accumulation of independent genetic alterations is essential for tumor development.

There is also increasing data on the prognostic value of molecular markers. Patients with a GBM with a 1p and 19q deletion generally have a significantly longer survival than patients with GBM that do not have these deletion.[32]Additionally, EGFR and p53 expression have been studied in GBM patients with the finding that EGFR overexpression (particularly when combined with normal p53 expression) may correlate with poorer survival in patients aged less than 55.[33]

Hegi et al. found that patients with GBM containing a methylated methylguaninemethyltransferase (MGMT) promoter benefited from radiation and temozolomide (TMZ) , whereas those without a methylated promoter did not have such a benefit (see treatment discussion) .[34] Specifically, patients with promoter region methylation achieved a 2-year survival rate of 46% with concurrent TMZ compared to 14% for those patients with unmethylated MGMT gene. Thus, it appears that the methylation status of MGMT is an important molecular marker for selecting TMZ as a first-line treatment. If so, then further research on specific inhibitors of MGMT could be valuable.[35, 36]

Many other factors other than histology have been investigated for their association with survival in GBM patients. Age continues to be strong a prognostic indicator, although the age range associated with more-favorable outcome varies between studies.[37, 38] In general, age less than 45 is associated with increased survival.[3] Stratifying patients into risk groups based on age is likely to lead to better prognostic information. For example, a retrospective study employing recursive partitioning of 832 glioblastoma patients who were enrolled into prospective clinical trials at the time of initial diagnosis established 3 risk groups based on age:≤40, 40 to 65, and ≥65.[39]Based on the commonly accepted belief that functional statusalso predicts longer survival, this study maintained that the 40 to 65 age group be subdivided by Karnofsky Performance Score (KPS) into >80 or <80, with the <80 group behaving similarly to the age ≥65 group.[40] KPS is summarized in Table 2.

Tumor location, size, and extent of resection are variables that have also been studied in relation to predicting survival. Multivariate analyses have not shown tumor location or size to be significant prognostic factors.[41] The benefit of extent of resection continues to be unresolved, though most of the neuro-oncology literature testifies to the benefit of extensive resection especially when compared to biopsy alone.[42] It must be noted, though, that these studies are retrospective in nature and subject to selection bias. They state that patients with surgically resectable tumors have a better survival than those who do not; this is not the same as stating that prognosis is improved by extensive resection. Nonetheless, in the absence of randomized clinical trials and prospectively collected data, this question will remain unanswered.

Table 2. Karnofsky Performance Score

SCORE	FUNCTION
100	Normal, no evidence of disease
90	Able to perform normal activity with only minor symptoms
80	Normal activity with effort, some symptoms
70	Able to care for self but unable to do normal activities
60	Requires occasional assistance, cares for most needs
50	Requires considerable assistance
40	Disabled, requires special assistance
30	Severely disabled
20	Very ill, requires active supportive treatment
10	Moribund

6. Treatment

Treatment of GBM can be divided into initial treatment and treatment at disease recurrence. New agents or treatment delivery techniques are typically tested in the recurrent disease setting where there are few approved treatment alternatives.

6.1. Initial Treatment

Standard treatment of GBM consists of cytoreductive surgery followed by radiation therapy in combination with temozolomide (TMZ) followed by adjuvant TMZ. The combination of radiation with TMZ followed by TMZ was shown to be significantly better than radiation therapy alone in a phase III clinical trial coordinated by the European Organization for Research and Treatment of Cancer (EORTC) and the National Cancer Institute of Canada (NCIC) .[43]Median overall survival in the chemoradiotherapy arm was 14.6 months, versus 12 months in the radiation arm. Perhaps more importantly, the percentage of patients remaining alive at 2 years increased from approximately 10% to approximately 26%.

A post-hoc analysis of tumor tissue in a subset of patients in the phase III trial demonstrated that patients whose tumors have methylation of the promoter region of the *MGMT* gene survived longer than those whose tumors were not methylated, and on average derived greater benefit from the addition of TMZ to radiation. However, TMZ did still provide modest benefit in the non-methylated group, with borderline statistical significance. There is currently no proven alternative treatment for patients with non-methylated tumors, so the combination of radiation and TMZ remains the treatment of choice for all patients with GBM at this time.[43-45]

6.2. Treatment at Progression

GBMs usually recur in spite of treatment. Once progression of a tumor occurs, treatment options include repeat surgical resection, radiosurgery, chemotherapy with standard agents, novel therapies as part of a clinical trial, or a combination of the above. Evaluating the efficacy of new modalities and agents is a challenge. Only a few randomized trials have been done at the time of progression. Most trials are single arm Phase II in design and are inherently limited in the number of patients treated. These trials assess efficacy endpoints such as response rate, which does not necessarily relate to overall survival. Six-month progression-free survival is now commonly used as a measure of efficacy instead.

6.2.1. TreatmentatProgression: Surgery

The same philosophy that pertains to aggressive resection at the time of initial presentation should apply at the time of progression. Important prognostic factors, such as age, performance status, and presumed extent of maximal safe resection should be considered. Surgery for recurrent GBM may also be considered if the diagnosis is in question, and for symptomatic relief from mass effect and cerebral edema. Surgical resection may increase survival in select patients with recurrent GBMs. Those patients with large mass effects may benefit the most. Increasing survival in this setting theoretically provides more time for adjuvant therapy to work. Decreasing tumor mass may also improve the efficacy of adjuvant therapy, as may the removal of hypoxic tissue which is resistant to chemotherapy. The lack of randomized trials evaluating the role of repeat resection and the obvious bias in the selection of patients for repeat surgery makes it difficult to assess the objective benefit of this strategy.

6.2.2. TreatmentatProgression: Radiation

Patients with recurrent GBM almost invariably underwent a previous full course of external beam radiotherapy, making re-irradiation more difficult and potentially more toxic. Various radiation techniques, including conventional radiotherapy, intensity-modulated radiotherapy (IMRT) , temporary or permanent brachytherapy, single- or multi-fraction radiosurgery, and photodynamic therapy may be used at progression. Data on re-irradiation of malignant gliomas using these techniques are limited.[46-47, 49, 50-57]. Given the difficulty and risk of toxicity of brain re-irradiation, it is offered to a relatively small minority of patients with recurrent GBM. It tends to be administered at centers with aggressive treatment philosophies, in highly selected patients with somewhat focal disease and good performance status. It is appropriate that salvage therapy be highly individualized, but the obvious selection bias makes it difficult to make conclusions regarding the benefit of re-irradiation. Additionally, both local failure and symptomatic radiation necrosis are common after re-irradiation.

6.2.3. TreatmentatProgression: Chemotherapy

Bevacizumab, a humanized monoclonal antibody against vascular endothelial growth factor (VEGF) , is approved for single agent use in recurrent GBM. Initial studies used bevacizumabin combination with irinotecan for patients with recurrent grade III or IV gliomas [58, 59]. Radiographic responses, defined as decreased contrast enhancement on MRI or CT, were noted in 63% of patients but improvements in progression free survival (PFS) and overall survival (OS) were less impressive. An identical follow up phase II study showed a response rate of 57% and 6M-PFS of 46% in a similar patient population. Based on 2 subsequent phase II studies, bevacizumab was approved by the FDA as a single agent for the treatment of recurrent GBM following prior therapy [60, 61]; this approval is based on an improvement in objective radiographic response rate (ORR) rather than an improvement in disease-related symptoms or survival. These data stand in contradistinction to the single digit radiographic response rates of several previous GBM studies.[62]

Clinical trials continue with bevacizumab in combination with cytotoxic and or targeted agents both in newly diagnosed and recurrent GBM patients [63-68]. Studies indicate that ultimately tumor progression occurs. There are, at present, two randomized phase III trials investigating the efficacy of upfront bevacizumab for newly diagnosed GBM—one is sponsored by the Radiation Therapy Oncology Group while the other is sponsored by Hoffman-La Roche in Europe. These trials, plus the non-randomized phase II studies, will provide information on whether dosing of traditional chemotherapy is abetter option for combination use with bevacizumaband whether bevacizumaband similar agents alter the recurrence pattern for GBMS [69, 70]. Additionally, imaging and biomarker studies are being performed in order to ascertain which patients may benefit the most from treatment with bevacizumaband whether such techniques can be used to predict survival [71, 72].

Beyond avastin, there is no consensus regarding the most appropriate salvage chemotherapeutic agent. Regardless of the lack of consensus on which chemotherapy agents to use, some patients will likely benefit from additional chemotherapeutic regimens.[73] Nitrosureas are the most commonly used second line agent, but carboplatin, etoposide, irinotecan, or a combination of these agents are also commonly used.[74-77]

In an attempt to improve the outcome of patients with GBM, novel molecular agents administered alone or in tandem with commercially available agents are being tested in clinical trials. More detailed information regarding these novel agents and how they may affect cell signaling pathways may be found elsewhere.[78-83]

Different agents work on specific targets that can influence cell growth, invasion/migration, angiogenesis, and apoptosis. A full discussion of the agents being tested is beyond the scope of this article. Moreover, none have yet to prove successful. However, clinical trials continue and involve tyrosine kinase inhibitors of the epidermal growth factor receptor (EGFR) , platelet derived growth factor (PDGF) , RAS/MAPK pathway, and PI3K/AKT/mTOR pathway. [79, 84-90]

In addition to the evaluation of novel chemotherapy agents, mechanisms of chemotherapy resistance gives insight into future therapeutic approaches. For example, methylation of the O(6) position of guanine is thought to be one mechanism of how TMZ affects tumor cells.

However, TMZ also alkylates the N(7) position of guanine and the N(3) position of adenine. These alkylated sites are repaired by the base excision repair pathway that depends on a group of enzymes in the poly (ADP-ribose) polymerase (PARP) family that provide the needed energy for base excision. PARP-1 inhibitors have been created and tested pre-clinically and have moved into Phase I testing.[91, 92]

6.2.4. Alternative DeliveryStrategies

The development of surgically-based drug delivery strategies specific for the central nervous system in combination with drugs that target molecules specific for gliomas is an exciting area of research.[93] Such approaches may improve the distribution of effective concentrations of agents and reduce systemic complications due to the compartmental specificity of a targeted therapy delivered locally. Additionally, such approaches may effectively contend with infiltrative tumor cells that lie beyond the surgical margin. One approach that has been approved for use is the placement of BCNU impregnated biodegradable polymers (Gliadel) at the time of surgical resection.[94] Convection enhanced drug delivery (CEDD) is a surgically-based method that can deliver large molecules which are soluble in the interstitial space and will have a long half life. CEDD delivers agents by slow direct infusion via stereo-tactically placed catheters. Several compounds have been created that can be delivered in this way.

6.2.5. OtherExperimentalTherapeuticApproaches

Clinical research in gene therapy utilizing replication incompetent versus competent (oncolytic) viruses is an exciting approach that is being evaluated in brain tumor patients. Recent progress has focused on improving gene delivery methodology, development of new delivery approaches such as stem cells and novel viruses, and increasing transgene potency.[95]As we learn more about the properties of neural stem cells, they may potentially be used as a direct antitumor agent, or a vehicle to deliver therapeutic agents or convert prodrugs within the tumor environment.[96]

There are several immunotherapy strategies that are being evaluated in brain tumor patients. These include non-specific activation of the immune system using cytokines, active specific therapy using vaccines, local adoptive immunotherapy with augmentation of cellular elements to enhance tumor cell kill, and passive immunotherapy approaches using antibodies directed at specific tumor antigens.[97]

Conclusion

An understanding of the epidemiologic, molecular, and genetic events regulating GBM is growing. Standard histopathology and epidemiology studies have helped us group patients into risk groups, which aide physicians in determining prognosis and treatment. Nonetheless, treatment results for most patients are unsatisfactory, likely due to the genetic and epidemiological heterogeneity. Continued advances in the use of genetic or molecular markers in conjunction with standard histopathological identification can lead to a more accurate tumor classification system that will allow improved assessment of prognosis and more standardized future studies and resulting data. Furthermore, the expanding amount of information on cell-growth signaling pathways and the role of oncogenes and tumor suppressor genes are critical to developing new molecular-based approaches to brain tumors. Appropriate evaluation of the efficacy of these novel agents requires the neuro-oncology community to continually redefine clinical trial design and strategy.

References

[1] Davis, F.G., et al., Prevalence estimates for primary brain tumors in the United States by behavior and major histology groups. *Neuro.Oncol*, 2001. 3(3): p. 152-8.

[2] Legler, J.M., et al., Cancer surveillance series [corrected]: brain and other central nervous system cancers: recent trends in incidence and mortality. *J. Natl. Cancer Inst,* 1999. 91(16): p. 1382-90.

[3] Wrensch, M., et al., Epidemiology of primary brain tumors: current concepts and review of the literature. *Neuro.Oncol*. 2002. 4(4): p. 278-99.

[4] Surawicz, T.S., et al., Descriptive epidemiology of primary brain and CNS tumors: results from the Central Brain Tumor Registry of the United States, 1990-1994. *Neuro.Oncol.* 1999. 1(1): p. 14-25.

[5] McKinley, B.P., et al., The impact of age and sex on the incidence of glial tumors in New York state from 1976 to 1995. *J.Neurosurg*. 2000. 93(6): p. 932-9.

[6] Gurney, J.G. and N. Kadan-Lottick, Brain and other central nervous system tumors: rates, trends, and epidemiology. *Curr.Opin.Oncol.* 2001. 13(3): p. 160-6.

[7] Osborne, R.H., et al., The genetic epidemiology of glioma. *Neurology*, 2001. 57(10): p. 1751-5.

[8] Malmer, B., et al., Genetic epidemiology of glioma. *Br. J. Cancer,* 2001. 84(3): p. 429-34.

[9] Cobbs, C.S., et al., Human cytomegalovirus infection and expression in human malignant glioma. *Cancer Res.*2002. 62(12): p. 3347-50.

[10] Cuomo, L., et al., Human herpesvirus 6 infection in neoplastic and normal brain tissue. *J. Med.Virol.* 2001. 63(1): p. 45-51.

[11] Gurney, J.G. and E. van Wijngaarden, Extremely low frequency electromagnetic fields (EMF) and brain cancer in adults and children: review and comment. *Neuro.Oncol.* 1999. 1(3): p. 212-20.

[12] Wrensch, M., et al., Adult glioma in relation to residential power frequency electromagnetic field exposures in the San Francisco Bay area. *Epidemiology*, 1999. 10(5): p. 523-7.

[13] Elwood, J.M., A critical review of epidemiologic studies of radiofrequency exposure and human cancers. *Environ. Health Perspect.* 1999. 107 Suppl 1: p. 155-68.

[14] Jauchem, J.R., A literature review of medical side effects from radio-frequency energy in the human environment: involving cancer, tumors, and problems of the central nervous system. *J.Microw. PowerElectromagn. Energy,* 2003. 38(2): p. 103-23.

[15] Inskip, P.D., et al., Incidence of intracranial tumors following hospitalization for head injuries (Denmark) . *Cancer Causes Control,* 1998. 9(1): p. 109-16.

[16] Inskip, P.D., et al., Cellular-telephone use and brain tumors. *N. Engl. J. Med,* 2001. 344(2): p. 79-86.

[17] Wrensch, M., et al., Environmental risk factors for primary malignant brain tumors: a review. *J.Neurooncol,* 1993. 17(1): p. 47-64.

[18] Sanai, N., A. Alvarez-Buylla, and M.S. Berger, Neural stem cells and the origin of gliomas. *N. Engl. J. Med.* 2005. 353(8): p. 811-22.

[19] Singh, S.K., et al., Cancer stem cells in nervous system tumors. *Oncogene,* 2004. 23(43): p. 7267-73.

[20] Shih, A.H. and E.C. Holland, Developmental neurobiology and the origin of brain tumors. *J.Neurooncol.* 2004. 70(2): p. 125-36.

[21] Vecht, C.J., G.L. Wagner, and E.B. Wilms, Treating seizures in patients with brain tumors: Drug interactions between antiepileptic and chemotherapeutic agents. *Semin.Oncol.,* 2003. 30(6 Suppl 19): p. 49-52.

[22] Forsyth, P.A., et al., Prophylactic anticonvulsants in patients with brain tumour. *Can. J. Neurol. Sci.*2003. 30(2): p. 106-12.

[23] Behin, A., et al., Primary brain tumours in adults. *Lancet,* 2003. 361(9354): p. 323-31.

[24] Henry, R.G., et al., Comparison of relative cerebral blood volume and proton spectroscopy in patients with treated gliomas. *AJNR Am. J.Neuroradiol.* 2000. 21(2): p. 357-66.

[25] Law, M., et al., Glioma grading: sensitivity, specificity, and predictive values of perfusion MR imaging and proton MR spectroscopic imaging compared with conventional MR imaging. *AJNR Am. J.Neuroradiol.* 2003. 24(10): p. 1989-98.

[26] Meyerand, M.E., et al., Classification of biopsy-confirmed brain tumors using single-voxel MR spectroscopy. *AJNR Am. J.Neuroradiol.* 1999. 20(1): p. 117-23.

[27] Rabinov, J.D., et al., In vivo 3-T MR spectroscopy in the distinction of recurrent glioma versus radiation effects: initial experience. *Radiology,* 2002. 225(3): p. 871-9.

[28] Jacobs, A.H., et al., Imaging in neurooncology. *NeuroRx.* 2005. 2(2): p. 333-47.

[29] Korshunov, A., A. Golanov, and R. Sycheva, Immunohistochemical markers for prognosis of cerebral glioblastomas. *J.Neurooncol.* 2002. 58(3): p. 217-36.

[30] Reavey-Cantwell, J.F., et al., The prognostic value of tumor markers in patients with glioblastomamultiforme: analysis of 32 patients and review of the literature. *J.Neurooncol.* 2001. 55(3): p. 195-204.

[31] Nutt, C.L., et al., Gene expression-based classification of malignant gliomas correlates better with survival than histological classification. *Cancer Res.* 2003. 63(7): p. 1602-7.

[32] Senger, D., J.G. Cairncross, and P.A. Forsyth, Long-term survivors of glioblastoma: statistical aberration or important unrecognized molecular subtype? *Cancer J.* 2003. 9(3): p. 214-21.

[33] Simmons, M.L., et al., Analysis of complex relationships between age, p53, epidermal growth factor receptor, and survival in glioblastoma patients. *Cancer Res.* 2001. 61(3): p. 1122-8.

[34] Hegi, M.E., et al., MGMT gene silencing and benefit from temozolomide in glioblastoma. *N. Engl. J. Med.* 2005. 352(10): p. 997-1003.

[35] Bobola, M.S., et al., O6-methylguanine-DNA methyltransferase, O6-benzylguanine, and resistance to clinical alkylators in pediatric primary brain tumor cell lines. *Clin. Cancer Res.*2005. 11(7): p. 2747-55.

[36] Kaina, B. and M. Christmann, DNA repair in resistance to alkylating anticancer drugs. *Int. J.Clin.Pharmacol.Ther.*2002. 40(8): p. 354-67.

[37] Curran, W.J., Jr., et al., Recursive partitioning analysis of prognostic factors in three Radiation Therapy Oncology Group malignant glioma trials. *J. Natl. Cancer Inst.*1993. 85(9): p. 704-10.

[38] Shiraishi, T. and K. Tabuchi, Genetic alterations of human brain tumors as molecular prognostic factors. *Neuropathology,* 2003. 23(1): p. 95-108.

[39] Lamborn, K.R., S.M. Chang, and M.D. Prados, Prognostic factors for survival of patients with glioblastoma: recursive partitioning analysis. *NeuroOncol.* 2004. 6(3): p. 227-35.

[40] Scott, J.N., et al., Which glioblastomamultiforme patient will become a long-term survivor? A population-based study. *Ann. Neurol.* 1999. 46(2): p. 183-8.

[41] Buckner, J.C., Factors influencing survival in high-grade *gliomas. Semin.Oncol,* 2003. 30(6 Suppl 19): p. 10-4.

[42] Schiff, D. and M.E. Shaffrey, Role of resection for newly diagnosed malignant gliomas. *Expert. Rev. Anticancer.Ther.* 2003. 3(5): p. 621-30.

[43] Stupp, R., et al., Radiotherapy plus concomitant and adjuvant temozolomide for glioblastoma. *N. Engl. J. Med.* 2005. 352(10): p. 987-96.

[44] Stupp, R., M.J. van den Bent, and M.E. Hegi, Optimal role of temozolomide in the treatment of malignant gliomas. *Curr. Neurol.Neurosci. Rep.*2005. 5(3): p. 198-206.

[45] Stupp, R., N. Pavlidis, and S. Jelic, ESMO Minimum Clinical Recommendations for diagnosis, treatment and follow-up of malignant glioma. *Ann.Oncol.* 2005. 16 Suppl 1: p. i64-5.

[46] Chan, T.A., et al., Treatment of recurrent glioblastomamultiforme with GliaSite brachytherapy. *Int. J.Radiat.Oncol. Biol. Phys.* 2005. 62(4): p. 1133-9.

[47] Gaspar, L.E., et al., Permanent 125iodine implants for recurrent malignant gliomas. *Int. J.Radiat.Oncol Biol. Phys.* 1999. 43(5): p. 977-82.

[48] Larson, D.A., et al., Permanent iodine 125 brachytherapy in patients with progressive or recurrent glioblastomamultiforme. *Neuro-oncol.* 2004. 6(2): p. 119-26.

[49] Patel, S., et al., Permanent iodine-125 interstitial implants for the treatment of recurrent glioblastomamultiforme. Neurosurgery, 2000. 46(5): p. 1123-8; discussion 1128-30.

[50] Shrieve, D.C., et al., Comparison of stereotactic radiosurgery and brachytherapy in the treatment of recurrent glioblastomamultiforme. Neurosurgery, 1995. 36(2): p. 275-82; discussion 282-4.

[51] Cho, K.H., et al., Single dose versus fractionated stereotactic radiotherapy for recurrent high-grade gliomas. *Int. J.Radiat.OncolBiol.Phys.* 1999. 45(5): p. 1133-41.

[52] Combs, S.E., et al., Stereotactic radiosurgery (SRS) . *Cancer*, 2005.

[53] Kondziolka, D., et al., Survival benefit of stereotactic radiosurgery for patients with malignant glial neoplasms. *Neurosurgery*, 1997. 41(4): p. 776-83; discussion 783-5.

[54] Hudes, R.S., et al., A phase I dose escalation study of hypofractionated stereotactic radiotherapy as salvage therapy for persistent or recurrent malignant glioma. *Int. J.Radiat.Oncol. Biol. Phys*. 1999. 43(2): p. 293-8.

[55] Lederman, G., et al., Treatment of recurrent glioblastomamultiforme using fractionated stereotactic radiosurgery and concurrent paclitaxel. *Am. J.Clin.Oncol.* 2000. 23(2): p. 155-9.

[56] Shepherd, S.F., et al., Hypofractionated stereotactic radiotherapy in the management of recurrent glioma. *Int. J.Radiat.Oncol. Biol. Phys.* 1997. 37(2): p. 393-8.

[57] Vordermark, D., et al., Hypofractionated stereotactic re-irradiation: treatment option in recurrent malignant glioma. BMC *Cancer*, 2005. 5(1): p. 55.

[58] Vredenburgh, J.J., et al., Phase II trial of bevacizumab and irinotecan in recurrent malignant glioma. *Clin. Cancer Res.* 2007. 13(4): p. 1253-9.

[59] Vredenburgh, J.J., et al., Bevacizumab plus irinotecan in recurrent glioblastomamultiforme. *J.Clin.Oncol*, 2007. 25(30): p. 4722-9.

[60] Friedman, H.S., et al., Bevacizumab Alone and in Combination WithIrinotecan in Recurrent Glioblastoma. *J.Clin.Oncol.* 2009.

[61] Kreisl, T.N., et al., Phase II trial of single-agent bevacizumab followed by bevacizumab plus irinotecan at tumor progression in recurrent glioblastoma. *J.Clin.Oncol.* 2009. 27(5): p. 740-5.

[62] Ballman, K.V., et al., The relationship between six-month progression-free survival and 12-month overall survival end points for phase II trials in patients with glioblastomamultiforme. *Neuro.Oncol.* 2007. 9(1): p. 29-38.

[63] Scott, B.J., et al., Bevacizumab salvage therapy following progression in high-grade glioma patients treated with VEGF receptor tyrosine kinase inhibitors. *Neuro.Oncol*. 12(6): p. 603-7.

[64] Bokstein, F., S. Shpigel, and D.T. Blumenthal, Treatment with bevacizumab and irinotecan for recurrent high-grade glial tumors. *Cancer,* 2008. 112(10): p. 2267-73.

[65] Lai, A., et al., Phase II Pilot Study of Bevacizumab in Combination WithTemozolomide and Regional Radiation Therapy for Up-Front Treatment of Patients With Newly Diagnosed GlioblastomaMultiforme: Interim Analysis of Safety and Tolerability. *Int. J.Radiat.Oncol Biol. Phys.* 2008.

[66] Gutin, P.H., et al., Safety and Efficacy of Bevacizumab with Hypofractionated Stereotactic Irradiation for Recurrent Malignant Gliomas. *Int. J.Radiat.Oncol. Biol. Phys*. 2009.

[67] Nghiemphu, P.L., et al., Bevacizumab and chemotherapy for recurrent glioblastoma: a single-institution experience. *Neurology*. 2009. 72(14): p. 1217-22.

[68] Quant, E.C., et al., Role of a second chemotherapy in recurrent malignant glioma patients who progress on bevacizumab. *Neuro.Oncol.* 2009.

[69] Bergsland, E. and M.N. Dickler, Maximizing the potential of bevacizumab in cancer treatment. Oncologist, 2004. 9 Suppl 1: p. 36-42.

[70] Norden, A.D., et al., Bevacizumab for recurrent malignant gliomas: efficacy, toxicity, and patterns of recurrence. *Neurology*. 2008. 70(10): p. 779-87.

[71] Chen, W., et al., Predicting treatment response of malignant gliomas to bevacizumab and irinotecan by imaging proliferation with [18F] fluorothymidine positron emission tomography: a pilot study. *J.Clin.Oncol.*2007. 25(30): p. 4714-21.

[72] Chamberlain, M.C., MRI in patients with high-grade gliomas treated with bevacizumab and chemotherapy. Neurology, 2006. 67(11): p. 2089; author reply 2089.

[73] Hau, P., et al., Salvage therapy in patients with glioblastoma: is there any benefit? *Cancer*, 2003. 98(12): p. 2678-86.

[74] Rosenthal, M.A., D.L. Ashley, and L. Cher, BCNU as second line therapy for recurrent high-grade glioma previously treated with Temozolomide. *J.Clin. Neurosci.*2004. 11(4): p. 374-5.

[75] Franceschi, E., et al., Phase II trial of carboplatin and etoposide for patients with recurrent high-grade glioma. *Br. J. Cancer*. 2004. 91(6): p. 1038-44.

[76] Reardon, D.A., et al., Phase II trial of irinotecan plus celecoxib in adults with recurrent malignant glioma. *Cancer,* 2005. 103(2): p. 329-38.

[77] Brandes, A.A., et al., Second-line chemotherapy with irinotecan plus carmustine in glioblastoma recurrent or progressive after first-line temozolomide chemotherapy: a phase II study of the GruppoItalianoCooperativo di Neuro-Oncologia (GICNO) . *J.Clin.Oncol*. 2004. 22(23): p. 4779-86.
[78] Butowski, N. and S.M. Chang, Small molecule and monoclonal antibody therapies in neurooncology. *Cancer Control.* 2005. 12(2): p. 116-24.
[79] Newton, H.B., Molecular neuro-oncology and development of targeted therapeutic strategies for brain tumors. Part 1: Growth factor and Ras signaling pathways. *Expert. Rev. Anticancer. Ther.*2003. 3(5): p. 595-614.
[80] Newton, H.B., Molecular neuro-oncology and development of targeted therapeutic strategies for brain tumors. Part 2: PI3K/Akt/PTEN, mTOR, SHH/PTCH and angiogenesis. *Expert Rev. Anticancer.Ther*. 2004. 4(1): p. 105-28.
[81] Newton, H.B., Molecular neuro-oncology and the development of targeted therapeutic strategies for brain tumors. Part 3: brain tumor invasiveness. *Expert Rev. Anticancer.Ther.* 2004. 4(5): p. 803-21.
[82] Newton, H.B., Molecular neuro-oncology and the development of targeted therapeutic strategies for brain tumors. Part 4: p53 signaling pathway. Expert Rev *Anticancer Ther.* 2005. 5(1): p. 177-91.
[83] Newton, H.B., Molecular neuro-oncology and the development of targeted therapeutic strategies for brain tumors. Part 5: apoptosis and cell cycle. Expert Rev *Anticancer Ther.* 2005. 5(2): p. 355-78.
[84] Raizer, J.J., HER1/EGFR tyrosine kinase inhibitors for the treatment of glioblastomamultiforme. *J.Neurooncol.* 2005. 74(1): p. 77-86.
[85] Rich, J.N., et al., Phase II trial of gefitinib in recurrent glioblastoma. *J.Clin.Oncol.*2004. 22(1): p. 133-42.
[86] Cloughesy, T.F., et al., Phase I trial of tipifarnib in patients with recurrent malignant glioma taking enzyme-inducing antiepileptic drugs: a North American Brain Tumor Consortium Study. *J.Clin.Oncol.* 2005. 23(27): p. 6647-56.
[87] Schmelzle, T. and M.N. Hall, TOR, a central controller of cell growth. *Cell*, 2000. 103(2): p. 253-62.
[88] Chang, S.M., et al., Phase I/pharmacokinetic study of CCI-779 in patients with recurrent malignant glioma on enzyme-inducing antiepileptic drugs. *Invest New Drugs,* 2004. 22(4): p. 427-35.
[89] Chang, S.M., et al., Phase II study of CCI-779 in patients with recurrent glioblastomamultiforme. *Invest New Drugs,* 2005. 23(4): p. 357-61.

[90] Galanis, E., et al., Phase II trial of temsirolimus (CCI-779) in recurrent glioblastomamultiforme: a North Central Cancer Treatment Group Study. *J.Clin.Oncol.* 2005. 23(23): p. 5294-304.

[91] Tentori, L., et al., Brain distribution and efficacy as chemosensitizer of an oral formulation of PARP-1 inhibitor GPI 15427 in experimental models of CNS tumors. *Int. J.Oncol.* 2005. 26(2): p. 415-22.

[92] Tentori, L. and G. Graziani, Chemopotentiation by PARP inhibitors in cancer therapy. *Pharmacol. Res.* 2005. 52(1): p. 25-33.

[93] Chiocca, E.A., et al., Neurosurgical delivery of chemotherapeutics, targeted toxins, genetic and viral therapies in neuro-oncology. *J.Neurooncol.*2004. 69(1-3): p. 101-17.

[94] Brem, H., et al., Placebo-controlled trial of safety and efficacy of intraoperative controlled delivery by biodegradable polymers of chemotherapy for recurrent gliomas. The Polymer-brain Tumor Treatment Group. *Lancet*, 1995. 345(8956): p. 1008-12.

[95] Lawler, S.E., P.P. Peruzzi, and E.A. Chiocca, Genetic strategies for brain tumor therapy. *Cancer Gene.Ther*, 2005.

[96] Westphal, M. and P.M. Black, Perspectives of cellular and molecular neurosurgery. *J.Neurooncol.*2004. 70(2): p. 255-69.

[97] Khan-Farooqi, H.R., R.M. Prins, and L.M. Liau, Tumor immunology, immunomics and targeted immunotherapy for central nervous system malignancies. *Neurol. Res.*2005. 27(7): p. 692-702.

In: Glioblastoma ISBN: 978-1-62100-858-3
Editors: M. F. Bezerra et.al pp. 101-115

Chapter 4

CO-AMPLIFIED ONCOGENES IN GLIOBLASTOMAS

Marie E. Beckner

ABSTRACT

It is well-established that *epidermal growth factor receptor* (*EGFR*) is often amplified in glioblastomas. Other oncogenes can be co-amplified with *EGFR* or amplified without its amplification. Many varieties of oncogene co-amplifications exist, including those involving genes within the same amplicon or in multiple amplicons. Many amplified oncogenes, including *EGFR*, are also frequently rearranged or mutated. Various functions in tumor cells are enhanced according to the specific combinations of genes amplified and/or mutated. Oncogenes mediate cell proliferation, protection from apoptosis, metabolic enhancements, etc. Elucidation of mechanisms that favor oncogene amplifications in the cancer cell genome is greatly needed to further understand malignancy. Also, application of multiplex techniques to detect oncogene amplifications in individual tumors is putatively an emerging need for selecting treatment combinations for patients with glioblastomas in clinical trials. This review highlights traditional oncogenes known to be amplified in glioblastomas. A focused view of copy number gains in known oncogenes provides a simplified approach to understand an important aspect of the complex genomic changes occurring in glioblastomas. Importantly, established amplified oncogenes are within the scope of potential cancer targets for the pharmaceutical industry to consider when designing cocktails of drugs to treat tumors in individual patients.

INTRODUCTION

Glioblastoma or glioblastoma multiforme (GBM) is the most common type of primary brain tumor in adults. These tumors resist all treatment modalities and are lethal within 15 months in most patients. Their genomic alterations are being examined with the goal of formulating targeted therapies that will improve prognosis. Therefore gains in the copy numbers of oncogenes are of interest to identify potential treatment targets. Our knowledge of a subset of genes in malignancy that serve as oncogenes has been established over the past several decades and can now be applied to individual tumors. Although the complete list of oncogenes remains unknown, there are at least a hundred or so of these genes that have been recognized and cited in the literature extensively. Many have drugs already developed to counteract activity of their encoded proteins or have ongoing pre-clinical studies and clinical trials being conducted to develop appropriate targeted drugs and biological agents. Thus, encoded proteins of established oncogenes are within the scope of potential cancer targets for the pharmaceutical industry to consider treating with cocktails of multiple drugs designed for individual patients. Reviewing established oncogenes reported as being amplified in GBMs is useful for determining whether there is a characteristic subset for these tumors, with the understanding that many variations will be present. If multiplex assays can be developed for the subset of amplified oncogenes common in glioblastomas, then individualized therapies can be designed for the targets discovered in each patient's tumor.

Initially genomic amplifications were detected with traditional cytogenetics and comparative genomic hybridization (CGH) . Whole chromosomes, their p and q arms, or portions of an arm were recognized as being amplified. Specific gene amplifications were determined by molecular techniques, such as Southern blots, quantitative polymerase chain reaction (PCR) , fluorescence in situ hybridization (FISH) , etc. More recently, gains in copy numbers of specific genes can now be detected with single nucleotide polymorphism (SNP) arrays and whole genome sequencing that generate massive amounts of information about each tumor. However, simpler multiplex techniques, such as real-time quantitative PCR and multiplex ligation dependent probe amplification, both performed with standard molecular biology laboratory equipment, can now offer quantitative data on 100 or so genes at a time with lower costs and relatively straightforward bioinformatics to interpret the results. Thus, a range of techniques can be used to analyze oncogenes in tumors.

Relatively large chromosomal regions of amplification occur in GBMS that may include amplification of one or more "driver" oncogenes and various numbers of "bystander" genes. Although the amplified bystander genes are often numerous, the driver oncogenes may be relatively few in number. Amplicons can be simple repetitions of intact genes or they can be complex and include rearrangements that involve driver oncogenes. Rearranged oncogenes can become constitutively activated. Some fusion products that result from rearrangements of two or more genes become more active than either of the wild type fusion partners.

CHROMOSOME 7 AND EGFR

Chromosome 7 is most commonly amplified in GBMs. In a series of 47 GBMs, 15 and 4 tumors had 3 and 4 centromeres per nucleus, respectively [Liu, et al., 1998]. The most commonly amplified oncogene, *epidermal growth factor receptor* (*EGFR*) , is located in the 7p12 amplicon. *EGFR* was amplified in 43% of the 206 adult primary GBMs surveyed in The Cancer Genome Atlas (TCGA) project [TCGA Research Network, 2008; Ozawa, et al., 2010]. In a subset of 91 GBMs studied for mutations, 24% had focal amplification of *EGFR* with no point mutations, 18% had point mutations, and 3% had *EGFR* point mutations but *EGFR* was not amplified [TCGA Research Network, 2008]. Another comprehensive study of 22 GBMs that searched for only focal amplifications of high amplitude (6-fold greater than diploid or 12 or more copies per nucleus) found these for *EGFR* in 23% of tumors [Parsons, et al., 2008]. In addition to being amplified in primary GBMs, *EGFR* is also frequently rearranged. Although 3 variants can be found in GBMs, the most common is variant III (*EGFRvIII*) . This variation imparts constitutive activation of EGFR resulting from the loss of 801 coding bases (exons 2-7) that encode the ligand-binding extracellular domain [Sugawa, et al., 1990]. When a gene is amplified, the extra copies permit mutations to occur without the cell risking loss of its wild type gene and protein. Accordingly, encoded proteins from both wild type and mutated forms of the gene can be produced and need to be considered in developing targeted therapy. Although amplification of *EGFR* correlates with more rapid growth in GBMs [Schlegel, et al., 1994], efforts to treat GBMs with EGFR-targeted therapies have not succeeded. Therefore, including other products of co-amplified oncogenes, as well as EGFR, as treatment targets should be considered in individually tailored clinical trials.

Adjacent genes in the 7p12 amplicon can be amplified in the absence of *EGFR* amplification. In one study, 12 of 190 GBMs had 7p12 amplicons that excluded the *EGFR* gene with loci both telomeric and centromeric to *EGFR* amplified. Some loci were found to be consistently overexpressed [Liu, et al., 2000]. A subsequent, more focused look at 2 Mb of the 7p11.2 region found several functional genes nearby, with *LANCL2* and *GASP* nearest to the centromeric (3') end of *EGFR* and *GBAS* and *L-3-PSP* slightly further from *EGFR*'s 3' end. No genes were found near the telomeric end of *EGFR*. In this study all these genes near *EGFR* were found to be consistent with a bystander status instead of being independent target genes due to the lack of their independent amplification [Eley, et al., 2002]. Nevertheless, other regions on chromosome 7 do amplify independently of *EGFR* and may include additional driver oncogenes on the same chromosome [Rossi, et al., 2005]. After focusing single therapeutic agents on *EGFR* without success, a more multidirectional approach is being taken [Gadji, et al., 2009]. Products of target oncogenes elsewhere on chromosome 7 and on other chromosomes are being considered.

Additional Oncogenes on Chromosome 7, Including CDK6 and MET

In some GBMs the long arm of chromosome 7 can have at least two amplicons, 7q21-22 and 7q31. Amplification of *CDK6*, 7q21-22, was found to occur in some gliomas separately from *EGFR* and also separately from *MET* at 7q31 [Costello, et al., 1997]. A study of pediatric GBMs also identified amplification at 7q21-22, including *CDK6* in 5 of 18 supratentorial tumors but not in any of the 6 adult GBMs that were also included. Amplification at 7q21-22 is also seen in a small percentage of the normal population [Qu et al., 2010] In the TCGA project, *CDK6* was found to be amplified in 1% of 206 adult GBMs [TCGA Research Network, 2008]. Amplification of *MET* (7q31) in GBMs was first detected as double minutes in a GBM cell line without concurrent *EGFR* amplification [Wullich, et al., 1993]. Another study of 18 gliomas from the same group found *MET* amplification in 3 GBMs [Fischer, et al., 1995]. Their later studies identified human *actin capping protein alpha-subunit (CAPZAZ)* and *glioma-amplified sequence (GAS) 7-1* and *GAS7-2* clustered in the *MET* amplicon. The prevalence of the *MET* amplification is now known to be 4% in primary adult GBMs [TCGA Research Network, 2008].

The 12q13-15 Amplicon Includes Multiple Oncogenes: CDK4, MDM2, CYP27B1, etc.

Following the *EGFR* amplicon at 7p12, the second most frequent GBM amplicon occurs at 12q13-15 (sometimes extended to 12q13-21) . Several oncogenes are located in this region and one or more of these most likely drives amplification of this region in GBMs or leads to maintenance of the amplicon when amplification occurs by chance. This is a complex amplicon and it can be co-amplified with *EGFR* or without concurrent 7p12 amplification. In an early study of the amplicon, *GLI* (12q13-14.3) was identified in a malignant glioma [Kinzler, et al., 1987]. Then *Murine double minute (MDM) 2* (12q13-14) was found to be amplified 8 to 70-fold and overexpressed 6-fold to greater than 100-fold in 6 of 75 GBMs in 1993. In one of these amplifications, *MDM2* had undergone a rearrangement. In one tumor, the extent of amplification and overexpression doubled in a recurrence. Two of the GBMs with *MDM2* amplification also had amplification of *EGFR*. Also *EGFR* amplification was detected in 69 GBMs without *MDM2* amplification [Reifenberger, et al., 1993]. Subsequently, *MDM2* was found to be co-amplified with *CDK4* and *SAS* in the 12q13-14 amplicon in 11 of 86 GBMs and amplified alone in one additional tumor. *CDK4* and *SAS* were amplified without *MDM2* in 17 of 86 GBMs. Other nearby genes, centromeric to *SAS*, were amplified less frequently, including *GADD153, GLI*, and *A2MR* in 9, 6, and 3 tumors, respectively. Amplification ranged from 8-fold to more than 70-fold. *EGFR* was amplified in 27 of the 86 GBMs and 5 of these had co-amplification at 12q13-14. A 5-fold threshold was used for detection of amplification in these studies. However, at least one additional *GLI* amplification at 4-fold was also documented. Overexpression of amplified genes was noted for *MDM2, CDK4*, and *SAS*, but was variably present for amplified *GADD153* and *GLI* and was absent for *A2MR*. For several reasons, including the expression results, *GADD153, GLI,* and *A2MR* were designated as bystanders in the amplicon [Reifenberger, et al., 1994].

Amplification of the 12q13-14 region was also detected by others in GBMs the following year with an incidence of 15% and the potential for rearrangements [Collins, 1995]. In the next year more extensive mapping of 12q13-15 found that *CDK4* and *MDM2* were located several megabases apart and new intervening loci were included in further investigation of 24 primary malignant gliomas and 2 GBM cell lines. Discontinuities were found between *CDK4* and *MDM2* to explain their independent amplification in some cases. Conversely, by this time *SAS* and *CDK4* were found to be very close, within 10 Kb, to explain their consistent co-amplification. Additional genes that co-amplified with *MDM2* included *RAP1B* (4 of 14 tumors) and *IFNG* in one tumor. *RAP1B* amplification (with overexpression) was considered to be possibly significant in individual tumors. *RAP1B* in one GBM also displayed evidence of rearrangement [Reifenberger, et al., 1996]. Studies reported the same year included *WNT1, OS-4, glioma amplified sequence (GAS) 16, GAS27, GAS41, GAS56, GAS64,* and *GAS89(CYP27B1)* in the amplicon, along with *CDK4, SAS, MDM2,* and *GLI* [Fischer, et al., 1996]. Amplification of *GAS41* was also found in low grade glioma [Fischer et al., 1997]. In a study of 110 primary malignant gliomas and 8 glioma cell lines, *CCND2* (12p13) amplification was also found in 2 GBMs but without significant overexpression of its transcripts [Buschges, et al., 1999]. TCGA results included amplification of *CCND2* in 2% of GBMs with RB pathway alterations (77% of 206 GBMs) [TCGA Research Network, 2008].

MDM2 amplifications in 13% of 75 GBMs were subsequently reported in a study that also showed that none of the *MDM2*-amplified tumors had *p53* mutations [Schiebe, et al., 2000]. Among the *glioma amplified sequence (GAS)* genes, *CYP27B1(GAS89)* was found to be amplified in 7 (25%) of 28 GBMs with various splice variants of it encoding truncated proteins. Overexpression was found for some of the *CYP27B1* splice variants. Also, *GAS41* was amplified in 23% of GBMs [Maas, et al., 2001]. In a later study 16 splice variants of *CYP27B1* in GBMs were found to result in truncated proteins lacking functional domains for enzymatic activity in vitamin D metabolism. Alternatively, a role in deregulation of transcription/translation of the *CYP27B1* enzyme was proposed with potential therapeutic implications [Diesel, et al., 2005]. *Glioma amplified sequence 64* was amplified in 5(10%) of 49 GBMs and was noted to have a very short open reading frame of only 191 bp and increased expression [Fischer, et al., 2002]. In a series of 97 primary GBMs, *phosphatidylinositol-3-kinase enhancer (PIKE*) was found to be co-amplified with the adjacent *CDK4* gene in 12 (12%) of tumors. *PIKE* was also overexpressed [Knobbe, et al., 2005].

Although early studies indicated at least two separate amplicons involving the 12q13-21 region, an amplicon-specific microarray applied to a set of gliomas revealed many amplified subregions, with at least one amplified in the 16 GBMs. Ten genes were overexpressed. In addition to *CDK4, MDM2, RAP1B, CTSP2 (OS-4)* , and *GAS41*, that have already been mentioned, *Ku70 binding protein 3 (KUB3) , OS-9, DCTN2, RAB31P*, and *FRS2*, were also reported. These were designated as being of greater interest among 50 genes in the 12q13.3-14 amplicon based on expression analysis. Amplification patterns among the amplicon's genes were diverse and indicated the possibilities for rearrangements. Maintenance of the amplicon was also noted in a GBM recurrence [Fischer, et al., 2008]. However, a subsequent study of recurrent GBMs found that 12q13-21 amplicons can be lost in recurrences. In regard to prognosis, patients with GBMs lacking amplifications of either *CDK4, CYP27B1, KUB3(XRCC6BP1)* , or *MDM2* had better survival [Fischer et al., 2010]. In the TCGA studies, *CDK4* and *MDM2* were amplified 14% and 11%, respectively, in 206 primary adult GBMs, according to the text, with slightly higher percentages given for tumors with specifically altered pathways [TCGA Research Network, 2008]. Another study that identified only high-level gene amplifications (6-fold) found amplified *CDK4* in 3 (14%) of 22 GBMs [Parsons, et al., 2008]. None of the other amplicons described in the literature for GBMs appear to have the complexity that has been found in 12q13-14. Several additional regions of amplification that include oncogenes are described as follows.

Oncogenes in the 4q12 Amplicon, Including PDGFRA, KDR, and KIT.

A role for platelet-derived growth factor (PDGF) signaling in low grade astrocytomas and some glioblastomas has been well-established for many years. Amplification of the *PDGF alpha receptor* gene, *PDGFRA*, 4q12, has been traditionally included in the genetic pathways leading to secondary GBMs. Analysis of 103 GBMs detected *PDGFRA* amplifications in 8% of tumors [Knobbe, et al., 2003]. In TCGA results, amplification of *PDGFRA* was reported for 11% of the GBMs. It was the third highest gene amplification and the second highest tyrosine kinase receptor amplification (after *EGFR*) [TCGA Research Network, 2008; Ozawa, et al., 2010]. In another study of 22 GBMs and 31 GBM cell lines, pooled with 456 other published cases, *PDGFRA* was amplified in 7.7% of cases and *EGFR* was amplified in 35.7%

[Rao, et al., 2010]. GBMs that are driven by PDGF signaling have recently been designated as "proneural" and approximately one third of this type show amplification of *PDGFRA* [Brennan, et al., 2009; Ozawa, et al., 2010]. An early study found that *PDGFRA* was amplified in normal cortex surrounding a GBM as well as in the GBM itself. However, only the GBM contained a rearranged version of *PDGFRA,* designated as *PDGFRA*$^{\Delta 8,9}$, that resulted in deletion of nucleotides encoding 81 amino acids in the extracellular region. Overproduction of structurally altered *PDGFRA* was proposed to take part in the onset and development of this GBM [Kumabe, et al., 1992]. Recently the same in-frame deletion of nucleotides encoding exons 8 and 9 of *PDGFRA* was detected in 6 (40%) of 15 GBMs in which *PDGFRA* was amplified, indicating that *PDGFRA*$^{\Delta 8,9}$ is a recurrent gene rearrangement in GBMs. Also, in one of the *PDGFRA*-amplified GBMs, a complex amplicon spanned *PDGFRA* and *KDR* genes with a novel fusion, *KP*, formed from the two genes. Breakpoints occurred within exon 10 of *PDGFRA* and intron 13 of *KDR* (cryptic in-frame exon) resulting in an in-frame fusion [Ozawa, et al., 2010]. Both *PDGFRA*$^{\Delta 8,9}$ and *KP* encode proteins with constitutive activation [Clarke, et al., 2003; Ozawa, et al., 2010]. Other *PDGFRA* mutations have also been occasionally observed [Ozawa, et al., 2010]. In addition to amplifications of *PDGFRA* and KDR, amplification of *KIT* has also been reported at 4q12 [Nobusawa, et al., 2010, 2011]. In a large series *PDGFRA*, *KIT*, and *KDR* were amplified in 33(8.5%) , 17 (4.4%) , and 13 (3.3%) , respectively, of 390 GBMs, with concurrent amplification of all three genes in 12 GBMs. An inverse association between amplification of *KIT* was found for *EGFR* amplification [Nobusawa, et al., 2011].

Oncogenes in the 1q32 Amplicon, Including MDM4, PIK3C2B, etc.

A complex amplicon exists at 1q32 in some GBMs. A major target in this region was found to be *MDM4* (structurally homologous to *MDM2* and encodes Mdm2-related protein) . Four (4%) of 106 GBMs demonstrated increased target:reference gene ratios with amplification levels on Southern blots that ranged from 5 to 25-fold and enhanced expression of *MDM4* transcripts was also present. A splice variant of *MDM4* (68-bp deletion) was also noted but its levels did not differ between GBMs harboring amplified *MDM4* versus GBMs lacking its amplification. In this study, other genes at 1q32 that co-amplified with *MDM4* included *glioma amplified chromosome 1*

(GAC1) , the *renin* gene (*REN*) , and *RBBP5*. Several other genes at 1q32, *ELF3, ELK4*, and *PTPN7*, did not co-amplify with *MDM4* [Riemenschneider et al., 1999]. MDM4 was amplified in 4% of 206 GBMs. Among 87% of tumors with altered p53 signaling, MDM4 was amplified in 7% [TCGA Research Network, 2008]. *PIK3C2B* is among other genes at 1q32 that have shown amplification. In a series of 103 GBMs, *PIK3C2B* was amplified in 6 tumors (6%) with overexpression found in 4 of these cases [Knobbe, et al., 2003]. Others have reported *PIK3C2B/MDM4* amplifications in 7.7% of GBMs (22 tumors, 8 cell lines, and 456 reported cases) [Rao, et al., 2010]. Amplification of *CNTN2 (TAX-1)* at 1q32.1 in GBMs has also been reported [Rickman, et al., 2001; Riemenschneider, et al., 2003].

Additional PIK3/AKT Oncogenes

Recently, *AKT3* (1q44) was found to be amplified in 2% of 206 GBMs [TCGA Research Network, 2008]. Earlier in a series of 103 GBMs no amplification of *AKT3* had been reported when 17 genes related to the PIK3/Akt pathway were surveyed [Knobbe, et al., 2003]. Also, *IRS2* (13q34) was rarely amplified in GBMs [TCGA Research Network, 2008]. The TCGA finding was supported by a prevalence of 2% amplification reported for *IRS2* in the series of 103 GBMs mentioned above [Knobbe, et al., 2003]. Others who also examined the PIK3/Akt pathway genes in GBMs found that in 107 primary and 32 secondary GBMs, *PIK3CA* (3q26.3) was amplified (greater than 3 copy numbers) in 14 (13%) and 3 (9%) of primary and secondary GBMs, respectively. Mutations in exons 9 and 20 of *PIK3CA* were detected in 5 (5%) and 1 (3%) of primary and secondary GBMs, respectively. In one GBM, *PIK3CA* was both mutated and amplified [Kita, et al., 2007]. A small percentage (~ 2%) of the 206 GBMs in TCGA project also demonstrated amplified *PIK3CA* [TCGA Research Network, 2008].

MYCN and CCND3

The *MYCN* (2p24.1) oncogene was also found to be amplified in a small number (~ 2%) of TCGA project's large series of GBMs [TCGA Research Network, 2008]. Earlier *MYCN* was found to be amplified (80 copies) in 1 of 4 GBMs that represented a tumor recurrence and its transcripts were also strongly expressed [Fujimoto, et al., 1989]. Others have also found amplified

MYCN in a small percentage of GBMs [Fuller, et al., 1992]. Lastly, there have been reports of *CCND3* (6p21) being amplified in GBMs. In a series of 110 primary malignant gliomas and 8 glioma cell lines, amplification of *CCND3* occurred in one primary GBM, one gliosarcoma, and in one GBM cell line [Buschges, et al., 1999]. *CCND3* was also amplified (50-fold) in 1 of 10 GBM cell lines in another study [Kuchiki, et al., 2000].

Ongoing Studies

In view of the potential for oncogenes to mediate key adaptations for the survival and competitive advantages of tumor cells, determining their amplifications is of great interest in GBMs. In ongoing studies we are attempting to correlate some of these amplifications with metabolic adaptations found in GBMs. Our focus is on identifying specific oncogenes that co-amplify with *EGFR* to influence ATP citrate lyase, a positive regulator of glycolysis (via cleavage of citrate, an inhibitor of phosphofructokinase 1) [Beckner, et al., 2011]. Other metabolic adaptations influenced by amplified oncogenes are also being investigated.

Conclusion

Certainly, this review is an incomplete listing of all amplified oncogenes in primary adult GBMs. However, it includes traditional oncogenes that already have therapeutic agents and strategies available or under development to counteract activities of their encoded proteins. For most of the oncogenes listed, their amplifications have been reported multiple times and occurred in the moderate to high range. Interestingly, a significant number of amplified oncogenes have also been shown to exist in rearranged as well as wild type versions in GBMs. Putatively, stratification to clinical trials with individualized combinations of therapies for patients will be aided by detection of the oncogene amplifications in each tumor. This can be done quickly with multiplex, PCR-based assays using simplified bioinformatics or by using more comprehensive and complex techniques, such as SNP arrays and whole genome sequencing. Currently, there appears to be sufficient information available to serve as a guide to begin developing clinical trials with combination therapies aimed at the proteins encoded by amplified oncogenes in individual tumors, with the understanding that the list of important oncogenes is not yet finalized. As new oncogenes are discovered, the subset of oncogenes potentially amplified in an individual's GBM will expand. This review focused on amplifications of oncogenes but activating mutations will also be important in planning future therapeutic strategies.

REFERENCES

Beckner, ME; Kant, JA; Pollack, IF; Nordberg, ML; Hamilton, RA. A potential role for co-amplification of other oncogenes with EGFR in the control of metabolism in glioblastomas. *FASEB J*, 2011 25, 1b318.

Brennan, C; Momota, H; Hambardzumyan, D; Ozawa, T; Tandon, A; Pedraza, A; Holland, E. Glioblastoma subclasses can be defined by activity among signal transduction pathways and associated genomic alterations. *PLoS ONE*, 2009 4, e7752.doi:10.1371/journal.pone.0007752.

Buschges, R; Weber, RG; Actor, B; Lichter, P; Collins, VP; Reifenberger, G. Amplification and expression of cyclin D genes (CCND1, CCND2 and CCND3) in human malignant gliomas. *Brain Pathol*, 1999 9, 435-442.

Clarke, ID; Dirks, PB. A human brain tumor-derived PDGFR-α deletion mutant is transforming. *Oncogene*, 2003 22, 722-733.

Collins, VP. Gene amplification in human gliomas. *Glia*, 1995 15, 289-96.

Costello, JF; Plass, C; Arap, W; Chapman, VM; Held, WA; Berger, MS; Su Huang, HJ; Cavenee, WK. Cyclin-dependent kinase 6 (CDK6) amplification in human gliomas identified using two-dimensional separation of genomic DNA. *Cancer Res*, 1997 57, 1250-1254.

Diesel, B; Rademacher, J; Bureik, M; Bernhardt, R; Seifert, M; Reichrath, J; Fischer, U; Meese, E. Vitamin D_3 metabolism in human glioblastoma multiforme: Functionality of CYP27B1 splice variants, metabolism of calcidiol, and effect of calcitriol. *Clin. Cancer Res*, 2005 11, 5370-5380.

Eley, GD; Reiter, JL; Pandita, A; Park, S; Jenkins, RB; Maihle, NJ; James, CD. A chromosomal region 7p11.2 transcript map: Its development and application to the study of EGFR amplicons in glioblastoma. *Neuro-Oncol*, 2002 4, 86-94.

Fischer, U; Heckel, D; Michel, A; Janka, M; Hulsebos, T; Meese, E. Cloning of a novel transcription factor-like gene amplified in human glioma including astrocytoma grade I. *Hum. Mol. Genet*, 1997 6, 1817-1822.

Fischer, U; Keller, A; Leidinger, P; Deutscher, S; Heisel, S; Urbschat, S; Lenhof, H-P; Meese, E. A different view on DNA amplifications indicates frequent, highly complex, and stable amplicons on 12q13-21 in glioma. *Mol. Cancer Res.*, 2008 6, 576-584.

Fischer, U; Leidinger, P; Keller, A; Folarin, A; Ketter, R; Graf, N; Lenhof, HP; Meese, E. Amplicons on chromosome 12q13-21 in glioblastoma recurrences. *Int. J. Cancer*, 2010 126, 2594-2602.

Fischer, U; Meltzer, P; Meese, E. Twelve amplified and expressed genes localized in a single domain in glioma. *Hum Genet*, 1996 98, 625-628.

Fischer, U; Muller, HW; Sattler, HP; Feiden, K; Zang, KD; Meese, E. Amplification of the MET gene in glioma. *Genes Chromosomes Cancer*, 1995 12, 63-65.

Fischer, U; Schutz, N; Hemmer, D; Meese, E. GAS64, the first amplified and putative non-translated gene. *Int. J. Oncol.*, 2002 20, 173-176.

Fujimoto, M; Sheridan, PJ; Sharp, ZD; Weaker, FJ; Kagan-Hallet, S; Story, JL. Proto-oncogene analyses in brain tumors. *J. Neurosurg.*, 1989 70, 910-915.

Fuller, GN; Bigner, SH. Amplified cellular oncogenes in neoplasms of the human central nervous system. *Mutat Res.,* 1992 276, 299-306.

Gadji, M; Crous, AM; Fortin, D; Krcek, J; Torchia, M; Mai, S; Drouin, R; Klonisch, T. EGF receptor inhibitors in the treatment of glioblastoma multiform: old clinical allies and newly emerging therapeutic concepts. *Eur. J. Pharmacol.*, 2009 625, 23-30.

Kinzler, KW; Bigner, SH; Bigner, DD; Trent, JM; Law, ML; O'Brien, SJ; Wong, AJ; Vogelstein, B. Identification of an amplified, highly expressed gene in a human glioma. *Science*, 1987 236, 70-73.

Kita, D; Yonekawa,Y; Weller, M; Ohgaki, H. PIK3CA alterations in primary (de novo) and secondary glioblastomas. *Acta Neuropathol*, 2007 113, 295-302.

Knobbe, CB; Reifenberger, G. Genetic alterations and aberrant expression of genes related to the phosphatidyl-inositol-3'-kinase/protein kinase B (Akt) signal transduction pathway in glioblastomas. *Brain Pathol*, 2003 13, 507-518.

Knobbe, CB; Trampe-Kieslich, A; Reifenberger, G. Genetic alteration and expression of the phosphoinositol-3-kinase/Akt pathway genes PIK3CA and PIKE in human glioblastomas. *Neuropathol Appl Neurobiol*, 2005 31, 486-490.

Kuchiki, H; Saino, M; Nobukuni, T; Yasuda, J; Maruyama, T; Kayama, T; Murakami, Y; Sekiya, T. Detection of amplification of a chromosomal fragment at 6p21 including the cyclin D3 gene in a glioblastoma cell line by arbitrarily primed polymerase chain reaction. *Int. J. Cancer*, 2000 85, 113-116.

Kumabe, T; Sohma, Y; Kayama, T; Yoshimoto, T; Yamamoto, T. Overexpression and amplification of α-PDGF receptor gene lacking exons coding for a portion of the extracellular region in a malignant glioma. *Tohoku J. Exp. Med*, 1992 168, 265-269.

Liu, L; Ichimura, K; Pettersson, EH; Collins, VP. Chromosome 7 rearrangements in glioblastomas; loci adjacent to EGFR are independently amplified. *J. Neuropathol Exp. Neurol.* 1998 57, 1138-1145.

Liu, L; Ichimura, K; Pettersson, EH; Goike, HM; Collins, VP. The complexity of the 7p12 amplicon in human astrocytic gliomas: detailed mapping of 246 tumors. *J. Neuropathol. Exp. Neurol.*, 2000 59, 1087-1093.

Maas, RM; Reus, K; Diesel, B; Steudel, W-I; Feiden, W; Fischer, U; Meese, E. Amplification and expression of splice variants of the gene encoding the P450 cytochrome 25-hydroxyvitamin D_3 1,α-hydroxylase (CYP27B1) in human malignant glioma. *Clin. Cancer Res.*, 2001 7, 868-875.

Nobusawa, S; Lachuer, J; Wierinckx, A; Kim, YH; Huang, J; Legras, C; Kleihaus, P, Ohgaki, H. Intratumoral patterns of genomic imbalance in glioblastomas. *Brain Pathol.*, 2010 20, 936-944.

Nobusawa, S; Stawski, R; Kim, YH; Nakazato, Y; Ohgaki, H. Amplification of the PDGFRA, KIT and KDR genes in glioblastoma: a population-based study. *Neuropathol.*, 2011 Mar 7. doi: 10.1111/j.1440-1789.2011.01204.x. [Epub ahead of print].

Ozawa, T; Brennan CW; Wang, L; Squatrito, M; Sasayama, T; Nakada, M; Huse, JT; Pedraza, A; Utsuki, S; Yasui, Y; Tandon, A; Fomchenko, EI; Oka, H; Levine, RL; Fujii, K; Ladanyi, M; Holland, EC. *PDGFRA* gene rearrangements are frequent genetic events in *PDGFRA*-amplified glioblastomas. *Genes and Develop*, 2010 24, 2205-2218.

Parsons, DW; Jones, S; Zhang, X; Lin, C-HJ; Leary, RJ; Angenendt, P; Mankoo, P; Carter, H; Siu,I-M; Gallia, GL; Olivi, A; McLendon, R; Rasheed, BA; Keir, S; Nikolskaya, T; Nikolsy, Y; Busam, DA; Tekleab, H; Diaz, LA, Jr; Hartigan, J; Smith, DR; Strausberg, RL; Marie, SKN; Shinjo, SMO; Yan, H; Riggins, GJ; Bigner, DD; Karchin, R; Papadopoulos, N; Parmigiani, G; Vogelstein, B; Velculescu, VE; Kinzler, KW. An integrated genomic analysis of human glioblastoma multiforme. *Science*, 2008 321, 1807-1812.

Qu, H-Q; Jacob, K; Fatet, S; Ge, B; Barnett, D; Delattre, O; Faury, D; Montpetit, A; Solomon, L; Hauser, P; Garami, M; Bognar, L; Hansely, Z; Mio, R; Farmer, J-P; Albrecht, S; Polychronakos, C; Hawkins, C; Jabado,

N. Genome-wide profiling using single-nucleotide polymorphism arrays identifies novel chromosomal imbalances in pediatric glioblastomas. *Neuro-Oncol*, 2010 12, 153-163.

Rao, SK; Edwards, J; Joshi, AD; Siu, IM; Riggins, GJ. A survey of glioblastoma genomic amplifications and deletions. *J. Neurooncol.*, 2010 96, 169-179.

Reifenberger, G.; Ichimura, K; Reifenberger, J; Elkahloun, AG; Meltzer, PS; Collins, VP. Refined mapping of 12q13-q14 amplicons in human malignant gliomas suggests CDK4/SAS and MDM2 as independent amplification targets. *Cancer Res.*, 1996 56, 5141-5145.

Reifenberger, G; Liu, L; Ichimura, K; Schmidt, EE; Collins, VP. Amplification and overexpression of the MDM2 gene in a subset of human malignant gliomas without *p53* mutations. *Cancer Res.*, 1993 53, 2736-2739.

Reifenberger, G; Reifenberger, J; Ichimura, K; Meltzer, PS; Collins, VP. Amplification of multiple genes from chromosomal region 12q13-14 in human malignant gliomas: Preliminary mapping of the amplicons shows preferential involvement of CDK4, SAS, and MDM2. *Cancer Res.* 1994 54, 4299-4303.

Rickman, DS; Tyagi, R; Zhu, X-X; Bobek, MP; Song, S; Blaivas, M; Misek, DE; Israel, MA; Kurnit, DM; Ross, DA; Kish, PE; Hanash, SM. The gene for the axonal cell adhesion molecule *TAX-1* is amplified and aberrantly expressed in malignant gliomas. *Cancer Res.*, 2001 61, 2162-2168.

Riemenschneider, M; Buschges, R; Wolter, M; Reifenberger, J, Bostrom, J; Kraus, JA; Schlegel, U; Reifenberger, G. Amplification an overexpression of the MDM4 (MDMX) gene from 1q32 in a subset of malignant gliomas without TP53 mutation or MDM2 amplification. *Cancer Res.*, 1999 59, 6091-6096.

Riemenschneider, MJ; Knobbe, CB; Reifenberger, G. Refined mapping of 1q32 amplicons in malignant gliomas confirms MDM4 as the main amplification target. *Int. J. Cancer*, 2003 104, 752-757.

Rossi, MR; La Duca, J; Matsui, S; Nowak, NJ; Hawthorn, L; Cowell, JK. Novel amplicons on the short arm of chromosome 7 identified using high resolution array CGH contain over expressed genes in addition to EGFR in glioblastoma multiforme. *Genes Chromosomes Cancer*, 2005 44, 392-404.

Schiebe, M; Ohneseit, P; Hoffmann, W; Meyermann, R; Rodemann, HP; Bamberg, M. Analysis of mdm2 and p53 gene alterations in glioblastomas and its correlation with clinical factors. *J. Neurooncol.*, 2000 49, 197-203.

Schlegel, J; Merdes, A; Stumm, G; Albert, FK; Forsting, M; Hynes, N; Kiessling, M. Amplification of the epidermal-growth-factor-receptor gene correlates with different growth behavior in human glioblastoma. *Int. J. Cancer*, 1994 56:72-77.

Sugawa, N; Ekstrand, AJ; James, CD; Collins, VP. Identical splicing of aberrant epidermal growth factor receptor transcripts from amplified rearranged genes in human glioblastomas. *Proc. Natl. Acad. Sci. USA*, 1990 87, 8602-8606.

The Cancer Genome Atlas (TCGA) Research Network. Comprehensive genomic characterization defines human glioblastoma genes and core pathways. *Nature*, 2008 455, 1061-1068.

Wullich, B; Muller, HW; Fischer, U; Zang, KD; Meese, E. Amplified met gene linked to double minutes in human glioblastoma. *Eur. J. Cancer*, 1993 29A, 1991-1995.

In: Glioblastoma ISBN: 978-1-62100-858-3
Editors: M. F. Bezerra et.al, pp. 117-131

Chapter 5

Mesenchymal Stem Cells: A Novel Therapeutic Delivery Vehicle for Glioblastoma

Candice A. Shaifer[1] and P. Charles Lin[2]
[1]Johns Hopkins University-School of Medicine, Baltimore
[2]National Cancer Institute, Frederick

Abstract

Each year 40,000 people are diagnosed with primary brain tumors, the majority of which are glioblastoma (GB) . [1] Glioblastoma is the most common brain tumor in adults and is the most malignant subtype. Despite best treatments with maximum surgical resection, radiation and chemotherapy, long-term survival of GB patients is rare (median survival is 14.6 months) . [2-4] Complete surgical resection is a challenge due to the diffusely infiltrative growth pattern of GB, and systemic therapy is limited by the selectivity of the blood brain barrier. Experimental evidence suggests that a subpopulation of cells called brain tumor stem cells (BTSCs) retain tumor initiating ability and are responsible for the invasive and chemo/radioresistant nature of malignant gliomas. [5-12] It is believed that BTSCs infiltrate into normal brain tissue of patients, resulting in distant disease recurrence and death. [13] As a result there is an increased impetus to find novel methods to eradicate the BTSC population. The use of mesenchymal stem cells (MSC) has become an attractive option. [14] MSCs are attractive for clinical use because they possess a natural affinity for tumors, can be easily isolated and expanded to the numbers required for application, and can be genetically modified through various means. Bone marrow-derived mesenchymal stem cells (BM-MSCs) can selectively home to gliomas as well as track disseminated nests of BTSCs in animal models. [15] Therefore, MSCs can serve as vehicles to deliver chemotherapeutic agents such as cytokines and oncolytic viruses to tumors. [16, 17]

Traditionally, MSCs are extracted from bone marrow, however the invasive harvesting procedure and decline in BM-MSC lifespan with increasing donor age highlight the need to find alternative sources of MSCs. [18] Human adipose tissue may become an excellent source of MSCs sharing many similarities with their bone marrow counterparts. [19] Acquisition of adipose tissue is less invasive and less expensive than bone marrow, making human adipose-derived mesenchymal stem cells (hAMSCs) an attractive alternative. hAMSCs express high levels of MSC surface markers implicated in cellmigration, and possess the potential for multi-lineage differentiation into adipocytes, osteoblasts, chondrocytes, myocytes, and neuron-like cells. [19-23] In acolon cancer model, genetically modified AMSCs were proven to be efficient gene delivery vehicles. [24] AMSCs not only homed to the site of colon cancer *in vitro,* but alsomediated an anti-tumor effect *in vivo*. Further supporting the potential for hAMSCs as therapeutic vehicles, the anti-tumoral efficacy of hAMSCs has been recently demonstrated in a murine model of brainstem glioma. [25] Thiscommentary will highlight the versatility of adipose derivedMSCs as vehicles for delivery oftherapeutic modalities, providing an avenue toovercome one of the major limitations ofchemotherapy for glioblastoma, getting thetreatment to the tumor.

INTRODUCTION

Malignant brain tumors remain virtually untreatable and lethal. [2-4] Based on histological analysis the most common brain tumors are astrocytomas (11.3%) , ependymomas (2.2%) , oligodendrogliomas (4%) and tumors with a mixture of two or more of these cell types (12.6%) . Of all the primary brain tumors, GB (23%) , which is a malignant astrocytoma, is the most devastating neoplasm of the central nervous system and maintains a dismal prognosis. [26-29] According to the World Health Organization, astrocytomas are classified as either localized or diffuse based on how they interact with their immediate microenvironment. Localized GB exhibit limited invasiveness and a restricted pattern of growth. [30] On the other hand, diffuse GBis invasive at the peritumoral edge and is able to metastasize to distant sites. The success of current therapies has been met with limitations due to the disseminated nature of these tumors. Currently, radio- and chemotherapies are utilized to eliminate the bulk brain tumor by targeting tumor angiogenesis, growth factor receptors, andaberrant intracellular signaling pathways. Within the past decade stem cells have been documented, through *in vitro* and *in vivo* studies, to possess a natural affinity towards tumors, including glioblastomas, [31-33] which has resulted in an impetus to find novel methods able to target the primary tumor as well as the microsatellites located distances away from the bulk tumor.

Two types of stem cells have been reported as cell carriers for cancer therapies: neural and mesenchymal stem cells. Neural stem cells (NSCs) are derived from fetal, neonatal, or postnatal tissues. [34] These cells are multipotent and can differentiate into neurons, astrocytes and oligodendrocytes. [35] Mesenchymal stem cells (MSCs) can be obtained from bone marrow [36-38] and adipose tissue. [39, 40] These cells are also multipotent and can differentiate into various mesenchymal lineage cells including adipocytes, osteocytes, and chondrocytes. [36, 41, 42] Severalgroups have reported on the ability of both stem cell populations to migrate great distances, home to the primary tumor as well disseminated tumor foci. [24, 25, 43, 44] However, before mesenchymal stem cells can be used as therapeutic delivery vehicles in human clinical trials, scientist must provethat the therapy will concurrently balance therapeutic efficacy while maintaining a safety profile to ensure increased survival with minimal complications. First, the agent must be highly potent to exhibit maximal anti-tumoral activity at low concentrations due to barriers imposed by immune, biochemical and physiological mechanisms. Secondly, the agent must continually produce the gene of interest (GOI) . Thirdly, the engineered stem cell-based carrier must remain present in the host. Lastly and most importantly any chemotherapeutic drug must effectively and selectively target brain tumor cells while sparing normal brain tissue.

Stem cell-mediated gene therapy has emerged as a potential strategy to improve the efficacy and minimize the toxicity of current gene therapy approaches. Multiple sources for clinically relevant and useful stem cells have been identified-adult cells, umbilical cord blood cells, and embryonic cells. However, this chapter will primarily discuss adult mesenchymal stem cells obtained from adipose tissue and the versatility of adipose-derivedMSCs as vehicles for delivery oftherapeutic modalities, providing an avenue toovercome one of the major limitations ofchemotherapy for glioblastoma.

MESENCHYMAL STEM CELLS AS DRUG DELIVERY SYSTEMS

Bone Marrow Derived-Mesenchymal Stem Cells

Mesenchymal stem cells exist in all tissues during human development, but in adults they are prevalent in bone marrow. In recent years interest has rapidly grown in the use of MSCs in treating caner. Balyasnikova, I.V. *et al.*, using antibody-mediated gene delivery, demonstrated that human MSCs engineered to express a single-chain antibody (scFv) on their cell surface against epidermal growth factor receptor variant III (EGFRvIII) showed improved binding to and displayed prolonged retention within EGFRvIII-expressing U87 gliomas. [43] The authors found that co-injection of human mesenchymal stem cells expressing a single chain antibody (scFv) against epidermal growth factor receptor variant III) (hMSC-scFvEGFRvIII) with U87 glioma cells expressing epidermal growth factor receptor variant III) (U87-EGFRvIII) delayed tumor growth, reduced CD31 positive staining of blood vessels and extended survival. This data was further supported by *in vitro* observations of pAKTdownregulation in U87-EGFRvIII glioma cocultured with hMSC-scFvEGFRvIII cells. [43] Interestingly, it has been reported that unmodified hMSCs inhibit Akt activity via direct cell-cell contact as well. [32] It is worth noting that although survival was prolonged for a week in the Balyasnikova*et al.* study, an additional injection of hMSC-scFvEGFRvIII in the established tumor was necessary to further extend the survival of the animal models. Also the effect of hMSC-scFvEGFRvIII on established EGFRvIII gliomas was dependent on initial tumor size. Large tumors were not affected by hMSCs-scFv.

The idea that the therapeutic potential of MSCs is heavily dependent upon their substantial tumoral presence has been observed and documented by others. Luetzkendorf, J. *et al.*, showed that TRAIL-expressing MSCs mediated caspase- and PARP-induced apoptosis in human colorectal cancer cells upon direct cell-to-cell contact. Additionally, the authors suggest that the number of TRAIL-MSC should exceed 10% of the tumor cells in order to see an obvious reduction in tumor size. [45] MSCs derived from umbilical cord blood engineered to secrete soluble TRAIL (hUCB-MSC TRAIL) were effective in tumor animal models by inhibiting tumor growth and enhancing the survival of glioma-bearing mice. However, in this studythe authors' note that a single intratumoral administration of MSC-TRAIL did not achieve complete regression. Clearly, repeated injections of a controlled number of TRAIL-MSCs at appropriate time intervals appear to be necessary to achieve efficacy for clinical application. [46]

Human Adipose-Derived Mesenchymal Stem Cells

Substantial findings support the use of BM-MSC as a cancer therapeutic delivery vehicle; however, some would argue that hAMSC is a better choice than BM-MSCs. The acquisition of adipose tissue is much easier than bone marrow, less invasive and available in larger quantities. Moreover, hAMSCs share many of the same characteristics as BM-MSCs including cell surface antigens, natural tropism for tumors, andmigratory capabilities. [47, 48]

Recently, the feasibility and efficacy of hAMSCs engineered to express the suicide gene, yeast fusion cytosine deaminase::uracil phosphoribosyltransferase, was examined in C6 rat glioblastoma. [49] The authors found that the effectiveness of adipose tissue-derived mesenchymal stem cells engineered to express yeast cytosine deaminase (CDy-AT-MSCs) relied on three factors. 1) The ability of the therapeutic stem cells to convert the non-toxic prodrug 5-fluorocytosine (5-FC) to its toxic form 5-fluorouracil (5-FU); 2) the ability of 5-FU to pass from the MSCs to the neighboring glioma cells (known as the bystander effect) and; 3) tumor cell apoptosis in the presence of CDy-AT-MSCs. In this study, tumor-free survival of animals directly correlated with the therapeutic stem cell dose. [49] The "bystander effect" has also been documented in the use of the Herpes simplex virus-thymidine kinase (HSV-*tk*) via gap junctions. [50] Kucerova, L. *et al*showed that direct coculture of hAMSCs with human glioma cells did not lead to proliferative support *in vitro*, but decreased tumor incidence in an 8-MG-BA glioma model. [51] In this case it suggests that even though hAMSCs and glioma cells express pro-tumorigenic markers, within this particular glioma model hAMSCs illicit a cancer inhibitory reaction. [52]

Neural Stem Cells

NSCs are a population of cells in the nervous system that have the ability to self-renew and give rise to various differentiated neural cell types such as astrocytes, neurons and oligodendrocytes. The subventricular zone (SVZ) [53, 54] of the brain ventricles and the subgranular zone (SGZ) of the hippocampal dentate gyrus [55] are the principal sources of NSCs in the adult human brain. NSC's application as delivery vehicles for glioma treatment was first documented in 2000. [31, 56, 57] Experimental studies have shown that NSCs are inherently attracted to gliomas supporting its potential as a reliable drug delivery vehicle to target the tumor bulk and disseminated microsatellites of glioblastoma and other brain neoplasms. NSCs have the ability to migrate to the tumor and decrease the size of the tumor. [32] However, one should proceed with caution. In some cases NSC contributes to tumor growth [33] and harvest and *ex vivo* expansion of NSCs has been met with difficulty thereby limiting its translational potential. [31]

SIGNALINGPATHWAYS THAT MEDIATEMSC TROPISM TO TUMORS

Human neural and mesenchymal stem cells have been used for cell-based therapies in regenerative medicine and as vehicles for delivering therapeutic agents to tumors. However, signals required for recruitment and homing of stem cells to disease sites are currently not well defined. Directed cell migration is initiated in response to chemoattractants. Therefore, it is imperative to identify various factors that regulate MSC migration towards gliomas. Numerous cytokines, growth factors, and their receptors have been shown to affect stem cell migration under normal and pathological conditions. Malignant gliomas secrete a plethora of growth factors to initiate the migration of cells into the tumor microenvironment such as hepatocyte growth factor (HGF) [58, 59] , epidermal growth factor (EGF) [60] , and vascular endothelial growth factor (VEGF) . [61] Cytokines such as stem cell factor-1 (SCF-1) [62, 63] , monocyte chemoattractant protein-1 (MCP-1) [64] , and stromal cell-derived growth factor-1 (SDF-1) [58, 65, 66] are well documented to be potent tumor-tropic agents as well.

In recent years, urokinase plasminogen activator/urokinase plasminogen activator receptor (uPA/uPAR) has gained interest in the tropism of MSCs to tumors due to its upregulation in invasive tumors and its involvement in chemotaxis and cell guidance during normal development. [67] Upon binding to uPAR, the plasminogen is activated and the extracellular matrix gets degraded. A study from Gutova, M *et al* showed that activation of uPA and uPAR in brain, lung, breast and prostate tumor augmented neural and mesenchymal stem cell tropism. On the other hand, depletion ofuPA from tumor conditioned-media blocked stem cell migration, whereas the presence of recombinant uPA stimulated migration. [68]

Overexpression of the SFD-1α receptor, CXCR4, onMSCs enhanced their migration towards an established tumor and primary glioma cell lines *in vitro*. [44] Interestingly, the SFD-1α/CXCR4 axis plays an important role in stem cell trafficking by regulating cell migration, homing/migration into bone marrow, and accumulation of immune cells in inflamed tissue. *In vivo* assessment of human mesenchymal stem cells expressing CXC chemokine receptor 4 (hMSC-CXCR4) demonstrated strong a migration towards distant intracranial gliomas compared to control MSCs. [44] The CXCR4 antagonist AMD3100 and anti-SDF-1α significantly inhibited chemotaxis toward SFD-1α, further confirming the role of SFD-1α/CXCR4 axis in the migratory response of MSCs. [44, 69] Thegrowth factor HGF has also been reported to regulate MSC migration. The chemotactic response of HGF was compared between human cord blood-derived MSCs (hUCB-MSCs) and human BM-MSCs. [69] The authors determined that hUCB-MSCs exhibited a stronger increase in migration towards HGF than BM-MSCs in an *in vitro* assay. Collectively, the findings support further exploitation of chemokines overexpressed in tumors, and whose corresponding receptors are expressed on stem cells, to subsequently enhance selective MSC migration towards gliomas.

DISCUSSION

Malignant gliomas are the most common primary brain tumor, and are hard to treat with combinatorial surgical resection, radiation and chemotherapy. These tumors possess the ability to extensively invade into surrounding tissue, making curative resection impossible. As a result, a curative approach would have to target tumor cell invaders residing outside the bulk of the tumor. Neural stem cells and bone marrow-derived mesenchymal stem cells have the capacity to home into gliomas and are able to migrate substantial distances to selectively target areas of malignancy. [15, 32,33] BM-MSCs have been utilized as carriers for cytokines and oncolytic viruses in experimental studies and could be translated into clinical use. [16, 17] However, concerns have arose with respect to the invasive nature of bone marrow aspiration which places the patient with additional surgical risks, the relatively low yield of BM-MSCs, and the decline in BM-MSC lifespan and differentiation capacity with donor age. [18] To alleviate these concerns and successfully treat glioblastomas using MSCs, one would need to harvest MSCs from accessible sources which pose less threat to the safety of the patient.

Recent work has demonstrated that the use of AMSCs, which share many similarities with BM-MSC, is a promising new strategy for the treatment of human gliomas. Yet, it remains to be seen whether these cells are applicable against the highly invasive nature of glioblastomas. [47, 48] Through experimental animal studies, what has been determined and supported is that constant therapeutic stem cell presence (via repeated injections) and direct contact between tumor cells and therapeutic stem cells is required to achieve a strong therapeutic benefit. [32, 45, 46] Additionally, human AMSCs have tremendous autologous therapeutic potential. [41] For example, an individual patient's MSCs would be harvested, expanded ex vivo, genetically modified and then administered back to the patient to target the glioma. An individual patient's MSCs can be tested for sensitivity to growth factors, cytokines, various drugs and inductive agents to maximize its therapeutic potential. Clearly, studies utilizing stem cell-mediated therapy are important steps toward translating AMSCs for use against intracranial gliomas.

One should proceed with MSC in cancer therapy with caution. MSCs have the potential to differentiate into bone [70, 71] , cartilage [71, 72] , fat [73] and various other connective tissues. [41] This property serves well in regenerative medicine, but would be detrimental to the cancer medicine community. One foreseeable problem is the potential enhancement of tumor growth with MSCs. The use of MSCs in tissue grafting, angiogenesis, heart infarction, cartilage and skeletal tissue repair and regeneration is extensive. Both hAMSC and BM-MSC have been reported to enhance tumorigenesis of human breast [74, 75] , colon [76] , cervical [74] , and brain [33] cancer cell lines. This could be a result of cytokines, chemokines and growth factors produced by MSCs to favor a proliferative burst within tumor cells or MSCs giving rise to endothelial-like cells contributing to the vasculature when recruited to tumors. [77] Cytokine arrays from hAMSC conditioned media have shown elevated production of GRO, interleukin-6 (IL-6) , IL-8, MCP-1, RANTES, transforming growth factor-β1 (TGF-β1) , metallopeptidase tissue inhibitor-2 (TIMP-2) , thrombopoietin, VEGF and urokinase plasminogen activator (uPAR) . [33]

The idea of AMSCs [33] and BM-MSCs [78, 79] being the source of factors supporting tumor angiogenesis has received mixed reviews. There have been reports that murine MSCs decreased angiogenesis in a B16F10 melanoma tumor model [80] , but rat MSCs did not affect angiogenesis in a rat glioma xenograft. [81] The effect of MSCs on angiogenesis and tumor growth appears to be context dependent, such as animal species and tumor types. Therefore, a thorough understanding of MSC biology is essential to ensure successful application of MSC in cancer therapy.

Although this commentary focuses on hAMSCs as a potential treatment for glioblastoma, it is feasible that the same idea could be applied to other types of primary brain tumors. The signaling mechanisms responsible for recruitment of hAMSCs towards glioblastoma could be shared by other malignant tumors. As a result, the application of hAMSCs would not solely be relevant to the 40,000 patients who are diagnosed with brain cancer each year, but also to patients who present with metastatic cancers to the brain.

REFERENCES

[1] Jemal, A., et al., Cancer statistics, 2002. CA *Cancer J.Clin.*, 2002. 52(1): p. 23-47.

[2] Stupp, R., et al., Radiotherapy plus concomitant and adjuvant temozolomide for glioblastoma.*N. Engl. J. Med.,* 2005. 352(10): p. 987-96.

[3] Affronti, M.L., et al., Overall survival of newly diagnosed glioblastoma patients receiving carmustine wafers followed by radiation and concurrent temozolomide plus rotational multiagent chemotherapy.*Cancer,* 2009. 115(15): p. 3501-11.

[4] Walker, M.D., et al., Randomized comparisons of radiotherapy and nitrosoureas for the treatment of malignant glioma after surgery. N. *Engl. J. Med,* 1980. 303(23): p. 1323-9.

[5] Sakariassen, P.O., H. Immervoll, and M. Chekenya, Cancer stem cells as mediators of treatment resistance in brain tumors: status and controversies.*Neoplasia,* 2007. 9(11): p. 882-92.

[6] Eramo, A., et al., Chemotherapy resistance of glioblastoma stem cells.*Cell Death Differ*, 2006. 13(7): p. 1238-41.

[7] Singh, S. and P.B. Dirks, Brain tumor stem cells: identification and concepts.*Neurosurg.Clin. N. Am.,* 2007. 18(1): p. 31-8, viii.

[8] Bao, S., et al., Glioma stem cells promote radioresistance by preferential activation of the DNA damage response.*Nature,* 2006. 444(7120): p. 756-60.

[9] Quinones-Hinojosa, A. and K. Chaichana, The human subventricular zone: a source of new cells and a potential source of brain tumors.*Exp. Neurol.,* 2007. 205(2): p. 313-24.

[10] Wei, J., et al., Glioma-associated cancer-initiating cells induce immunosuppression.*Clin. Cancer Res.,* 2010. 16(2): p. 461-73.

[11] Bleau, A.M., et al., PTEN/PI3K/Akt pathway regulates the side population phenotype and ABCG2 activity in glioma tumor stem-like cells.*Cell Stem. Cell,* 2009. 4(3): p. 226-35.

[12] Murat, A., et al., Stem cell-related "self-renewal" signature and high epidermal growth factor receptor expression associated with resistance to concomitant chemoradiotherapy in glioblastoma.*J.Clin.Oncol.,* 2008. 26(18): p. 3015-24.

[13] Zaidi, H.A., et al., Origins and clinical implications of the brain tumor stem cell hypothesis.*J.Neurooncol.,* 2009. 93(1): p. 49-60.

[14] Dazzi, F. and N.J. Horwood, *Potential of mesenchymal stem cell therapy.Curr.Opin.Oncol.,* 2007. 19(6): p. 650-5.

[15] Nakamizo, A., et al., Human bone marrow-derived mesenchymal stem cells in the treatment of gliomas.*Cancer Res.,* 2005. 65(8): p. 3307-18.

[16] Kosztowski, T., H.A. Zaidi, and A. Quinones-Hinojosa, Applications of neural and mesenchymal stem cells in the treatment of gliomas. Expert. Rev. Anticancer.*Ther.,* 2009. 9(5): p. 597-612.

[17] Jiang, H., et al*., Examination of the therapeutic potential of Delta-24-RGD in brain tumor stem cells: role of autophagic cell death.J. Natl. Cancer Inst.,* 2007. 99(18): p. 1410-4.

[18] Redmond, K.J., et al., A radiotherapy technique to limit dose to neural progenitor cell niches without compromising tumor coverage.*J.Neurooncol.,* 2011.

[19] Kern, S., et al., Comparative analysis of mesenchymal stem cells from bone marrow, umbilical cord blood, or adipose tissue.*Stem. Cells,* 2006. 24(5): p. 1294-301.

[20] Momin, E.N., et al., Mesenchymal stem cells: new approaches for the treatment of neurological diseases.*Curr. Stem. Cell Res.Ther.,* 2010. 5(4): p. 326-44.

[21] Anghileri, E., et al., Neuronal differentiation potential of human adipose-derived mesenchymal stem cells.*Stem. Cells Dev.,* 2008. 17(5): p. 909-16.

[22] Matsumoto, T., et al., Mature adipocyte-derived dedifferentiated fat cells exhibit multilineage potential.*J. Cell Physiol.,* 2008. 215(1): p. 210-22.

[23] Lamfers, M., et al., Homing properties of adipose-derived stem cells to intracerebral glioma and the effects of adenovirus infection.*Cancer Lett.,* 2009. 274(1): p. 78-87.

[24] Kucerova, L., et al., Adipose tissue-derived human mesenchymal stem cells mediated prodrug cancer gene therapy.*Cancer Res.,* 2007. 67(13): p. 6304-13.

[25] Choi, S.A., et al., Therapeutic efficacy and safety of TRAIL-producing human adipose tissue-derived mesenchymal stem cells against experimental brainstem glioma. *Neuro.Oncol.,* 2011. 13(1): p. 61-9.

[26] Davis, F.G., B.J. McCarthy, and M.S. Berger, Centralized databases available for describing primary brain tumor incidence, survival, and treatment: Central Brain Tumor Registry of the United States; Surveillance, Epidemiology, and End Results; and National Cancer Data Base.*Neuro.Oncol.,* 1999. 1(3): p. 205-11.

[27] McGirt, M.J., et al., Independent association of extent of resection with survival in patients with malignant brain astrocytoma.*J.Neurosurg.,* 2009. 110(1): p. 156-62.

[28] McGirt, M.J., et al., Gliadel (BCNU) wafer plus concomitant temozolomide therapy after primary resection of glioblastoma multiforme.*J.Neurosurg.,* 2009. 110(3): p. 583-8.

[29] Thuppal, S., J.M. Propp, and B.J. McCarthy, Average years of potential life lost in those who have died from brain and CNS tumors in the USA.*Neuroepidemiology,* 2006. 27(1): p. 22-7.

[30] Kleihues, P., et al., The WHO classification of tumors of the nervous system. *J.Neuropathol. Exp. Neurol.,* 2002. 61(3): p. 215-25; discussion 226-9.

[31] Aboody, K.S., et al., Neural stem cells display extensive tropism for pathology in adult brain: evidence from intracranial gliomas. *Proc. Natl. Acad. Sci. USA,* 2000. 97(23): p. 12846-51.

[32] Khakoo, A.Y., et al., Human mesenchymal stem cells exert potent antitumorigenic effects in a model of Kaposi's sarcoma.*J. Exp. Med.,* 2006. 203(5): p. 1235-47.

[33] Yu, J.M., et al., Mesenchymal stem cells derived from human adipose tissues favor tumor cell growth in vivo.*Stem. Cells Dev.,* 2008. 17(3): p. 463-73.

[34] Ehtesham, M., C.B. Stevenson, and R.C. Thompson, *Stem cell therapies for malignant glioma.Neurosurg. Focus,* 2005. 19(3): p. E5.

[35] Brustle, O., et al., In vitro-generated neural precursors participate in mammalian brain development. *Proc. Natl. Acad. Sci. USA,* 1997. 94(26): p. 14809-14.

[36] Pittenger, M.F., et al., Multilineage potential of adult human mesenchymal stem cells.*Science,* 1999. 284(5411): p. 143-7.

[37] Colter, D.C., I. Sekiya, and D.J. Prockop, Identification of a subpopulation of rapidly self-renewing and multipotential adult stem cells in colonies of human marrow stromal cells.*Proc. Natl. Acad. Sci. USA,* 2001. 98(14): p. 7841-5.

[38] Prockop, D.J., I. Sekiya, and D.C. Colter, Isolation and characterization of rapidly self-renewing stem cells from cultures of human marrow stromal cells.*Cytotherapy,* 2001. 3(5): p. 393-6.

[39] Zuk, P.A., et al., Human adipose tissue is a source of multipotent stem cells.*Mol. Biol. Cell,* 2002. 13(12): p. 4279-95.

[40] Zuk, P.A., et al., Multilineage cells from human adipose tissue: implications for cell-based therapies.*Tissue Eng.,* 2001. 7(2): p. 211-28.

[41] Caplan, A.I., The mesengenic process.*Clin.Plast. Surg.,* 1994. 21(3): p. 429-35.

[42] Gregory, C.A., J. Ylostalo, and D.J. Prockop, Adult bone marrow stem/progenitor cells (MSCs) are preconditioned by microenvironmental "niches" in culture: a two-stage hypothesis for regulation of MSC fate.*Sci. STKE,* 2005. 2005(294): p. pe37.

[43] Balyasnikova, I.V., et al., Mesenchymal stem cells modified with a single-chain antibody against EGFRvIII successfully inhibit the growth of human xenograft malignant glioma.*PLoS One,* 2010. 5(3): p. e9750.

[44] Park, S.A., et al., CXCR4-transfected human umbilical cord blood-derived mesenchymal stem cells exhibit enhanced migratory capacity toward gliomas.*Int. J.Oncol.,* 2010. 38(1): p. 97-103.

[45] Luetzkendorf, J., et al., Growth inhibition of colorectal carcinoma by lentiviral TRAIL-transgenic human mesenchymal stem cells requires their substantial intratumoral presence.*J. Cell Mol. Med.,* 2009. 14(9): p. 2292-304.

[46] Kim, S.M., et al., Gene therapy using TRAIL-secreting human umbilical cord blood-derived mesenchymal stem cells against intracranial glioma.*Cancer Res.,* 2008. 68(23): p. 9614-23.

[47] Lee, R.H., et al., Characterization and expression analysis of mesenchymal stem cells from human bone marrow and adipose tissue.*Cell Physiol.Biochem.,* 2004. 14(4-6): p. 311-24.

[48] Dominici, M., et al., Minimal criteria for defining multipotent mesenchymal stromal cells. The International Society for Cellular Therapy position statement. *Cytotherapy,* 2006. 8(4): p. 315-7.

[49] Altanerova, V., et al., Human adipose tissue-derived mesenchymal stem cells expressing yeast cytosinedeaminase::uracil

phosphoribosyltransferase inhibit intracerebral rat glioblastoma.*Int. J. Cancer,* Epub ahead of print.

[50] Matuskova, M., et al., HSV-tk expressing mesenchymal stem cells exert bystander effect on human glioblastoma cells.*Cancer Lett.,*2010. 290(1): p. 58-67.

[51] Kucerova, L., et al., Tumor cell behaviour modulation by mesenchymal stromal cells. *Mol. Cancer.,* 2010. 9: p. 129.

[52] Mantovani, A., et al., Cancer-related inflammation.*Nature,* 2008. 454(7203): p. 436-44.

[53] Doetsch, F., et al., Subventricular zone astrocytes are neural stem cells in the adult mammalian brain.*Cell,* 1999. 97(6): p. 703-16.

[54] Sanai, N., et al., Unique astrocyte ribbon in adult human brain contains neural stem cells but lacks chain migration.*Nature,* 2004. 427(6976): p. 740-4.

[55] Eriksson, P.S., et al., Neurogenesis in the adult human hippocampus.*Nat. Med.,* 1998. 4(11): p. 1313-7.

[56] Aboody, K.S., et al., Targeting of melanoma brain metastases using engineered neural stem/progenitor cells.*Neuro.Oncol.,* 2006. 8(2): p. 119-26.

[57] Kim, S.K., et al., PEX-producing human neural stem cells inhibit tumor growth in a mouse glioma model.*Clin. Cancer Res.,* 2005. 11(16): p. 5965-70.

[58] Takeuchi, H., et al., Intravenously transplanted human neural stem cells migrate to the injured spinal cord in adult mice in an SDF-1- and HGF-dependent manner.*Neurosci.Lett.,* 2007. 426(2): p. 69-74.

[59] Kendall, S.E., et al., Neural stem cell targeting of glioma is dependent on phosphoinositide 3-kinase signaling.*Stem. Cells,* 2008. 26(6): p. 1575-86.

[60] Boockvar, J.A., et al., Constitutive EGFR signaling confers a motile phenotype to neural stem cells. *Mol. Cell Neurosci.,* 2003. 24(4): p. 1116-30.

[61] Schmidt, N.O., et al., Brain tumor tropism of transplanted human neural stem cells is induced by vascular endothelial growth factor.*Neoplasia,* 2005. 7(6): p. 623-9.

[62] Erlandsson, A., J. Larsson, and K. Forsberg-Nilsson, Stem cell factor is a chemoattractant and a survival factor for CNS stem cells.*Exp. Cell Res.,* 2004. 301(2): p. 201-10.

[63] Sun, L., J. Lee, and H.A. Fine, Neuronally expressed stem cell factor induces neural stem cell migration to areas of brain injury.*J.Clin. Invest.,* 2004. 113(9): p. 1364-74.
[64] Widera, D., et al., MCP-1 induces migration of adult neural stem cells. *Eur. J. Cell Biol.,* 2004. 83(8): p. 381-7.
[65] Imitola, J., et al., Directed migration of neural stem cells to sites of CNS injury by the stromal cell-derived factor 1alpha/CXC chemokine receptor 4 pathway.*Proc. Natl. Acad. Sci. USA,* 2004. 101(52): p. 18117-22.
[66] Kokovay, E., et al., *A*dult SVZ lineage cells home to and leave the vascular niche via differential responses to SDF1/CXCR4 signaling. *Cell Stem. Cell,* 2010. 7(2): p. 163-73.
[67] Eagleson, K.L., A. Bonnin, and P. Levitt, Region- and age-specific deficits in gamma-aminobutyricacidergic neuron development in the telencephalon of the uPAR(-/-) mouse.*J. Comp. Neurol.,* 2005. 489(4): p. 449-66.
[68] Gutova, M., et al., Urokinase plasminogen activator and urokinase plasminogen activator receptor mediate human stem cell tropism to malignant solid tumors. *Stem. Cells,* 2008. 26(6): p. 1406-13.
[69] Son, B.R., et al., Migration of bone marrow and cord blood mesenchymal stem cells in vitro is regulated by stromal-derived factor-1-CXCR4 and hepatocyte growth factor-c-met axes and involves matrix metalloproteinases. *Stem. Cells,* 2006. 24(5): p. 1254-64.
[70] Ducy, P., T. Schinke, and G. Karsenty, The osteoblast: a sophisticated fibroblast under central surveillance.*Science,* 2000. 289(5484): p. 1501-4.
[71] Cancedda, R., et al., Developmental control of chondrogenesis and osteogenesis.*Int. J. Dev. Biol.,* 2000. 44(6): p. 707-14.
[72] de Crombrugghe, B., et al., Transcriptional mechanisms of chondrocyte differentiation.*Matrix Biol.,* 2000. 19(5): p. 389-94.
[73] Rosen, E.D. and B.M. *Spiegelman, Molecular regulation of adipogenesis.Annu. Rev. Cell Dev. Biol.,* 2000. 16: p. 145-71.
[74] Grisendi, G., et al., Adipose-derived mesenchymal stem cells as stable source of tumor necrosis factor-related apoptosis-inducing ligand delivery for cancer therapy.*Cancer Res.,* 2011. 70(9): p. 3718-29.
[75] Zimmerlin, L., et al., Regenerative therapy and cancer: in vitro and in vivo studies of the interaction between adipose-derived stem cells and breast cancer cells from clinical isolates.*Tissue Eng.* Part A, 2011. 17(1-2): p. 93-106.

[76] Zhu, W., et al., Mesenchymal stem cells derived from bone marrow favor tumor cell growth in vivo. *Exp. Mol.Pathol.,* 2006. 80(3): p. 267-74.

[77] Roorda, B.D., et al., Bone marrow-derived cells and tumor growth: contribution of bone marrow-derived cells to tumor micro-environments with special focus on mesenchymal stem cells. *Crit. Rev.Oncol.Hematol.,* 2009. 69(3): p. 187-98.

[78] Kinnaird, T., et al., Marrow-derived stromal cells express genes encoding a broad spectrum of arteriogenic cytokines and promote in vitro and in vivo arteriogenesis through paracrine mechanisms.*Circ. Res.,* 2004. 94(5): p. 678-85.

[79] Honczarenko, M., et al., Human bone marrow stromal cells express a distinct set of biologically functional chemokine receptors.*Stem. Cells,* 2006. 24(4): p. 1030-41.

[80] Otsu, K., et al., Concentration-dependent inhibition of angiogenesis by mesenchymal stem cells.*Blood,* 2009. 113(18): p. 4197-205.

[81] Bexell, D., et al., Bone marrow multipotent mesenchymal stroma cells act as pericyte-like migratory vehicles in experimental gliomas.*Mol.Ther.,* 2009. 17(1): p. 183-90.

In: Glioblastoma ISBN: 978-1-62100-858-3
Editors: M. F. Bezerra et.al, pp. 133-148

Chapter 6

Targeting Fibroblast Growth Factor (FGF) Signals in Glioblastoma

Pedro Cuevas[1], Fernando Carceller[2], Javier Angulo[1], Rocío González-Corrochano[3], Adrián Cuevas-Bourdier[4], and Guillermo Giménez-Gallego[3]

[1]Departamento de Investigación, Servicio de Histología, IRYCIS, Hospital Universitario Ramón y Cajal
[2]Servicio de Neurocirugía, Hospital Universitario La Paz
[3]Departamento de Estructura y Función de Proteínas, Centro de Investigaciones Biológicas, Consejo Superior de Investigaciones Científicas, (CSIC)
[4]Servicio de Anatomía Patológica, Hospital Universitario Ramón y Cajal, Madrid

In Memoriam
"Yo sólo pretendo estar en el lugar donde pueda ser útil" Carlos Revilla

Abstract

Glioblastoma multiforme (GBM) is the most malignant form of human astrocytoma with a survival for the majority of patients less than two years. Glioblastoma exhibits a rapid, progressive and infiltrative growth, which renders the tumor unressectable at the time of diagnosis.

Current treatment modalities include maximal surgical debulking, followed by focal radiotherapy and adjuvant chemotherapy. Glioblastoma is highly vascularized and, therefore, antiangiogenic agents aimed to the inhibition of vascular endothelial cell growth factor (VEGF) signalling are increasingly being explored as therapeutic options. However, patients succumb in a very high number of cases because of chemoresistance development and the appearance of mechanisms circumventing the effects of VEGF-targeted antiangiogenic drugs. The fibroblast growth factor (FGF) signalling network plays a key role in glioma growth. In addition, FGF plays an important role in the overcoming of chemotherapy and the failures of anti-VEGF therapies. This review summarizes laboratory and clinical research on glioblastoma angiogenesis and discusses the potential use of new safe and efficient FGF inhibitors for the treatment of glioblastoma.

INTRODUCTION

Glioblastoma (GBM) are the most common primary brain tumors, with a worldwide annual incidence of around 7 cases per 100,000 individuals (Furnari et al., 2007) . More than 20,000 cases are diagnosed every year in USA. Gliomas display disproportionately a high mortality rate. The high malignancy of GBM is due to their intense cell proliferation, diffuse infiltration, high resistance to apoptosis and robust angiogenesis (Giese and Westphal 1996) . Although probably it is not an exclusive case, it has been observed that in gliomal angiogenesis, tumoral cells incorporate to the neovessels after a process of genetic reprogramming (vascular mimicry) (Ricci-Vitiani et al., 2001; Wang et al., 2010) . The primary therapy for GBM consists in surgery followed by radio- and chemotherapies with temozolomide (TMZ) (Aoki et al., 2007) . Despite this multimodal therapy the prognosis has only slightly improved, and patients with high-grade gliomas show a median survival of 14 months for grade 4 and 36 months for grade 3 gliomas according to the World Health Organization (WHO) (Stupp et al., 2005; Furnari et al., 2007) . The understanding of molecular pathology of cancers in general and in glioma in particular led, lately, to new opportunities for glioma therapy. Several growth factors such as epidermal growth factor (EGF) , vascular endothelial growth factor (VEGF) and fibroblast growth factor (FGF) and its cognate receptors have been implicated in gliomagenesis (Onishi et al., 2011) . The feasibility of inhibiting these well characterized growth factors has recently attracted considerable clinical interest.

ANGIOGENESIS PROCESS

Angiogenesis is a complex biological process that involves the activation, proliferation and directed migration of endothelial cells to form new capillaries from existing blood vessels. This sprouting of capillaries from pre-existing vessels occurs during embryonic and foetal development. Transient angiogenesis occurs also in adult tissues during the female reproductive cycle and during wound healing. Angiogenesis is finely regulated by pro-angiogenic and anti-angiogenic stimuli. Pathological angiogenesis occurs when these two factors extemporaneously misbalance. Pathological angiogenesis is a prominent feature of a high number of diseases, including many sort of tumours, age-related wet macular degeneration, diabetic retinopathy, rheumatoid arthritis, endometriosis, psoriasis and rosacea (Folkman, 1995) . The induction of new blood vessel growth is necessary if tumors are to grow beyond a minimal size, as in the example of relatively thin melanomas residing entirely above the epidermis that are avascular and therefore rarely metastasize. Tumoral neovessels promote tumor growth by supplying nutrients and oxygen, and removing waste products, and, in addition, contribute to metastasis by dissolving their surrounding extracellular matrix (ECM) when the activated endothelial cells migrate toward the tumor to form the new vascular network (Presta et al., 2005) .

The first proangiogenic agents to be isolated were fibroblast growth factor (FGF) (Giménez-Gallego et al., 1985; Esch et al., 1985) and vascular endothelial growth factor (VEGF) (Leung et al., 1989) . Epidermal growth factor (EGF) , vascular endothelial growth factor (VEGF) and fibroblast growth factor (FGF) contribute strongly to the growth and promotion of glioblastoma (Auguste et al., 2001; Loilome et al., 2009) . As angiogenic growth factors play a key role in tumor growth and metastasis, their inhibition has gained great interest in the last years as a targeted molecular therapy for treatment of cancers.

FIBROBLAST GROWTH FACTOR SIGNALLING

The fibroblast growth factor (FGF) constitutes one of the largest families of polypeptide growth factors. A wealth of studies carried out since its initial discovery has shown that FGF constitutes a complex growth factor signalling pathway, reflecting the multitude of physiological functions that are controlled by FGF signalling. The mammalian FGF family comprises 18 ligands, which exert their actions through 4 highly conserved tyrosine kinase receptors (FGFR1-4) (Olsen et al., 2003) . These receptors have common features including a cytoplasmic conserved tyrosine kinase (TK) domain, a transmembrane domain, and an extracellular ligand binding domain, which contains either two or three immunoglobulin-like domains. A number of splice variants with these different receptor families have been also additionally described. In addition to the effects on cell replication, FGF regulates cell survival, differentiation, ECM composition, chemotaxis, cell adhesion, and migration. Different cell types or even the same cell may display alternate and sometimes opposing responses to FGF, depending on their state of differentiation, biochemical status, or the cellular, physical and chemical environment of the cell (Szebenyi and Fallon, 1999) . These activities govern a wide variety of developmental and physiological processes, since in addition to endothelial cells, practically, all cell lineages derived from the embryonic mesoderm and neuroectoderm are under the control of these proteins.

FGF, at times expressed at very high levels remain sequestered at the extracellular matrix (ECM) after reaching the outer cell space by their heparan sulphate proteoglycans (HSPGs) components (Olsen et al., 2003) . FGF are released from the ECM by heparinases, proteases or specific FGF-binding proteins. Obviously, the subversion of this powerful signalling system and any defects in the tight control of its activity, either through uncontrolled synthesis or the continuous mobilization of the ECM bound FGF, cause serious physiological disturbances (Powers et al., 2000) .

FGF seems to be directly involved in tumorigenesis by the autocrine, paracrine, and intracrine induction of cancer cell proliferation. Furthermore, FGF signalling may affect processes other than growth associated to tumor progression. For example, they can be involved in the creation of profuse blood irrigation networks to sustain the intense metabolism of the tumor cells, which subsequently favours their dissemination throughout the organism. Tumor metastasis is additionally favoured by the activation of enzymes that degrade the vascular basement membrane, remodelate ECM and enhance cell motility by FGF. Moreover, it is also involved in inhibiting apoptosis, enhancing the survival of tumor cells, promoting the resistance of tumors to chemotherapeutic drugs and radiation, controlling tumor dormancy, and controlling the self-renewal of cancer stem cells (Turner and Grose, 2010) . Cancer dormancy is defined as an unusually long-time between removal of the primary tumor and subsequent relapse in a patient who is clinically disease-free.

DEREGULATION OF FGF AND FGFR SIGNALLING IN GBM

Accumulating evidence implicates specific FGFs and FGFRs as components of autocrine and paracrine signalling pathways involved in glioma growth (Auguste et al., 2001) . As anti-angiogenic therapy may require long-term treatment, it is useful to identify safe small synthetic compounds to reduce production cost and eventually to increase bioavailability. The optimal lead drug for anti-angiogenic therapy should be a substance that exerts its anti-angiogenic effects at the remote site of vascular vessels growth if delivered systemically.

Based on a relatively wide screening of naphthalene sulphonate derivatives (Fernández-Tornero et al., 2003) and on three-dimensional structural studies, we performed a series of systemic studies to develop FGF inhibitors. We found that dobesilate (2,5-dihydroxyphenylsulfonate) and gentisic acid (2,5-dihydroxybenzoic acid) inhibit relevant activities of FGF. Dobesilate is the active principle of Doxium that has been used for many years for treating diabetic retinopathy and chronic venous insufficiency (Haritoglou et al., 2009) . Gentisic acid is a widespread plant secondary metabolite involved in pest defense and a catabolite of aspirin. We also showed that these compounds recognize both the growth factors and their plasmalemmal receptors, displacing heparin from its binding site in FGF, change the three-dimensional structure of the growth factor at their receptor recognizing site, and are capable of dissociating the receptor growth factor signalling complex (Fernández et al., 2010) .

Using the rat sponge assay of FGF induced angiogenesis, we showed that intraperitoneal administration of any of these lately characterized FGF inhibitors is sufficient to suppress the angiogenic response in the FGF containing sponge compared with rat treated with vehicle alone (Fernández et al., 2010) . The efficiency of an angiogenesis inhibitor should therefore ideally be reflected by an inhibition of ERK-1/2 phosphorylation. When FGF-stimulated C6 glioma cells were treated with dobesilate, a strong inhibition of ERK-1/2 phosphorylation occurred parallel with attenuation of glioma cell proliferation (Cuevas et al., 2006a) . We checked whether cell motility, an important pre-requisite for angiogenesis and metastasis, was affected by dobesilate. In a bioassay of FGF-induced cell migration, complete inhibition was achieved by dobesilate at concentrations close to those that produced a maximal effect in the mitogenesis assay (Fernández et al., 2010) .

The diverse growth factor signalling pathways converge at specific transcription factors, including signal transducer and activator of transcription-3 (STAT-3) . STAT-3 gene targets affect proliferation, growth and apoptosis. Aberrant activation of STAT-3 has been identified in glioblastoma (Brantley and Benveniste, 2008) and its inhibition has significant potential as therapeutical target of glioblastoma. In this context, we have demonstrated that treatment of C6 glioma cells with dobesilate *in vitro* triggered apoptosis and growth arrest (Cuevas et al., 2005) . Further studies in glioma cells showed that dobesilate significantly inhibited constitutive activation of STAT-3 (tyrosine phosphorylated) , and expression of the prosurvival proteins Bcl—xL and cyclin D1 by attenuating the upstream FGF/FGFR pathway (Cuevas et al., 2006b) .

Development of resistance to chemotherapeutic agents represents a serious obstacle to effective therapy. FGF inhibition may constitute a strategy to overcome such limitations, as in tumoral cells the development of broad spectrum resistance to anticancer drugs following repeated chemotherapeutic treatments is FGF-dependent (Song et al., 2000; Zhang et al., 2001) . Indeed, a FGF inhibitor (suramin) which was the starting point in the search that identified the new family of inhibitors headed by dobesilate, induces a significant enhancement of doxorubicin efficiency against prostate cancer (Zhang et al., 2001) . Recently, we have reported that, in an established rat orthotopic glioma model, comparative NMRI studies revealed a dramatic increase in tumor mass after irinotecan treatment and a much smaller increase after combinatory therapy (dobesilate plus irinotecan) (Cuevas et al., 2011) . Parallel to inhibition of glioma growth dobesilate administration normalizes tumor vascular perfusion, eliminating permeable vessels and reducing blood vessel number (Figure 1) .

The “vascular normalization” is characterized by attenuation of hyperpermeability, increased vascular pericyte coverage, a more normal basement membrane, and a resultant reduction in tumor hypoxia and interstitial fluid pressure. These in turn can lead to an improvement in the metabolic profile of the tumor microenvironment, the delivery and efficacy of exogenously administered therapeutic, and a reduction in the number of glioma cell satellitosis (Cuevas et al., 2011) .

Taken together, our results demonstrate that dobesilate shows important features of potent FGF inhibitors. These features include inhibition of FGF binding to its receptor, downstream ERK-signalling, STAT-3 inhibition, attenuation of cell migration, cell proliferation, angiogenesis, promotion of cell apoptosis and chemosensitization (Figure 2).

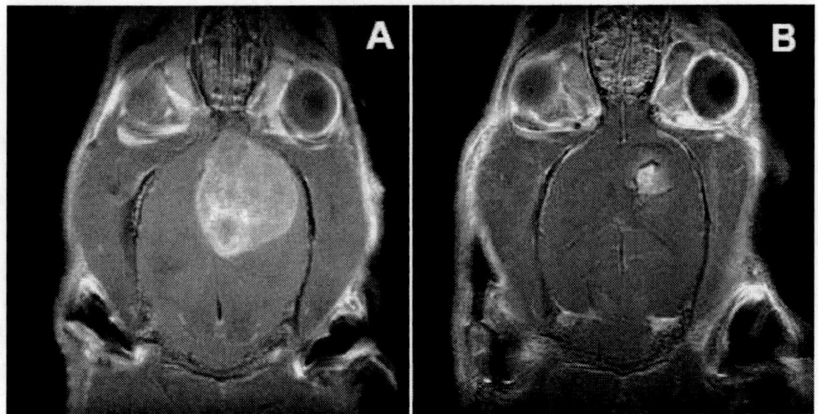

Figure 1. Strong contrast accumulation, suggesting an anomalous tumor hyperpermeability, was observed in rats treated with irinotecan (A) . Contrarily, no gadolinium contrast, indicating a normalization of tumor vasculature, was detected in rats treated with a combination of dobesilate and irinotecan (B) . Note the small tumor volume in combinatory therapy compared to treatment with irinotecan alone.

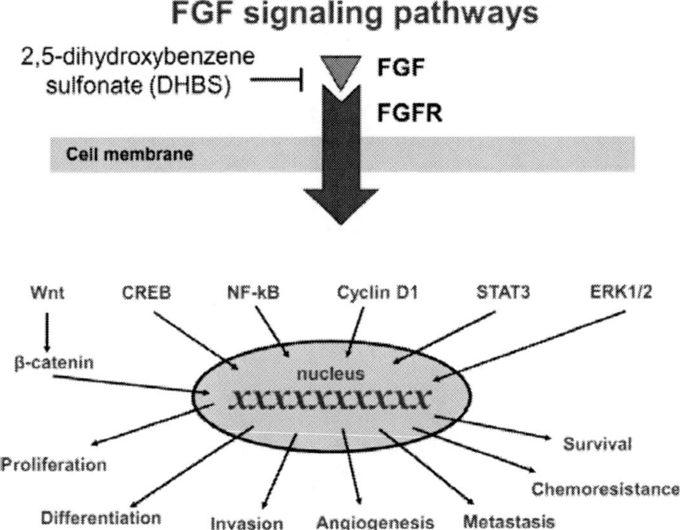

Figure 2. Schematic drawing of the inhibition of FGF/FGFR signalling pathways. FGF initiates signals when they bound to their receptor. Pharmacologic inhibitors as dobesilate attenuate several biological responses regulated by FGF in cancer cells.

FGF PARTICIPATES IN THE INTRINSIC RESISTANCE TO ANTI-EGF/EGFR THERAPY

The epidermal growth factor receptor (EGFR) is dysregulated in various tumor types such as GBM (Raizer, 2005) . As the intracellular (TK) of the EGFR activates signalling cascades leading to cell proliferation, angiogenesis and inhibition of apoptosis, the EGFR represents an attractive target in cancer therapy. In GBM, the EGFR is overexpressed in about 40 to 50% of cases, and almost half of these co-express the mutant receptor subtype EGFRvIII (Loew et al., 2009) . This EGFR variant is constitutively activated and thereby may contribute to the aggressive and refractory course of GBM which is associated with a median survival of only 40 to 60 weeks from diagnosis. Two available HER1/EGFR tyrosine kinase inhibitors (TKIs) are gefitinib (Iressa) and erlotinib (Tarceva); both show antitumor and radiosensitization effects in vitro and in animal models of GBM. Various trials are ongoing focussing on EGFR and EGFRvIII as new therapeutic targets in GBM. Preliminary results from trials of gefitinib in recurrent GBM show no increased time to progression or overall survival (OS) compared with historical control (Loew et al., 2009) . Studies with erlotinib show greater antitumor activity in patients with GBM than with gefitinib (Loew et al., 2009) , although the impact of both agents on OS remains unclear. Recently, it has been reported that the FGF/FGFR signalling pathway may participate on the intrinsic resistance to EGFR tyrosine kinase inhibitors (TKIs) (Kono et al., 2009) . Thus, FGF/FGFR signal pathway inhibitors should be quickly tested as therapeutics in combination with EGFRTKIs, in glioma patients.

GLIOBLASTOMA CANCER STEM CELLS

Epidemiological data suggest that the incidence of gliomas is rising (Hess et al., 2004) . This is surprising because the brain is partially protected from the environment factors by the blood-brain barrier (BBB) and has a low proliferative potential compared with other organs. Recent advances from the stem cell biology field have impacted on our understanding of brain carcinogenesis and tumor types (Stiles and Rowitch, 2008) . Normal neural human stem cells are thought to reside within the brain mostly in the subventricular zone (SVZ) lining the lateral ventricles and within the dentate gyrus of the hippocampus (Mckay, 1997) . These stem cells persist throughout adulthood into old age and may divide symmetrically for self-renewal and asymmetrically to produce neurons, astrocytes and oligodendrocytes (Uchida et al., 2000) . In contrast, glioma stem cells are a population within a glioma that can divide infinitely, has the capacity to show neuronal, astrocytic and oligodendroglial differentiation and can recapitulate the whole tumor when transplanted into the brain of a nude mouse (Galli et al., 2004) . Clinically, glioma stem cells are of great interest, because they may represent the population of cells within a tumor that may be resistant to therapy and responsible for tumor relapse (Bao et al., 2006) . GBM stem cells seem to be dependent on ones from aberrant vascular niches that mimic the normal neural stem cell niche. Glioblastoma cancer stem cells are in contact with tumoral blood vessels attracted to niche by secretion to the extracellular matrix (ECM) of several angiogenic growth factors as FGF and VEGF (Calabrese et al., 2007; Hsu et al., 2010) .

This has given rise to speculation that more effective therapies will result from approaches aimed at targeting the stem-cell-like component of GMB. Using coimmunefluorescence and multiphoton laser scanning microscopy it has been reported that $CD133^{+}$/$nestin^{+}$ glioma cells are closely associated with vasculature. $Nestin^{+}$ cells were found in every stage of glioma development, whereas $CD133^{+}$ cells were only present since intermediates stages corresponding with VEGF overexpression. Nestin, a class VI intermediate filament protein is expressed in gliomas, and its expression levels are higher in gliomas with high WHO histopathological classification grades than in those with low grades. Nestin plays important roles in cell growth, migration and invasion of glioma cells (Ishiwata T, 2011) and serve as a novel candidate for molecular-targeted therapy for gliomas, including glioblastomas. Furthermore, increasing the number of endothelial cells and blood vessels in experimental glioma augmented the glioma stem cell population and the rate of tumor growth (Calabrese et al., 2007) . The presence of VEGF in glioblastoma stem cell niche implies that anti-VEGF therapy might function to disrupt stem cell maintenance. In this regard, treating glioma-bearing animals with anti-VEGF therapy depleted tumor blood vessels and caused a significant reduction both in the glioma stem cell population and tumor growth rate (Calabrese et al., 2007) . This treatment did not alter the proliferation or survival of most of the glioma cells, suggesting that the drug was specifically acting on the glioma stem cells. Since dobesilate inhibits malignant marker, nestin expression in C6 glioma cells (unpublished results) and because FGF participate in the maintenance of glioblastoma stem cells (Hsu et al., 2010) and also in the resistance of these cells to radiation therapy (Firat, 2011) , this FGF inhibitor may play a role in glioma stem cell inhibition.

FGF Particpates in the Resistance to Anti-VEGF Therapy

With the discovery of vascular endothelial growth factor (VEGF) as a major driver of tumor angiogenesis, efforts have focussed on novel therapies aimed at inhibiting VEGF activity, with the goal of regressing tumors by starvation. In 2004 the humanized version of a monoclonal antibody to VEGFA, bevacizumab (Avastin, Genetech, South San Francisco, CA) , became the first Food and Drug Administration (FDA) -approved antiangiogenic drug in the United States. It was approved as a first-line treatment agent for metastatic colorectal cancer, in combination with 5-flurouracil, and was subsequently approved for treatment of unressectable, recurrent or metastatic non-squamous-cell lung cancer, breast cancer and GBM. The antibody recognizes all isoforms of VEGFA and has a circulating half-life of as long as 21 days after intravenous infusion. However, the randomized phase II BRAIN study in GBM showed that the median survival rate (MSR) after Avastin treatment is limited and it was only 2-3 months longer compared to other treatments (Junk, 2011) . Moreover, Avastin use is costly and could cause serious side effects such as gastrointestinal perforation, bleeding and hypertension. Although the mechanism of action is unknown it is postulated that the anti-VEGF antibody may play a role in "normalization" of the tumor vasculature, making it more susceptible to drugs administered subsequently (Jain , 2005) .

Tumor vessels are structurally and functionally abnormal. This abnormality impairs effective delivery of therapeutic agents to all regions of tumors, creates an abnormal oedematous microenvironment in which hypoxia may play a key role that reduces the effectiveness of therapy. Anti-VEGF therapy has the potential to normalize structurally and functionally abnormal tumor vasculature and improve the tumor microenvironment (Jain, 2005) . However, although anti-VEGF therapy normalizes tumor vasculature and alleviates vasogenic oedema in glioblastoma patients, its clinical efficacy is unclear. GBM progression during anti-VEGF treatment correlated with significant increases in plasma FGF (Batchelor et al., 2007) . Recent clinical and experimental studies showed that tumor recurrence and accelerated formation of metastases was associated with anti-VEGF therapy (Ebos et al., 2009a,b; Paez-Ribes et al., 2009) (Figure 3) .

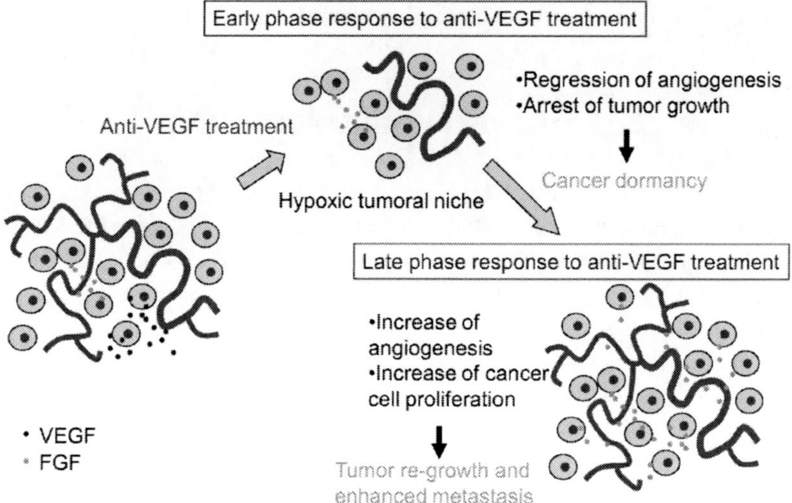

Figure 3. FGF upregulation is implicated in the inefficacy of anti-angiogenesis targeting of VEGF in late stage of tumorigenesis.

The suppression of abnormal glioma angiogenesis by inhibiting FGF rather than VEGF is likely a more suitable approach, given that FGF inhibition itself also suppresses VEGF induced angiogenesis (Jonca et al., 1997) , and FGF activation seems responsible of the medium/long-term inefficiency of VEGF inhibition-based antitumoral therapies (Casanovas et al., 2005) . Moreover, VEGF inhibition is associated with serious side effects that may be avoided using dobesilate, since despite its limited therapeutic use to date, it has been employed clinically for many years without any reported side effects.

CONCLUSION

Gliomas are one of the most devastating and incurable tumors. Sustained excessive angiogenesis by glioma cells is the major reason for their uncontrolled growth and resistance toward conventional therapies, resulting in high mortality. Therefore, targeting angiogenesis should be a logical strategy to prevent or control glioma cell growth. Since the FGF/FGFR system participates in glioma growth and plays an important role in the overcoming of chemotherapy and the failures of anti-VEGF therapies, its inhibition is of great clinical interest. The 2,5-dihydroxyphenylic acids define a new class of safe and efficient FGF inhibitors, and they constitute new leads to search for drugs to treat GBM showing an uncontrolled synthesis/release of FGF.

ACKNOWLEDGMENTS

The authors thank Begoña Cuevas and Argentina Fernández Ayerdi for their participation in animal studies referred in this work, and M. Chantal Bourdier for her contribution in editorial work. This work was supported by the CONSOLIDER Project CSD2009-00088 from the Spanish Ministry of Science and Innovation and by Action Medicines S.L.

REFERENCES

Aoki T, Hashimoto N, Matsutani M. Management of glioblastoma. *Expert Opin. Pharmacother,* 2007; 8:3133-3146.

Auguste P, Gürsel DB, Lemière S, Reimers D, Cuevas P, Carceller F, Di Santo JP, Bikfalvi A. Inhibition of fibroblast growth factor/fibroblast growth factor receptor activity in glioma cells impedes tumor growth by both angiogenesis-dependent and -independent mechanisms. *Cancer Res.,* 2001; 61:1717-1726.

Bao S, Wu Q, McLendon RE, Hao Y, Shi Q, Hjelmeland AB, Dewhirst MW, Bigner DD, Rich JN. Glioma stem cells promote radioresistance by preferential activation of the DNA damage response. *Nature,* 2006; 444:756-760.

Batchelor TT, Sorensen AG, di Tomaso E, Zhang WT, Duda DG, Cohen KS, Kozak KR, Cahill DP, Chen PJ, Zhu M, Ancukiewicz M, Mrugala MM, Plotkin S, Drappatz J, Louis DN, Ivy P, Scadden DT, Benner T, Loeffler JS, Wen PY, Jain RK. AZD2171, a pan-VEGF receptor tyrosine kinase inhibitor, normalizes tumor vasculature and alleviates edema in glioblastoma patients. *Cancer Cell.* 2007;11:83-95.

Brantley EC, Benveniste EN. Signal transducer and activator of transcription-3: a molecular hub for signaling pathways in gliomas. *Mol. Cancer Res.* 2008;6:675-684.

Calabrese C, Poppleton H, Kocak M, Hogg TL, Fuller C, Hamner B, Oh EY, Gaber MW, Finklestein D, Allen M, Frank A, Bayazitov IT, Zakharenko SS, Gajjar A, Davidoff A, Gilbertson RJ. A perivascular niche for brain tumor stem cells. *Cancer Cell,*. 2007;11: 69-82.

Casanovas O, Hicklin DJ, Bergers G, Hanahan D. Drug resistance by evasion of antiangiogenic targeting of VEGF signaling in late-stage pancreatic islet tumors. *Cancer Cell,* 2005;8: 299-309.

Cuevas P, Díaz-González D, Giménez-Gallego G, Dujovny M. Dihydroxy-2,5 benzenesulphonate (dobesilate) elicits growth arrest and apoptosis in glioma cells. *Neurol Res.,* 2005; 27: 797-800.

Cuevas P, Díaz-González D, García-Martín-Córdova C, Sánchez I, Lozano RM, Giménez-Gallego G, Dujovny M. Dobesilate diminishes activation of the mitogen- activated protein kinase ERK1/2 in glioma cells. *J. Cell Mol. Med.,* 2006a; 10:225-230.

Cuevas P, Díaz-González D, Sánchez I, Lozano RM, Giménez-Gallego G, Dujovny M. Dobesilate inhibits the activation of signal transducer and activator of transcription 3, and the expression of cyclin D1 and bcl-XL in glioma cells. *Neurol. Res.*, 2006b; 28: 127-130.

Cuevas P, Carceller F, Angulo J, González-Corrochano R, Cuevas-Bourdier A, Giménez-Gallego G. Antiglioma effects of a new, low molecular mass, inhibitor of fibroblast growth factor. *Neurosci. Lett.,* 2011, 10; 491:1-7.

Ebos JM, Lee CR, Kerbel RS. Tumor and host-mediated pathways of resistance and disease progression in response to antiangiogenic therapy. *Clin. Cancer Res.,* 2009;15: 5020-5025.

Ebos JM, Lee CR, Cruz-Munoz W, Bjarnason GA, Christensen JG, Kerbel RS. Accelerated metastasis after short-term treatment with a potent inhibitor of tumor angiogenesis. *Cancer Cell,* 2009;15: 232-9.

Esch F, Baird A, Ling N, Ueno N, Hill F, Denoroy L, Klepper R, Gospodarowicz D, Böhlen P, Guillemin R. Primary structure of bovine pituitary basic fibroblast growth factor (FGF) and comparison with the amino-terminal sequence of bovine brain acidic FGF. *Proc. Natl. Acad. Sci. U S A,* 1985; 82:6507-11.

Fernández IS, Cuevas P, Angulo J, López-Navajas P, Canales-Mayordomo A, González-Corrochano R, Lozano RM, Valverde S, Jiménez-Barbero J, Romero A, Giménez-Gallego G. Gentisic acid, a compound associated with plant defense and a metabolite of aspirin, heads a new class of in vivo fibroblast growth factor inhibitors. *J. Biol. Chem.,* 2010; 285:11714-11729.

Fernández-Tornero C, Lozano RM, Redondo-Horcajo M, Gómez AM, López JC, Quesada E, Uriel C, Valverde S, Cuevas P, Romero A, Giménez-Gallego G. Leads for development of new naphthalenesulfonate derivatives with enhanced antiangiogenic activity: crystal structure of acidic fibroblast growth factor in complex with 5-amino-2-naphthalene sulfonate. *J. Biol. Chem.,* 2003;278:21774-21781.

Firat E, Gaedicke S, Tsurumi C, Esser N, Weyerbrock A, Niedermann G. Delayed cell death associated with mitotic catastrophe in γ-irradiated stem-like glioma cells. *Radiat. Oncol.,* 2011;6: 71.

Folkman J. Angiogenesis in cancer, vascular, rheumatoid and other diseases. *Nat. Med.,* 1995, 1: 27-31

Furnari FB, Fenton T, Bachoo RM, Mukasa A, Stommel JM, Stegh A, Hahn WC, Ligon KL, Louis DN, Brennan C, Chin L, DePinho RA, Cavenee WK. Malignant astrocytic glioma: genetics, biology, and paths to treatment. *Genes Dev.*, 2007;21: 2683-2710.

Galli R, Binda E, Orfanelli U, Cipelletti B, Gritti A, De Vitis S, Fiocco R, Foroni C, Dimeco F, Vescovi A. Isolation and characterization of tumorigenic, stem-like neural precursors from human glioblastoma. *Cancer Res.*, 2004, 1;64: 7011-7021.

Giese A, Westphal M. Glioma invasion in the central nervous system. *Neurosurgery,* 1996; 39:235-250.

Giménez-Gallego G, Rodkey J, Bennett C, Rios-Candelore M, DiSalvo J, Thomas K. Brain-derived acidic fibroblast growth factor: complete amino acid sequence and homologies. *Science*, 1985;230: 1385-1388.

Haritoglou C, Gerss J, Sauerland C, Kampik A, Ulbig MW; CALDIRET study group. Effect of calcium dobesilate on occurrence of diabetic macular oedema (CALDIRET study): randomised, double-blind, placebo-controlled, multicentre trial. *Lancet,* 2009; 373: 1364-1371.

Hess KR, Broglio KR, Bondy ML. Adult glioma incidence trends in the United States, 1977-2000. *Cancer,* 2004;101: 2293-2299.

Hsu YC, Liao WC, Kao CY, Chiu IM. Regulation of FGF1 gene promoter through transcription factor RFX1. *J. Biol. Chem.*, 2010;285: 13885-13895.

Ishiwata T, Teduka K, Yamamoto T, Kawahara K, Matsuda Y, Naito Z. Neuroepithelial stem cell marker nestin regulates the migration, invasion and growth of human gliomas. *Oncol. Rep.*, 2011; 26: 91-99.

Jain RK. Normalization of tumor vasculature: an emerging concept in antiangiogenic therapy. *Science,* 2005;307: 58-62.

Jonca F, Ortéga N, Gleizes PE, Bertrand N, Plouët J. Cell release of bioactive fibroblast growth factor 2 by exon 6-encoded sequence of vascular endothelial growth factor. *J. Biol. Chem.,* 1997; 272: 24203-24209.

Junck L. Bevacizumab antiangiogenic therapy for glioblastoma. *Neurology,* 2011;76: 414-415.

Kono SA, Marshall ME, Ware KE, Heasley LE. The fibroblast growth factor receptor signaling pathway as a mediator of intrinsic resistance to EGFR-specific tyrosine kinase inhibitors in non-small cell lung cancer. *Drug Resist. Updat.,* 2009;12: 95-102.

Leung DW, Cachianes G, Kuang WJ, Goeddel DV, Ferrara N. Vascular endothelial growth factor is a secreted angiogenic mitogen. *Science.* 1989;246: 1306-1309.

Loew S, Schmidt U, Unterberg A, Halatsch ME. The epidermal growth factor receptor as a therapeutic target in glioblastoma multiforme and other malignant neoplasms. *Anticancer Agents Med. Chem.*, 2009;9: 703-715.

Loilome W, Joshi AD, Rhys CM, Piccirillo S, Vescovi AL, Gallia GL, Riggins GJ. Glioblastoma cell growth is suppressed by disruption of fibroblast growth factor pathway signaling. *J. Neurooncol.,* 2009;94: 359-366.

McKay R. Stem cells in the central nervous system. *Science,* 1997; 276: 66-71.

Olsen SK, Garbi M, Zampieri N, Eliseenkova AV, Ornitz DM, Goldfarb M, Mohammadi M. Fibroblast growth factor (FGF) homologous factors share structural but not functional homology with FGFs. *J. Biol. Chem.,* 2003; 278: 34226-36.

Onishi M, Ichikawa T, Kurozumi K, Date I. Angiogenesis and invasion in glioma. *Brain Tumor Pathol.,* 2011;28: 13-24.

Pàez-Ribes M, Allen E, Hudock J, Takeda T, Okuyama H, Viñals F, Inoue M, Bergers G, Hanahan D, Casanovas O. Antiangiogenic therapy elicits malignant progression of tumors to increased local invasion and distant metastasis. *Cancer Cell.* 2009;15: 220-231.

Powers CJ, McLeskey SW, Wellstein A. Fibroblast growth factors, their receptors and signaling. *Endocr. Relat. Cancer,* 2000;7: 165-197.

Presta M, Dell'Era P, Mitola S, Moroni E, Ronca R, Rusnati M. Fibroblast growth factor/fibroblast growth factor receptor system in angiogenesis. *Cytokine Growth Factor Rev.,* 2005;16: 159-178.

Raizer JJ. HER1/EGFR tyrosine kinase inhibitors for the treatment of glioblastoma multiforme. *J. Neurooncol.,* 2005;74: 77-86.

Ricci-Vitiani L, Pallini R, Biffoni M, Todaro M, Invernici G, Cenci T, Maira G, Parati EA, Stassi G, Larocca LM, De Maria R. Tumour vascularization via endothelial differentiation of glioblastoma stem-like cells. *Nature,* 2010;468: 824-828.

Song S, Wientjes MG, Gan Y, Au JL. Fibroblast growth factors: an epigenetic mechanism of broad spectrum resistance to anticancer drugs. *Proc. Natl. Acad. Sci. U S A,* 2000; 18;97: 8658-8663.

Stiles CD, Rowitch DH. Glioma stem cells: a midterm exam. *Neuron,* 2008; 58: 832-846.

Stupp R, Mason WP, van den Bent MJ, Weller M, Fisher B, Taphoorn MJ, Belanger K, Brandes AA, Marosi C, Bogdahn U, Curschmann J, Janzer RC, Ludwin SK, Gorlia T, Allgeier A, Lacombe D, Cairncross JG, Eisenhauer E, Mirimanoff RO; European Organisation for Research and Treatment of Cancer Brain Tumor and Radiotherapy Groups; National Cancer Institute of Canada Clinical Trials Group. Radiotherapy plus concomitant and adjuvant temozolomide for glioblastoma. *N. Engl. J. Med.,* 2005; 352: 987-996.

Szebenyi G, Fallon JF. Fibroblast growth factors as multifunctional signaling factors. *Int. Rev. Cytol.,* 1999; 185: 45-106.

Turner N, Grose R. Fibroblast growth factor signalling: from development to cancer. *Nat. Rev. Cancer,* 2010;10: 116-129.

Uchida N, Buck DW, He D, Reitsma MJ, Masek M, Phan TV, Tsukamoto AS, Gage FH, Weissman IL. Direct isolation of human central nervous system stem cells. *Proc. Natl. Acad. Sci. U S A* 2000; 97: 14720-14725.

Wang R, Chadalavada K, Wilshire J, Kowalik U, Hovinga KE, Geber A, Fligelman B, Leversha M, Brennan C, Tabar V. Glioblastoma stem-like cells give rise to tumour endothelium. *Nature,* 2010;468: 829-833.

Zhang Y, Song S, Yang F, Au JL, Wientjes MG. Nontoxic doses of suramin enhance activity of doxorubicin in prostate tumors. *J. Pharmacol. Exp. Ther.,* 2001;299: 426-433.

In: Glioblastoma ISBN: 978-1-62100-858-3
Editors: M. F. Bezerra et.al, pp. 149-162 © 2012 Nova Science Publishers, Inc.

Chapter 7

HOW TO STOP GLIAL NEOPLASTIC BRAIN DEVELOPMENT: ANTISENSE STRATEGY

Jerzy Trojan*[1*]*, Heliodor Kasprzak*[2]
***and Donald D. Anthony*[3]**

[1]INSERM U602, Paul Brousse Hospital, Paris XI University, 94007 Villejuif, France, and Gene Therapy Lab., Faculty of Medicine, Cartagena´s University, Cartagena de Indias, Colombia
[2]Dept. Neurosurgery, Collegium Medicum, Nicolas Copernic University, 85067 Bydgoszcz, Poland
[3]Dept. General Medicine, School of Medecine, CWRU University, Cleveland, 44106 OH, USA

ABSTRACT

Antisense technique was particularly used to target tumour antigens, which arrest of expression was not efficiently stopped using antibodies or other inhibitors. Antisense is working not only as an anti – gene stopping tool, but especially indirectly by inducing apoptosis and a strong immune in vitro and in vivo anti tumour response, verified in murine models i. e. of glioma or teratocarcinoma containing neuro-glial derivatives. Antisense strategy targeting principal growth factors as IGF-I, TGFbeta and their receptors, but also their downstream signalling effectors,

---

* Address for correspondence: Faculty of Medicine, Campus Zaragocilla, Cartagena´s University, Cartagena de Indias, Colombia. E-mail: jerzytrojan@hotmail.com

particularly glycogenesis, has given satisfactory experimental results for treatment of different malignant tumours including human glial tumour - glioblastoma.

Keywords: glioma, gene therapy, antisense, growth factors, IGF-I

1. Introduction

One of the most trying pathological conditions of the central nervous system is the malignant glial development of the brain. The brain stem cells which have persisted after birth can differentiate in malignant tumour - glioblastoma multiforme [1]. The mortality of this tumour is still close to 100 %, and the survival, using an immune or chemotherapy (temozolomid) [2] is rarely more than 18 months.

Gene expression during neoplastic development of the brain concern different growth factors as IGF-I, EGF, FGF, VEGF, TGF alpha and beta, and their signal transduction pathway PI3K/AKT elements including glycogen synthetase [3]. Among growth factors, IGF-I plays a principal role during development of the brain reappearing in malignant glial differentiation [4].

This hypothesis has strongly underlined the usefulness of techniques permitting to target and stop the expression of growth factors present in tumoural development by anti – gene strategies, particularly antisense approach. The "discovery" of the antisense approach was made in 1984/1985 [5,6]. The antisense approach, as a concept, was created to study basic problems of gene regulation, particularly useful in developmental biology investigations, bypassing inherent limitations of functional studies dependent upon natural mutant cells or artificially mutagenized cells. The demonstration of antisense technology as a totally performing tool, simultaneously suppressing the targeted protein expression, changing a morphologic phenotype of cultured neoplastic cells, and stopping *in vivo* a growth of experimentally established tumours in 100% cases, was done for the first time in 1992/93 using antisense anti IGF-I approach for glioma treatment [7]. The *in vitro* mechanism of anti - gene approach (antisense and triple helix techniques) , including both immune and apoptotic phenomena, was demonstrated in 1996/2001 [8]. The promising clinical results of IGF-I antisens treatment of malignant glioma – the survival of patients between 18 – 24 months, were published in 2003/2009 [9,10]. Recently, other targets than IGF-I, as TGFbeta and their downstream signal transduction pathway elements as glycogen synthase among others, were proposed for treatment of malignant gliomas using antisense technology [11,12]. Treatment of gliobastoma using antisense TGFbeta has entered in phase II clinical trial [13]. During the last years, we observe an increase of antisense approach for the treatment of tumours and especially of gliomas, the last presenting almost 100 publications in 2008-2010. Other technologies suppressing gene expression like "knock out", si RNA or miRNA knockdown, and PNA approach did not demonstrate yet the expected clinical results. Recent neuroscience research on different growth factors as a common target in glioma cell treatment, underlines a focus on the role of growth factors transduction pathway mediated by tyrosine kinase, TK [3].

2. Neoplastic Glial Development

During the development of the central nervous system including the regionalization of the central nervous system human stem cells that have persisted in matrix areas and are still active after birth, could give both tumour type neuroblastic - neuroblastoma, as glial type - gliomas [14]. Glial cells are involved in regulating various functions in the brain, which control neurogenesis and synaptogenesis, and the regulation of neurons [15], their dysfunction leads to different neuropathologies: a malignancy can lead to very serious consequences - the development of malignant gliomas - glioblastoma multiforme [1].

Gene expression during the neoplastic development of the brain, and especially during the appearance of malignant glioma, concerns various growth factors and their receptors (IGF-I, EGF, FGF, VEGF, TGF alpha and beta and their signaling pathways PI3K/AKT including glycogen synthase [3,9]. The IGF-I playing a special role among the growth factors is involved not only in neuro and gliogenesis but also in glucose metabolism and growth. IGF-I functions through its receptor IGF-IR (tyrosine kinase) that is specifically expressed during the formation of the neural tube. IGF-I decreases after birth similar to other transitional antigens, such as AFP. During postnatal period, IGF- I mRNA is localized in the anterolateral ventricle of the subventricular zone, suggesting a potential role in promoting the proliferation of neoplastic glial cells [4,9,16].

One of the main models to study the development of malignant central nervous system of mammals is the mouse teratocarcinoma. Teratocarcinoma is a tumour involving a totipotent embryonal carcinoma in various tissues including neuroectoblast tracing the successive stages of the histogenesis from the matrix cells [14,17]. The mouse teratocarcinoma model was used to study the development of human CNS tumours. The mouse teratocarcinoma reproduces caricaturally the development of primitive neural tube in which neuroectoblastic cells are differentiating roughly into two distinct populations: one consisting of glial cells that specialize in building a framework, and the other consisting by neuroblasts. Using AFP as a conventional marker in cells undergoing differentiation, the two emerging populations give positive results. For this reason, to distinguish between glial cells and neuroblasts, we used as the marker IGF-I. In this case, glial cells characterized by immunocytochemistry gave positive reaction and neuroblastic cells, negative [7]. This observation suggested that targeting the IGF-I present in the glial cell framework of neuroectoblastic derivatives of murine teratocarcinoma or of human or murine gliomas, we could stop the development neoplastic at least glial of the nervous system. This assumption led us to develop techniques for gene therapy of glioma targing IGF-I gene, the anti – gene strategy, particularly antisense approach [5,7].

3. Antisense

New anti-tumoural therapies including the glioma tumour, offer techniques of gene-therapy, particularly immuno-gene-therapy [9,18]. These are often related to the use of inhibitors or the anti - gene techniques either of antisense type or of triple helix type, "discovered" in 1984 and 1994, respectively [5,19,20].

The "antisense therapy" is generally applied as gene therapy in the strict sense - the use of antisense oligonucleotides injected directly into the cells of tissue, or as cell gene therapy - injecting the cells transfected with a vector expressing antisense RNA (usually with the help of cationic lipids) . In both cases - antisense RNA or antisense oligonucleotides - they inhibit the translation of messenger RNA on which they are directed. If the antisense RNA, forming a double-stranded RNA blocks the ribosomal machinery, antisense oligonucleotides induce a ribonuclease RNase H recognizing the hybrid oligonucleotide / mRNA, which degrades the strand ribonucleic [6,19]. To increase the biological effect of antisense oligonucleotides in their intracellular penetration, and make them more efficient against biological nucleases, they are modified chemically using phosphorothioate or phosphoramidate 13]. The antisense approach constitutes since 1992/93 a technique of choice for gene therapy of malignant glioma [5]. With regard to recently introduced siRNA technique [21], the role of 21-23 double-stranded RNA oligonucleotides in siRNA is similar to that played in the mechanism of triple helix DNA containing oligonucleotides as 23 RNA [20]. In terms of miRNA (non-coding RNA composed of 21 to 24 molecules) , its high rate was reported in glioma [22]. To make tools-drugs more powerful than antisense RNA, it means binding more readily to DNA or RNA, there was also the development of small molecules of acid peptidonucléique, APN, the use of which has brought the first satisfactory results in animal tests [23]. At the moment we have no experimental and clinical evidence showing that siRNA, miRNA or APN can effectively replace antisense technology [22]. As for the triple helix, its use in anti IGF-I therapy seems less well controlled in vivo than the antisense because of its molecular mechanism dependent on the promoter of IGF-I gene undergoing mutagenesis [8,9].

Antisense technology directed against IGF-I and other growth factors and their receptors ie TGFbeta, is not exclusive for the treatment of glioma and is in the process of expending to the treatment of other malignancies (cancers of the liver, pancreas, colon, melanoma) [9,13].

4. Antisense Therapy of Glioma

Among the various approaches used in antisense therapy of glioma, that of antisense anti growth factors, their receptors and related signal transduction pathway elements seem very promising. If growth factors, mainly IGF-I and its receptor may be considered as the first link in the signaling pathway PI3K/AKT/GWK, the glycogen synthase, GS, is the last link in the chain [3,9,12]. Malignant glial cells transfected either with antisense anti-IGF-I or with anti GS, have expressed an MHC-I antigen. In addition, in the case of glioma and embryonal carcinoma (the latter developing in vivo in teratocarcinoma) , the transfected lines have expressed B7 antigen. Cells transfected with antisense anti IGF-I also become apoptotic [8,12]. The transfected antisense anti IGF-I or anti GS cells, injected in animals bearing glioma, induce a decrease or disappearance of established tumours; this phenomenon being due to the immune response mediated by anti-tumour CD8 T. The CD8 T cells in the context of the transfected cells becoming in turn apoptotic, activate dendritic cells. B7 molecules can be included together with MHC-I in this mechanism because both antigens are needed to activate T CD8 [8,9,24] (Figure 1) . For this reason too, the absence of B7 in glial cells transfected with antisense anti GS, could explain the partial response of glioma treatment (tumour reduction) compared to therapy with antisense anti IGF-I (total cessation of tumour development) . Similar experimental results were obtained using the antisense approach directed against other growth factors [9]. Which is not surprising, knowing that growth factors have the same signaling pathway that IGF-I (Figure 1) . If the experimental results obtained with antisense anti IGF-I appear to be more efficient in the suppression of tumours, this could be explained by its role as the "supervisor" of mitogenesis of other growth factors (EGF, PDGF etc) [4,16].

If there are approximately 400 articles on IGF-I each year, there are also nearly 2,000 articles dedicated to the relationship between growth factors and glioma, and moreover, between 2008-10, almost 100 articles relating to antisense and glioma. Experimental studies of glioma therapy, using either antisense oligonucleotides or vectors expressing antisense explored particularly IGF-IR, EGF-R, FGF, VEGF, TGF alpha and beta, PI3K, AKT2, Bcl-2, c-myb, c -Met (receptor tyrosine kinase) [9,13,16] (Table 1.) .

In terms of clinical research in the past five years: 2006-2011, the very promising results of gene therapy of glioma (and other tumours) were demonstrated using the antisense anti TGF beta (TGF-beta2, being included in the mechanism of proliferation, metastasis and angiogenesis, plays an important role in tumour progression) [11,13]. Currently 140 patients are included in Phase II / III glioma grade III and IV (GBM) treated with antisense anti TGF beta (modified oliogodeoxynucléotides - phosphorothioate antisense TGF beta2 - AP 12009) . The treatment is well tolerated by patients. In 2007 the survival reached 28.6 months, and in two cases complete remission was observed [11]. In another strategy of antisense anti TGF beta2 (cell gene therapy) , median survival has reached 78 weeks and stabilization of the cancer process was observed [25]. In addition, in antisense anti TGF beta approach, the elements indicating mechanism of cellular immune response were observed [13,25].

The clinical results obtained with antisense anti TGF beta2 are very similar to those described recently by using the cell gene therapy approach of antisense anti IGF-I. The median survival for patients treated with antisense anti IGF-I was 19-20 months. The immune response was shown after each "vaccination" against IGF-I. There was an increase in the expression of molecules CD8 + CD28 + in PBL cells removed from treated patients (Figure 1) . Also a characteristic change in the phenotype - "switch" CD8 + CD11b + / CD8 + CD11b-a has accompanied every rate increase of CD8 +. Treatment was well tolerated and no secondary symptoms were reported. In two patients treated pharmacologically (temozolomide) , followed by antisense anti IGF-I, the average survival exceeded 21 months [9].

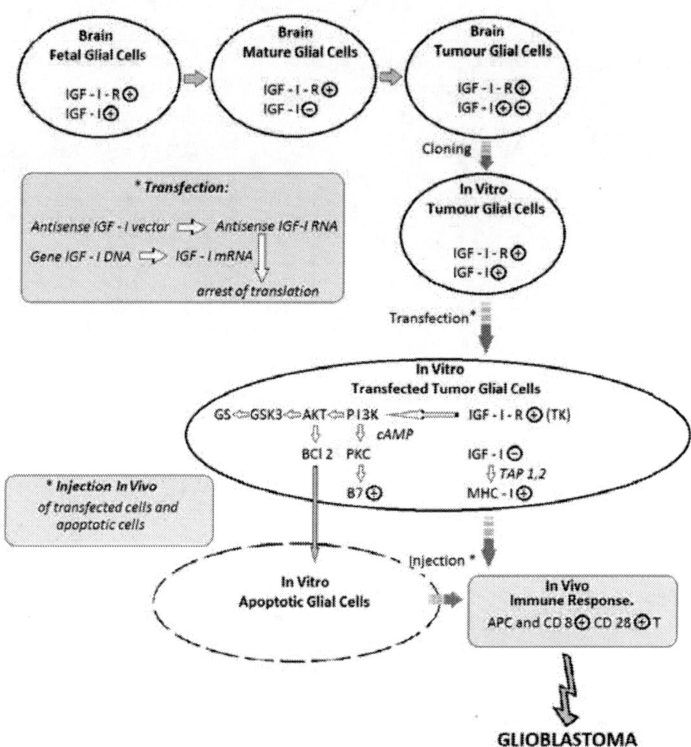

Figure 1. Antisense therapy. Example of antisense anti IGF-I treatment of glial malignant tumour – glioblastoma. The occurrence of IGF-I in different glial cells, from foetal to tumour cells, is demonstrated. The schema of therapy shows transfected in vitro brain tumour glial cells using a vector containing cDNA of IGF-I in antisense orientation. After transfection the cells express IGF-I RNA antisense stopping the IGF-I synthesis characteristic for tumour cells. They become MHC-I [+] and B7 [+], and partially apoptotic. The signal transduction pathway (related to IGF-I receptor) involved in immune and apoptotic mechanism of antisense approach, is common also for other growth factors as EGF, VEGF, TGF-beta or PDGF. The transfected cells, together with apoptotic cells and APC cells induced in vivo, activate T lymphocytes (CTL $CD8^{+}CD28^{+}$) [3,8,9,10,24]. Abreviations: TK (tyrosine kinase of growth factors receptor); PI3K (phosphatidyinositol 3 kinase); AKT (PKB, protein kinase B); GSK3 (glycogene synthetase kinase 3; GS (glycogene synthetase); PKC (protein kinase C); Bcl 2 (key molecule of apoptosis); TAP 1,2 (transporter associated with antigen processing antigen); APC (antigen presenting cell) .

Table 1. Treatment of gliomas using antisense approach. Examples of targeted growth factors and related elements. Selection of articles from last five years

PI3K regulated integrin-linked kinase (ILK)	Antisense oligodeoxynucleotide Experimental therapy	Edwards et al. Mol Cancer Ther 2006; 5(3): 645.
AKT2	Antisense (vector) Experimental therapy	Pu et al. J Neuro Oncol 2006; 76(1): 1.
VEGF	Antisense oligodeoxynucleotide Experimental therapy	Hong et al. Cancer Letters 2006; 2361: 39.
EGF-R (receptor tyrosine kinase)	Antisense (vector) Experimental therapy	Kang et al. Cancer Gene Ther 2006; 13: 530.
TGF beta 2	Antisense (vector) Clinical trial	Fakhrai et al. Cancer Gene Ther 2006; 13: 1052.
IGF-I	Antisense and Triple helix(vector) Clinical trial	Kasprzak et al. Neurol Neurochir 2006; 40(6): 509.
IGF-I	Antisense and Triple helix(vector) Clinical trial	Trojan et al. Int. J. Cancer Prevent. 2007; 2(4): 227.
IGF-I and IGF-I-R (receptor tyrosine kinase)	Antisense and Triple helix(vector) Experimental therapy and Clinical trial	Trojan et al. Neuroscience 2007; 145: 795.
TGF beta 2	Antisense oligodeoxynucleotide (AP 12009) Clinical trial	Hau et al. Oligonucleotides 2007; 17(2): 201.
Glycogen synthase (GS)	Antisense (vector) Experimental therapy	Ardourel et al. Cancer Biol Ther 2007; 6(5): 719.
c-Met (receptor tyrosine kinase)	Antisense oligonucleotide Experimental therapy	Chu et al. J Surg Res 2007; 141(2): 284.
TGF beta and specific. immun. activation	Antisense oligonucleotide (NPs) Experimental therapy	Schneider et al. J Neuroimmun 2008; 195(1-2): 21.
TGF beta and immun. activation	Antisense oligonucleotide Experimental therapy	Vega et al. Future oncol 2008; 4(3): 433
VEGF	Antisense (vector) Experimental therapy	Lin et al. Cancer Sci 2008; 99(12): 2540
TGF beta 2	Antisense oligodeoxynucleotide Clinical trial	Schlingensiepen et al. Rec Res Cancer Res 2008; 177: 137.
IGF-I	Antisense (vector) Clinical trial	Trojan et al. JAC 2009; 1: 21.

TGF beta 2	Antisense oligodeoxynucleotide Clinical trial	Hau et al. Expert Rev Anticancer Ther 2009; 9(11):1663.
IGF BP2	Antisense (vector) Experimental therapy	Moore et al. Proc Natl Acad Sci USA 2009; 106(39): 16675
EGFR	Antisense oligonucleotide Experimental therapy	Loew et al. Anticancrer Agents Med Chem 2009; 9(6): 703.
TGF beta	Antisense oligodeoxynucleotide Clinical trial	Vallieres IDrugs 2009; 12(7): 445.
IGF-I	Antisense (vector) Clinical trial	Trojan et al. Biomed and Pharmaother 2010; 64(8): 576.
c-Met (receptor tyrosine kinase)	Antisense oligonucleotide Experimental therapy	Chu et al. Oncol Rep 2010; 24(1):189.
AKT2	Antisense oligonucleotide Experimental therapy	Zhang et al. Oncol Rep 2010; 24(1):65.
EGFR	Antisense oligonucleotide Experimental therapy	Li et al. Oncol Rep 2010; 23(6): 1585.
PED/PEA-15 (ERK1/2-interacting protein)	Antisense oligonucleotide Experimental therapy	Botta et al. Hum Gene Ther 2010; 21(9): 1067.
EGFR	Antisense oligonucleotide Experimental therapy	Kang et al. J Biomed Mater Res A 2010; 93(2): 585.
TGFbeta and T cell therapy	Antisense oligodeoxynucleotide Clinical trial	Dietrich et al. Curr Opin Oncol 2010; 22(6):604.
VEGF	Antisense (vector) Experimental therapy	Yang et al. J Neurooncol 2011; 103(1): 33.

The IGF-I receptor and PKC, the latter included in the signaling pathway, constituted also the targets for clinical treatment of glioma [9]. If the antisense targeting anti PKC did not give the expected results, the treatment of glioblastoma by antisense anti IGF-I receptor, IGF-IR, done in 2001, opened the door to clinical research of different tumours [26]. Clinical results of the approach of antisense anti IF-IR, less spectacular than those obtained in the case of IGF-I or TGF beta-2, are due to the fact that over-expression of IGF-IR during tumour development is less important than of other receptors, such as the EGF receptor. Moreover, taking into account other factors involved in the PI3K/AKT signaling pathway, the signal of IGF-IR may be inappropriate or exaggerated during neoplastic development to be controlled by its blocking [4].

5. Approval of Clinical Trial

The approval for the gene therapy clinical trial of glioblastoma using IGF-I antisense approach (based on NIH clinical protocol n°1602, Bethesda, Maryland, 24. 11. 1993) was administrated by the Bioethical Commissions of the L. Rydygier Medical University, Bromberg (Bydgoszcz) , Jagiellonian University, Cracow, Poland (n° KB/176/2001, 28. 06. 2002, and n°KBET/184/L/2000, 21. 09. 2000) , La Sabana University, Chia, Colombia, no P 004-10, 15. 12. 2010, and registered by international Wiley Gene Therapy Clinical Trial database, Stockholm, n° 635 and 636 (J Gene Med, updated 2002) . The protocol was verified by Ministry of Health, AFSSAPS Committee, Paris, France, 03. 06. 2005, and by NATO Science program 2003 - 2007 (n° LST 980517) .

6. Conclusion

According to Baserga and Pollak [4, 7, 16], IGF-I is one of the most important growth factors related to normal to normal and neoplastic differentiation, being expressed in about 17 different tumours. Since the symposium "IGFs and Cancer", held in Halle in Germany (15–17. 09.2000) , IGF-I is admitted as a diagnostic marker signalling precancerous step of different types of tumours especially of malignant brain tumour – glioblastoma [27]. The study of risc factors and of the treatment of glioblastoma are in constant progress from some years [1, 2, 28].

Despite the considerable effort of clinical research, especially recent very successful application of chemotherapy (temozolomide) , and inhibitors and antibodies (imatinib, getifinib, vastin) [2,9,29], the mortality of patients with glioblastoma is still important. If survival gradually reached two years, we are quite far from a won battle [1,2,13,30]. Treatment approaches, which generally target growth factors, are recently focusing on the use of antisense. The tendency to use antisense technology, goes with the recent proposals of the research pathway TK (tyrosine kinase growth factor) / PI3K/GS in glial cells, constituting the target in the treatment of malignant glioma [3,12]. Given that the mentioned signal pathway is common to various growth factors, an arrest using antisense or inhibitors techniques, of at least two growth factors simultaneously (IGF-I, TGF beta2 or EGF) could constitute a direction for future clinical research of malignant gliomas.

We can conclude that the future belongs to the complex therapy. As the example given, the combination of anti IGF-IR either IGF-I or TGF beta antisense with chemotherapy would be a possible opportunity; taking into account the signaling pathway in the complex therapy, there isalso a relationship between the receptor for IGF-I and estrogen [4,16]. In the future in progress, the complex therapy will include pharmacological treatment (temozolomide) , followed by the use of immunotherapy and techniques of inhibitors including inhibitors and antisense strategies [31,32,33]; the immunotherapy being strictly related to the anti-immune response is also present in the antisense approach [7,10,18].

ACKNOWLEDGEMENTS

We thank Jean-François Nicolas (Institut Pasteur, Paris) for his critical review of this manuscript, Tom Philips from Thomson Scientific Lim., London, for the references related to the development of AP-12OO9 (TGF-beat2 antisense oligonucleotide in phase III clinical trial of malignant tumours) , and Annabelle Trojan for professional corrections.

REFERENCES

[1] M. Sanson, F. Laigle-Donadey, A. Benouaich-Amiel, Molecular changes in brain tumours: prognostic and therapeutic impact, *Curr. Opin. Neurol.* 18 (2006) 623-630.

[2] R. Stupp, M.E. Hegi, M.J. van den Bent, W.P. Masson, M. Weller, R.O. Mirimanof, J.G. Caincross, Changing paradigms--an update on the multidisciplinary management of malignant glioma, *Oncologist* 11 (2006) 165-180.

[3] M.E. Beckner, G.T. Gobbel, R. Abounader, F. Burovic, N.R. Agostino, J. Laterra, I.F. Pollack, Glycolytic glioma cells with active glycogen synthase are sensitive to PTEN and inhibitors of PI3K and gluconeogenesis, *Lab. Invest.* 85 (2005) 1457-1470.

[4] M.N. Pollak, E.S. Schernhammer, E. Hankinson, Insulin-like growth factors and neoplasia, *Nat. Rev. Cancer* 4 (2004) 505-518.

[5] J.L. Rubenstein, J.F. Nicolas, F. Jacob, Nonsense RNA: a tool for specifically inhibiting the expression of a gene in vivo, *C. R. Acad. Sci.* III 299 (1984) 271-274.

[6] N. Dias, C.A. Stein, Basic concepts and antisense oligonucleotides mechanisms, *Mol. Cancer Therapeutics* 1 (2002) 347-355.

[7] J. Trojan, T.R. Johnson, S. Rudin, Ju. Ilan, M.L. Tykocinski, J. Ilan, Treatment and prevention of rat glioblastoma by immugenic C6 cells expressing antisense insulin-like growth factor I RNA, *Science* 259 (1993) 94-97.

[8] A. Ly, H.T. Duc, M. Kalamarides, L.A. Trojan, Y. Pan, A. Shevelev, J.-C. François, T. Noël, A. Kane, D. Henin, D.D. Anthony, J. Trojan, Human glioma cells transformed by IGF-I triple-helix technology show immune and apoptotic characteristics determining cell selection for gene therapy of glioblastoma, *J. Clin. Pathol.* (*Molec. Pathol.)* 54(4) (2001) 230-239.

[9] J. Trojan, J.-F. Cloix, M. Ardourel, M. Chatel, D.D. Anthony, IGF-I biology and targeting in malignant glioma, *Neuroscience* 145(3) (2007) 795-811.

[10] J. Trojan, A. Ly, M.X. Wei, M. Bierwagen, P. Kopinski, Y. Pan, M-Y. Ardourel, T. Dufour, A. Shevelev, L.A. Trojan, J-C. François, C. Andres, T. Popiela, M. Chatel, H. Kasprzak, D.D. Anthony, H.T. Duc, Antisense anti IGF-I cellular therapy of malignant tumours: immune response in cancer patients, *Biomed. and Pharmacother*. 64(8) (2010) 576-578.

[11] P. Hau, P. Jachimczak, R. Schlingensiepen, I. Schulmeyer, F. Jauch, A. Steinbrecher, Inhibition of TGF-beta2 with AP 12009 in recurrent malignant gliomas: from preclinical to phase I/II studies, *Oligonucleotides* 17(2) (2007) 201-212.

[12] M.-Y. Ardourel, M. Blin, J.-L.Moret, T. Dufour, H.T. Duc, T. Hevor, J. Trojan, J.-F. Cloix, A new putative target for antisense gene therapy of glioma: glycogen synthetase, *Cancer Biol. Ther*. 6(5) (2007) 719-723.

[13] K.H. Schlingensiepen, B. Fischer-Blass, S. Schmaus, S. Ludwig, Antisense therapeutics for tumor treatment: the TGF-beta2 inhibitor AP 12009 in clinical development against malignant tumors, *Recent Results Cancer Res.* 177 (2008) 137-150.

[14] J. Gaillard, J.M. Caillaud, R. Maunoury, H. Ohayon, J. Trojan, Expression of neuro-ectoblast in murine teratocarcinomas: electron-microscopic and immunocytochemical studies, applications in

embryology and in tumor pathology of central nrvous system (in french) , Bull. Inst. Pasteur 82 (1984) 335-385.

[15] B.A. Barres, What is a glial cell ?, *Glia* 43 (2003) 4-5.

[16] R. Baserga, The insulin-like growth factor-I receptor as a target for cancer therapy, *Expert. Opin. Ther. Targets* 9 (2005) 753-768.

[17] J. Trojan, T.R. Johnson, S.D. Rudin, B.K. Blossey, K.M. Kelley, A. Shevelev, F.W. Abdul Karim, D.D. Anthony, M.L. Tykocinski, Ju. Ilan, J. Ilan, Gene therapy of murine teratocarcinoma: Separate functions for insulin-like growth factors I and II in immunogenicity and differentiation. *Proc. Natl. Acad. Sci. USA* 91 (1994) 6088-6092.

[18] E.A. Vega, M.W. Graner, J. H. Sampson, Combating immunosuppression in glioma, *Future Oncol.* 4(3) (2008) 433-442.

[19] H. Weintraub, J. Izant, R. Harland, Antisense RNA as a molecular tool for genetic analysis, *Trends Gene.* 1(1) (1985) 23-25.

[20] C. Hélène, Control of oncogene expression by antisense nucleic acid, *Eur. J. Cancer* 30A (1994) 1721-1726.

[21] R.J. Boado, RNA interference and nonviral targeted gene therapy of experimental brain cancer. *NeuroRx.* 2(1) (2005) 139-150.

[22] M.F. Corsten, R. Miranda, R. Kasmieh, A.M. Krishevsky, R. Weisslederer, R. Shak, MicroRNA-21 knockdown disrupts glioma growth in vivo and displays synergistic cytotoxicity with neural precursor cell delivered S-TRAIL in human gliomas, *Cancer Res.* 67(19) (2007) 8994-9000.

[23] L. Orgel, Prebiotic chemistry and the origin of the RNA world, *Critical Rev. Biochem. Mol. Biol.* 39 (2004) 99-123.

[24] J.F. Fonteneau, M. Larsson, N. Bhardwaj, Interactions between dead cells and dendritic in the induction of antiviral CTL responses, *Curr. Opin. Immunol.* 14 (2002) 471-477.

[25] H. Fakhrai, J.C. Mantil, L. Liu, G.L. Nicholson, C.S. Murphy-Satter, J. Ruppert, Phase I clinical trial of a TGF-beta antisense-modified tumor cell vaccine in patients with advanced glioma, *Cancer Gene Ther.* 13(12) (2006) 1052-1060.

[26] D. Sachdev, D. Yee, Disrupting insulin-like growth factor signalling as a potential cancer therapy, *Mol. Cancer Ther.* 6(1) (2007) 1-12.

[27] W. Zumkeller, IGFs and IGF-binding proteins as diagnostic markers and biological modulators in brain tumors, *Expert. Rev. Mol. Diagn.*, 2 (2002) 473-477.

[28] R. Jiang, C. Mircean, I. Shmulevich I, D. Cogdell, Y. Jia, I. Tabus, K. Aldape, R. Sawaya, J. M. Bruner, G.N. Fuller, W. Zhang, Pathway

alterations during glioma progression revealed by reverse phase protein lysate arrays, *Proteomics* 6 (2006) 2964-2971.

[29] P.Y. Wen, W.K. Yung, K.R. Lamborn, P.L. Dahia, Y. Wang, B. Peng, L.E. Abrey, J. Raizer, T.F. Cloughesy, K. Fink, M. Gilbert, S. Chang, L. Junck, D. Schiff, M.D. Prados, Phase I/II study of imatinib mesylate for recurrent malignant gliomas: Norty American Brain Tumour Consortium Study 99-08, *Clin. Cancer Res.* 12 (2006) 4899-4907.

[30] T. Gorlia, M.J. van den Bent, M.E. Hegi, Nomograms for predicting survival of patients with newly diagnosed glioblastoma: prognostic factor analysis of EORTC and NCIC trial 26981-22981/CE.3, *Lancet Oncol.* 9(1) (2008) 29-38.

[31] R. K. Goudar, Q. Shi, M. D. Hjelmeland, S.T. Keir, R.E. McLendon, C.J. Wikstrand, E.D. Reese, C.A. Conrad, P. Traxler, H.A: Lane, D. A. Reardon, W.K. Cavenee, X.F. Wan, D.D. Bigner, H.S. Friedman, J.N. Rich, Combination therapy of inhibitors of epidermal growth factor receptor/vascular endothelial growth factor receptor 2 (AEE788) and the mammalian target of rapamycin (RAD001) offers improved glioblastoma tumor growth inhibition, *Mol. Cancer Ther.* 4 (2005) , 101-112.

[32] F. M. Lemoine, M. Cherai, C. Giverne, D. Dimitri, M. Rosenzwajg, H. Trebeden-Negre, N. Chaput, B. Barro, N. Thioun, B. Gattegnio, F. Selles, A. Six, N. Azar, J.P. Lotz, A. Buzyn, M. Sibony, A. Delcourt, O. Boyer, S. Herson, D. Klatzmann, R. Lacave, Massive expansion of regulatory T-cells following interleukin 2 treatment during a phase I-II dendritic cell-based immunotherapy of metastatic renal cancer, Internat. *J. Oncol.* 35(3) (2009) 569-581.

[33] M. Cavazzana-Calvo, S. Hacein-Bey-Abina and A. Fischer A, Ten years of gene therapy: thoughts and perspectives, *Med. Sci.* (Paris) 26(2) (2010) 115-118.

In: Glioblastoma ISBN: 978-1-62100-858-3
Editors: M. F. Bezerra et.al, pp. 163-172

Chapter 8

CHANGE IN EXPRESSION OF 06-METHYLGUANINE-DNA METHYLTRANSFERASE (MGMT) FOLLOWING CHEMOTHERAPY FOR MALIGNANT GLIOMA

Satoshi Utsuki[1], Hidehiro Oka[1], Chihiro Kijima[1], Yoshiteru Miyajima[1], Kiyotaka Fujii[1], Toshihide Matsumoto[2], and Yuichi Sato[2]

[1]Department of Neurosurgery, Kitasato University School of Medicine, Kanagawa, Japan

[2]Department of Molecular Diagnostics, School of Allied Health Sciences, Kitasato University, Kanagawa, Japan

ABSTRACT

It has been reported that the therapeutic response to certain drugs such as temozolomide and nimustine hydochloride (ACNU) correlates with the expression of the O6-methylguanine-DNA methyltransferase (MGMT) protein. Studies further indicate that MGMT expression may be suppressed by various anticancer agents or interferon-beta (IFN-β) . We examined a cohort of patients with malignant glioma to determine the influence of chemotherapy on MGMT expression.

Tissue samples from 24 patients were collected, each documenting a recurrence of tumor following chemotherapy. The histologic diagnoses recorded prior to chemotherapy were anaplastic oligodendroglioma (3 cases) , anaplastic astrocytoma (5 cases) , and glioblastoma (16 cases) . Biopsy confirmation of a second recurrence, unchanged in type, was also obtained from four patients with diagnoses including anaplastic oligodendroglioma (2 cases) , anaplastic astrocytoma (1 case) , and glioblastoma (1 case) .

As initial chemotherapy, the patients received one of three treatments: IAV combination treatment (IFN-β, ACNU, and vincristine, 17 cases) , IPE combination treatment (IFN-β, cisplatin, and etoposide, 3 cases) , or temozolomide monotherapy (4 cases) . All patients underwent irradiation (60 Gy) in addition to initial chemotherapy. Second-line chemotherapy with IPE or temozolomide was administered to two patients each. Expression of MGMT was evaluated histochemically in 52 sequential specimens from 24 tumors.

A qualitative decrease in MGMT expression was found in 2 of 17 tumors after treatment with IAV, in 4 of 5 tumors after an IPE regimen, and in 2 of 6 tumors after single-agent temozolomide treatment.

These results suggest that expression of MGMT protein in malignant glioma may be suppressed by IPE chemotherapy.

INTRODUCTION

Even if chemotherapy is initially effective against malignant glioma, there may be subsequent acquisition of drug resistance. Temozolomide is used as the first line treatment for malignant glioma [1], and the manifestation of the O6-methylguanine-DNA methyltransferase (MGMT) protein has the greatest effect on drug resistance [2].

It has been reported that MGMT in tumor cells increases following temozolomide therapy and radiotherapy [3, 4], and that this increase in MGMT promotes resistance to treatment of the tumor. In contrast, it has been reported that anticancer drugs such as O6-benzylguanine (BG) [5], cisplatin [6-8] and interferon-beta (IFN-β) [9, 10] inhibit manifestation of the MGMT protein, and that these drugs may potentially be used as new combination therapy for the treatment of malignant glioma. The aim of this study is to investigate changes in the expression of MGMT protein following chemotherapy.

MATERIAL AND METHODS

Twenty four patients with recurrent malignant melanoma were enrolled in this study. These patients included 12 males and 12 females ranging in age from 12 to 74 years (mean 47 years) . Each underwent two or more tumor resections following chemotherapy between August, 2007 and January, 2009. Histological diagnosis was done in all cases, including four secondary recurrences of malignant glioma. The survey included 52 specimens in total: 24 specimens before chemotherapy, the first 24 recurrent specimens after chemotherapy, and the second four recurrent specimens after a second round of chemotherapy. The diagnoses at the primary operation were anaplastic astrocytoma (5 cases) , anaplastic oligodendroglioma (3 cases) , and glioblastoma (16 cases) . The diagnoses at the third surgery were anaplastic astrocytoma (2 cases) , anaplastic oligodendroglioma (1 case) , and glioblastoma (1 case) . In all cases, pathological diagnosis was unchanged from the initial diagnosis to the diagnosis at the first and second recurrence.

All patients received irradiation of 60 Gy with initial chemotherapy. Two courses of IAV treatment (IFN-β, nimustine hydrochloride (ACNU) and vincristine) or IPE treatment (interferon-beta, cisplatin, etoposide) , were given as initial chemotherapy until August, 2006. These initial treatments were combined with radiotherapy. After September of 2006, temozolomide became available to use in Japan and was used as initial chemotherapy. The second round of chemotherapy was provided two months after the initial chemotherapy. The intravenous IAV chemotherapy regimen consisted of vincristine (1 mg/m2) on the first day, two doses of ACNU (100 mg/m2) on the second day, followed by IFN-β (600 × 104 IU) three times a week for six weeks. The intravenous IPE chemotherapy regimen consisted of cisplatin (20mg/m2) and etoposide (60mg/m2) for five days, followed by IFN-β (600 × 104 IU) three times a week for six weeks. Temozolomide treatment (75 mg/m2) was given in addition to radiotherapy for 42 days, followed by 200 mg/m2 for the first five days of every four weeks. After recurrence temozolomide was given at 150 mg/m2 for five days, and 200 mg/m^2 for the first five days of every four weeks, as long as possible.

The specimens were immunostained for expression of MGMT. Specimens were scored as having one of three possible results: negative (no MGMT-positive cells) , slightly positive (<30% MGMT-positive cells) , or strongly positive (>30% MGMT-positive cells) . Changes in MGMT expression were evaluated pre- and post-chemotherapy. Specimens were compared between the first and second recurrence. The expression of MGMT was considered to be "decreased" when immunostaining of MGMT changed between pre- and post-chemotherapy from strongly positive to slightly positive, or from slightly positive to negative. On the contrary, MGMT was considered to be "increased" when immunostaining changed from negative to slightly positive, or from slightly positive to strongly positive. If the level of immunostaining remained the same pre- and post-chemotherapy, MGMT expression was considered unchanged.

RESULTS

At the primary operation, 6 specimens were MGMT negative, 8 specimens were slightly positive and 10 were strongly positive. The 24 patients were treated with either IAV (17 patients) , IPE (3 patients) or temozolomide (4 patients) as initial chemotherapy.

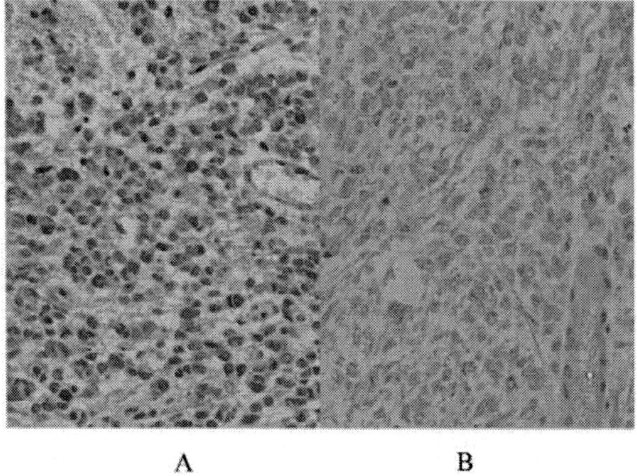

A B

Figure 1. A: Photomicrographs showing immunohistochemical staining for MGMT in anaplastic astrocytoma before chemotherapy. This tumor was judged to be strongly positive since almost all tumor cells were immunopositive for MGMT. (original magnification X200) B: Photomicrographs showing immunohistochemical staining for MGMT in recurrent anaplastic astrocytoma after IPE therapy. This tumor was judged to be slightly positive since few tumor cells were immunopositive for MGMT. The change in MGMT expression was judged to be a decrease. (original magnification X200) .

All four of the patients who had a second recurrence were treated with IAV as initial chemotherapy. Two patients were treated with IPE and two patients were treated with temozolomide as the second chemotherapy. For the 5-day temozolomide administration, 5-10 courses (median 8 courses) were performed.

MGMT expression was decreased in 2/17 specimens after IAV therapy, 4/5 specimens after IPE therapy (Figure 1) and 2/6 specimens after temozolomide therapy. Reduction of MGMT expression was most common in IPE treatment (Table 1) . Expression of MGMT was increased in 3/17 specimens after the IAV treatment (Figure 2) .

In the remaining cases, expression of MGMT was equal in pre- and post-chemotherapy specimens. In 3/4 cases in which the patients underwent a third surgery, the expression of MGMT protein after the second chemotherapy treatment was equal. However, in the other case of a third surgery, treated with IPE as the second chemotherapy, the expression of MGMT decreased. In this case MGMT expression was unchanged after IAV treatment as the first chemotherapy (Figure 3) .

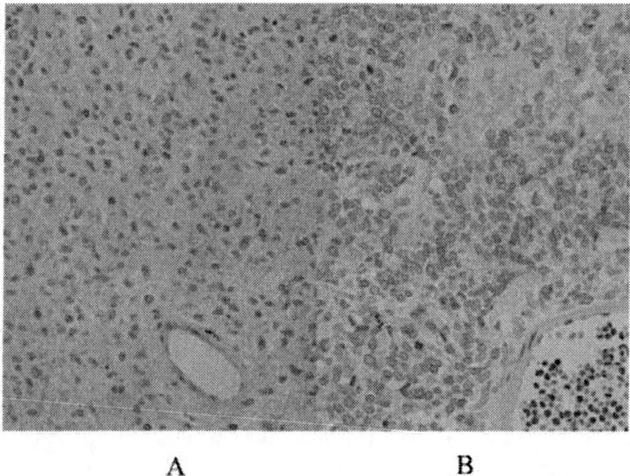

A B

Figure 2. A: Photomicrographs showing immunohistochemical staining for MGMT in anaplastic oligodendroglioma before chemotherapy. This tumor was judged to be slightly positive since a small number of tumor cells (<30%) were immunopositive for MGMT. (original magnification X200) B: Photomicrographs showing immunohistochemical staining for MGMT in recurrent anaplastic oligodendroglioma after IAV therapy. This tumor was judged to be strongly positive since almost all tumor cells were immunopositive for MGMT. The change in MGMT expression was judged to be an increase. (original magnification X200) .

Table 1. Change of the MGMT protein after the chemotherapy

	Decrease	Not change	Increase
After IAV	2/17	12/17	3/17
After IPE	4/5	1/5	0/5
After temozolomide	2/6	4/6	0/6

IAV: interferon-beta, ACNU and vincristine combination treatment. IPE: interferon-beta, cisplatin and etoposide combination treatment. Decrease: immunostaining of MGMT changed between pre- and post-chemotherapy from strongly positive to slightly positive, or from slightly positive to negative. Not change: the level of immunostaining remained the same pre- and post-chemotherapy. Increase: immunostaining changed from negative to slightly positive, or from slightly positive to strongly positive.

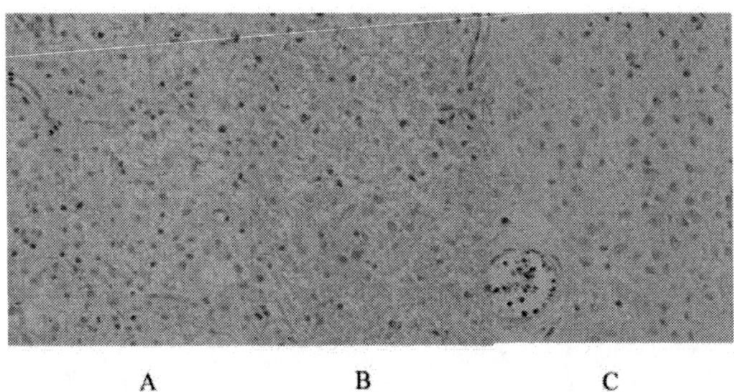

A B C

Figure 3. A: Photomicrographs showing immunohistochemical staining for MGMT in anaplastic astrocytoma before chemotherapy. This tumor was judged to be strongly positive since approximately 35% of tumor cells were immunopositive for MGMT. (original magnification X200) . B: Photomicrographs showing immunohistochemical staining for MGMT in recurrent anaplastic astrocytoma after IAV therapy. The ratio of MGMT-positive tumor cells did not change. (original magnification X200) . C: Photomicrographs showing immunohistochemical staining for MGMT of second recurrent anaplastic astrocytoma after IPE therapy. This tumor was judged to be slightly positive since few tumor cells were immunopositive for MGMT. The change in MGMT expression was judged to be a decrease. (original magnification X200) .

DISCUSSION

Various types of chemotherapeutic drugs are used in the treatment of malignant brain tumors, including alkylating agents. However, there are differences in patient susceptibility to chemotherapeutic agents, even if the gliomas are of equal grade. In addition, for the tumor of an individual patient, the susceptibility to each chemotherapeutic agent may change due to epigenetic changes during the treatment process. Temozolomide is used as a standard chemotherapy for malignant gliomas [1], but the activation of the DNA repair enzyme MGMT is well known as one of the factors to attenuate the effect of temozolomide [2]. One of the mechanisms of action by which temozolomide exerts its antitumor effect is by methylation of nucleotides of DNA. MGMT offsets the antitumor effect of temozolomide by interfering this methylation. MGMT expression is regarded as the main factor in drug resistance to temozolomide, and expression of MGMT is found in approximately 70% of malignant gliomas [11]. When temozolomide is the primary chemotherapeutic treatment, a method to inactivate or attenuate the function of MGMT is considered [12]. Chemotherapeutic drugs such as BG [5], cisplatin [6-8] and IFN-β [9, 10] have been reported to attenuate the function of MGMT. Results of phase II trial are reported in BG for their ability to attenuate MGMT, and it was reported that cisplatin was effective for 20% for recurrent glioblastoma [13], and the results of phase II trial are reported [14]. Preliminary experiments with IFN-β show that transcription of MGMT is inhibited by IFN-β, and clinical trials have reported that the antitumor effect of temozolomide is reinforced by IFN-β [15].

The results of the present study have demonstrated that the expression of MGMT before initiation of chemotherapy was 18/24 (75%) strongly positive or slightly positive, regardless of past report. Although the number of cases was small, the expression of MGMT decreased in 80% of cases (4/5) after IPE therapy, and the degree of loss of MGMT was greater than in a case after IAV and temozolomide therapy. Therefore, IPE treatment was one of the most effective combination drugs to inhibit expression of MGMT in this study.

There are many reports showing that cisplatin decreases expression of MGMT. The mechanism is thought to be repression of transcription from the MGMT promoter [11] and the down-regulation of MGMT mRNA expression [8].

Therefore, it is likely that cisplatin is the primary drug responsible for the decrease of MGMT in IPE therapy. Also, cisplatin may enhance the effect of temozolomide, where MGMT is regarded as the primary factor in drug-resistance, if cisplatin decreases expression of MGMT. There are many reports regarding the efficacy of the combination of cisplatin and temozolomide in the treatment of malignant tumors such as melanoma [16], adenocarcinoma [17], and acute leukemia [18], with the exception of malignant glioma. In cases of malignant glioma in which MGMT expression is high, the administration of cisplatin inhibited expression of MGMT and was thought to improve the efficacy of temozolomide.

Conclusion

IPE chemotherapy may inhibit expression of MGMT in tumor cells. The IPE therapy may improve the effect of chemotherapeutic drugs such as temozolomide where MGMT is a factor in drug resistance.

References

[1] Stupp, R.; Mason, W. P.; van den Bent, M. J.; Weller, M.; Fisher, B.; Taphoorn, M. J.; Belanger, K.; Brandes, A. A.; Marosi, C.; Bogdahn, U.; Curschmann, J.; Janzer, R. C.; Ludwin, S. K.; Gorlia, T.; Allgeier, A.; Lacombe, D.; Cairncross, J. G.; Eisenhauer, E. and Mirimanoff, R. O. (2005) . For the European Organization for Research and Treatment of Cancer Brain Tumor and Radiotherapy Groups and National Cancer Institute of Canada Clinical Trials Group. Radiotherapy plus concomitant and adjuvant temozolomide for glioblastoma. *N. Engl. J. Med. 352,* 987-996.

[2] Hegi, M. E.; Diserens, A. C.; Gorlia, T.; Hamou, M. F.; de Tribolet, N.; Weller, M.; Kros, J. M.; Hainfellner, J. A.; Mason, W.; Mariani, L.; Bromberg, J. E.; Hau, P.; Mirimanoff, R. O.; Cairncross, J. G.; Janzer, R. C. and Stupp, R. (2005) . MGMT gene silencing and benefit from temozolomide in glioblastoma. *N. Engl. J. Med, 352,* 997-1003.

[3] Brandes, A. A.; Franceschi, E.; Tosoni, A.; Bartolini, S.; Bacci, A.; Agati, R.; Ghimenton, C.; Turazzi, S.; Talacchi, A.; Skrap, M.; Marucci, G.; Volpin, L.; Morandi, L.; Pizzolitto, S.; Gardiman, M.; Andreoli, A.; Calbucci, F. and Ermani, M. (2010) . O(6) -methylguanine DNA-methyltransferase methylation status can change between first surgery

for newly diagnosed glioblastoma and second surgery for recurrence: clinical implications. *Neuro. Oncol. 12,* 283-288.

[4] Jung, T. Y.; Jung, S.; Moon, K. S.; Kim, I. Y.; Kang, S. S.; Kim, Y. H.; Park, C. S. and Lee, K. H. (2010) . Changes of the O6-methylguanine-DNA methyltransferase promoter methylation and MGMT protein expression after adjuvant treatment in glioblastoma. *Oncol. Rep. 23,* 1269-1276.

[5] Quinn, J. A.; Jiang, S. X.; Reardon, D. A.; Desjardins, A.; Vredenburgh, J. J.; Rich, J. N.; Gururangan, S.; Friedman, A. H.; Bigner, D. D.; Sampson, J. H.; McLendon, R. E.; Herndon, J. E. 2nd.; Walker, A. and Friedman, H.S. (2009) . Phase II trial of temozolomide plus o6-benzylguanine in adults with recurrent, temozolomide-resistant malignant glioma, *J. Clin. Oncol. 27,* 1262-1267.

[6] Park, C. K.; Park, S. H.; Lee, S. H.; Kim, C. Y.; Kim, D. W.; Paek, S. H.; Kim, D. G.; Heo, D. S.; Kim, I. H. and Jung, H. W. (2009) . Methylation status of the MGMT gene promoter fails to predict the clinical outcome of glioblastoma patients treated with ACNU plus cisplatin. *Neuropathology. 29,* 443-449.

[7] Sato, K.; Kitajima, Y.; Nakagawachi, T.; Soejima, H.; Miyoshi, A.; Koga, Y. and Miyazaki, K.(2005) . Cisplatin represses transcriptional activity from the minimal promoter of the O6-methylguanine methyltransferase gene and increases sensitivity of human gallbladder cancer cells to 1-(4-amino-2-methyl-5-pyrimidinyl) methyl-3-2-chloroethyl) -3-nitrosourea. *Oncol. Rep. 13,* 899-906.

[8] Tanaka, S.; Kobayashi, I.; Utsuki, S.; Oka, H.; Yasui, Y. and Fujii, K. (2005) . Down-regulation of O6-methylguanine-DNA methyltransferase gene expression in gliomas by platinum compounds. *Oncol. Rep. 14,* 1275-1280.

[9] Motomura, K.; Natsume, A.; Kishida, Y.; Higashi, H.; Kondo, Y.; Nakasu, Y.; Abe, T.; Namba, H.; Wakai, K. and Wakabayashi, T. (2011) . Benefits of interferon-β and temozolomide combination therapy for newly diagnosed primary glioblastoma with the unmethylated MGMT promoter: A multicenter study. *Cancer. 117,* 1721-1730.

[10] Natsume, A.; Wakabayashi, T.; Ishii, D.; Maruta, H.; Fujii, M.; Shimato, S.; Ito, M. and Yoshida, J. (2008) . A combination of IFN-beta and temozolomide in human glioma xenograft models: implication of p53-mediated MGMT downregulation. *Cancer Chemother. Pharmacol. 61,* 653-659.

[11] Silber, J. R.; Bobola, M. S.; Ghatan, S.; Blank, A.; Kolstoe, D. D. and Berger, M. S. (1998) . O6-methylguanine-DNA methyltransferase activity in adult gliomas: relation to patient and tumor characteristics. *Cancer Res. 58,* 1068-1073.

[12] Liu, L. and Gerson, S. L. (2006) . Targeted modulation of MGMT: clinical implications. *Clin. Cancer Res. 12,* 328-331.

[13] Silvani, A.; Eoli, M.; Salmaggi, A.; Lamperti, E.; Maccagnano, E.; Broggi, G. and Boiardi, A.(2004) . Phase II trial of cisplatin plus temozolomide, in recurrent and progressive malignant glioma patients. *J. Neurooncol. 66,* 203-208.

[14] Zustovich, F.; Lombardi, G.; Della Puppa, A.; Rotilio, A.; Scienza, R. and Pastorelli, D. (2009) . A phase II study of cisplatin and temozolomide in heavily pre-treated patients with temozolomide-refractory high-grade malignant glioma. *Anticancer. Res. 29,* 4275-4279.

[15] Wakabayashi, T.; Kayama, T.; Nishikawa, R.; Takahashi, H.; Yoshimine, T.; Hashimoto, N.; Aoki, T.; Kurisu, K.; Natsume, A.; Ogura, M. and Yoshida, J. (2008) . A multicenter phase I trial of interferon-beta and temozolomide combination therapy for high-grade gliomas (INTEGRA Study) . *Jpn. J. Clin. Oncol. 38,* 715-718.

[16] Wierzbicka-Hainaut, E.; Sassolas, B.; Mourey, L.; Guillot, B.; Bedane, C.; Guillet, G. and Tourani, J. M. (2010) . Temozolomide and cisplatin combination in naive patients with metastatic cutaneous melanoma: results of a phase II multicenter trial. *Melanoma. Res. 20,* 141-146.

[17] Lombardi, G.; Zustovich, F.; Della Puppa, A.; Borgato, L.: Orvieto, E.; Manara, R.; Cecchin, D.; Berti, F.; Farina, P.; Gardiman, M. P.; Scienza, R. and Zagonel, V. (2010) . Cisplatin and temozolomide combination in the treatment of leptomeningeal carcinomatosis from ethmoid sinus intestinal-type adenocarcinoma.*J. Neurooncol.* [Epub ahead of print].

[18] Seiter, K.; Katragadda, S.; Ponce, D.; Rasul, M. and, Ahmed, N. (2009) . Temozolomide and cisplatin in relapsed/refractory acute leukemia. *J. Hematol. Oncol. 2,* 21.

In: Glioblastoma ISBN: 978-1-62100-858-3
Editors: M. F. Bezerra et.al, pp. 173-199© 2012 Nova Science Publishers, Inc.

Chapter 9

The Role of Immunohistochemistry in the Diagnosis and Prognosis of Glioblastoma Patients

Aline Paixão Becker[1], Gisele Caravina[1], Carlos Clara[2], and Rui Manuel Reis[3,4]

[1]Department of Pathology; [2]Department of Neurosurgery;
[3]Molecular Oncology Research Center, Barretos Cancer Hospital, Barretos, São Paulo, Brazil
[4]Life and Health Sciences Research Institute (ICVS) , Health Sciences School, University of Minho, Braga, Portugal

Abstract

Glioblastoma, astrocytoma grade IV, is the most frequent and aggressive primary brain tumor. According to the WHO, it presents two major histological variants: giant cell glioblastoma and gliosarcoma, however it can also exhibit different patterns of differentiation such as small cell, oligodendroglial component and lipidized cells. Due to the aggressive behavior, this tumor has been extensively studied, in order to better understand the phenomena underling the morphological features of neoplastic and microvascular proliferation, necrosis, and so on. The immunohistochemistry is an auxiliary diagnostic tool that has been used for a long time in the routine diagnosis and is being increasingly used to determine patient prognosis and therapeutic response. In the present chapter we will address the main immunohistochemical markers used currently in the differential diagnosis of glioblastoma and its variants, like GFAP, vimentin and galectins 1 and 3. Furthermore, we will discuss the growing role of immunohistochemical markers, for instance EGFR, MGMT, PTEN and CD133, in patient survival and treatment resistance.

1. Introduction

Glioblastoma (GBM) is the most frequent and aggressive primary brain tumor [1;2] , classified as grade IV by the World Health Organization (WHO) in its last edition [1]. There are two main described variants of GBM with known different outcome and prognosis: giant cell GBM (GC-GBM) and gliosarcoma (GSM) [1]. Although GBM is a rare tumor, with incidence of about 3.2/100,000 person-years in the United States and Europe [3], it has a very poor prognosis, about 12 months, with five-year survival rate less than 5%, being one of the most lethal human neoplasms [3].

Regarding the histogenesis, clinical course and biological behavior of the tumor, GBMs can be classified as primary (*de novo*) – without precursor lesions, which affects older patients and present fast clinical evolution – or secondary – that evolve from a previous grade II or III astrocytoma, which affects younger individuals and presents a longer clinical history [1;2;4]. Although these two subtypes share common histological aspects, their molecular profiles are different: primary GBMs are characterized by *EGFR* amplification/overexpression, *PTEN* mutation/deletion, *p16* deletions or *MDM2* overexpression; while the main genetic markers for secondary GBM are *TP53* and *IDH1* mutations [4;5]. These distinct genetic pathways could explain the different clinical behavior, survival rates and possible response to the current available treatments [1;2].

In the past decades, great efforts are being made in diagnostic (radiological, histopathological, and more recently molecular methods) , clinical and surgical areas in order to achieve a better response to the current therapeutic options, and as a result, improvements in both progression-free and overall survival have been reported [6], especially after the recent use of temozolomide in addition to the surgery and radiotherapy treatment [7]. In this setting, the histopathological analysis is still a crucial step, being mandatory for definite diagnosis [8] , and the immunohistochemistry (IHC) techniques became an attractive tool to determine diagnostic, prognosis and response to the therapeutic agents, alternative and complementary to the current sophisticated molecular analysis [8].

GBM is a predominantly astrocytic tumor, characterized by nuclear atypia and pleomorphism, mitotic activity, microvascular proliferation and necrosis (Figure 1A,B) [1;2;9]. Although some earlier classifications do not consider necrosis as an essential feature for this diagnosis [2], its importance in the diagnostic and prognosis of GBM is widely accepted [8]. The histological heterogeneity is remarkable, with some tumors showing striking pleomorpism and others being monotonous and densely cellular [2] (Figure 1C) , however, the astrocytic nature of the tumor can be easily identified, at least focally [1]. In rare examples, some heterologous differentiation, for instance, epithelial (glandular and squamous – Figure 1D) or mesenquimal, as noted in GSM, can be seen [1;2]. In addition, GBM can show different patterns of differentiation such as small cells, lipidized cells and even an oligodendroglial component [1].

The detection of oligodendroglial differentiation is important in the outcome of GBM [8].

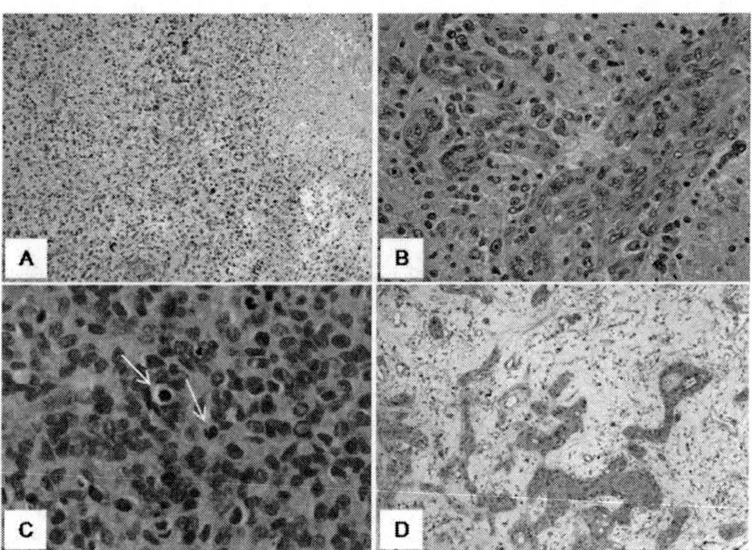

Figure 1. Morphological features of glioblastoma: A) High cellular pleomorphism and areas of necrosis (upper right) -H E 40x.B) Microvascular proliferation-H E 400×.C) Monomorphic cells, with high mitotic activity(arrows) -H E 400×. D) Epithelial component(squamous differentiation) -H E 100×.

At present time, this is the main diagnostic dilemma of GBM, for two reasons: 1) Anaplastic oligodendrogliomas (AO) - grade III (WHO) , may share similar histopathological and radiological features with GBM, which can make distinction difficult, especially in minute specimens or in the absence of classical morphological characteristics [1;2;10], nevertheless, AO may have a better response to chemotherapy and longer survival time [10]; 2) In the last WHO classification, anaplastic oligoastrocytomas (AOA) with necrosis is classified as "GBM with oligodendroglial component - WHO grade IV" (GBM-O) [1], and it is well known that these patients have an intermediate prognosis between patients with AOA grade III and ordinary GBM [1;8].

2. IMMUNOHISTOCHEMISTRY

The use of antigen-antibody mechanism for detecting proteins in a given tissue, was initially used in frozen tissue, as described by Coons [11] in 1940s, and later in 1974, Taylor and colleagues, demonstrated that the detection of at least some antigens from processed tissue was also possible [11]. In surgical pathology, the use of IHC has grown since the 1990s [11], and beyond the use merely in the diagnosis of tumors, IHC is also used to determine stage and grade of tumors, and as an important aid for biological research and drug development [12], where it can help to validate the findings of molecular studies, at protein level (expression, subcellular localization and tissue distribution) .

In surgical pathology, the IHC reactions are usually performed in formalin-fixed, paraffin-embedded (FFPE) tissue. Processing and staining may be performed manually or in automated equipments [12] (Figure 2) . The samples can be disposed in individual slides or in multiple series in a single slide, as in tissue microarrays (TMAs) [12].

Concerning the technique of IHC, there are several steps for making this method feasible for adequate analysis [11]: a) use of adequate fixative substances, in order to preserve the antigenicity of the tissue. Buffered formalin is the most widely and the best fixative reagent used; b) adequate samples, with representative areas in a slide selected by an experienced pathologist; c) correct removal of the paraffin of the paraffin-embedded tissue; d) pre-treatment of the tissue with enzymatic digestion (trypsin) , for "unmasking" antigens altered by formalin [13] or antigen retrieval, by heating the tissue at high temperatures before the IHC reaction, which could preclude the trypsin treatment and enables the use of IHC in long-term formalin-fixed tissues [14]; e) blocking the endogenous targets for IHC, by means of biotin-avidin complex, peroxidase-antiperoxidase or alkaline phosphatase to prevent high background detection; f) use of a buffer solution, (normal serum, non-fat dry milk, BSA or gelatin, and commercial blocking buffers with proprietary formulations) [12] to reduce the background staining; g) couterstaining with hematoxylin; h) analysis at light microscopy.

The antibodies used in IHC can be polyclonal or monoclonal, which increases the specificity of the reactions. However, false negative and false positive results may persist. Causes of false negativity are due to several issues, such as wrong concentrations or a damaged antibody, and alteration of the tissue antigenicity [15]. The main causes of false positivity are the cross-reactivity and nonspecific binding of the antibody to the tissue, and release of soluble proteins from the cytoplasm of normal cells invaded by tumor [15]. It is important to note that a careful light microscopy analysis needs to be made, concerning the subcellular localization of the antigen in an IHC reaction and the type of cell that is immunopositive, which can also lead to misinterpretation of the results.

Currently, IHC is a tool of utmost importance in the routine of the neuropathologist. Although the current WHO classification tries to avoid defining tumor entities solely by IHC [1;6], the use of this technique has made possible, for example, to adequately classify GBM as an astrocytic, instead of a poorly differentiated and embryonal tumor [4], as previously believed. In the following sections, we will describe some of the most frequently used antibodies in neuropathology.

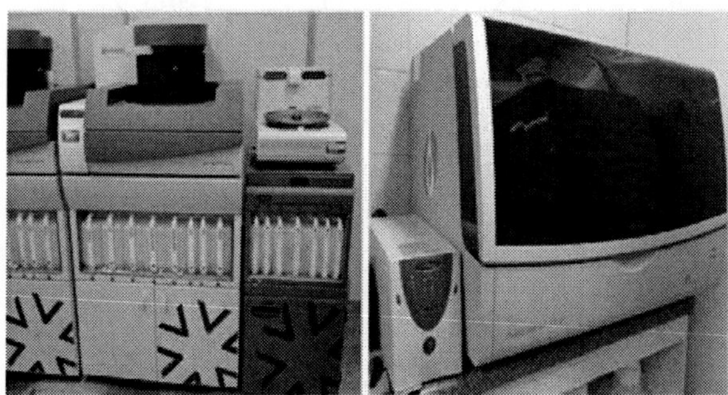

Figure 2. Automated equipment for immunohistochemical reactions. There are several commercial trademarks available.

As the list of available antibodies is growing every day, we choose to describe the ones with the main impact on the diagnosis and prognosis, describing the antibodies according to their most important functions.

3. IMMUNOHISTOCHEMISTRYI IN DIAGNOSIS OF GLIOBLASTOMA

3.1. Glial Fibrillary Acidic Protein (GFAP)

GFAP is a class of intermediate filaments of the cytoskeleton of glial astrocytic cells that is expressed in the cytoplasm of differentiated glial cells, both in normal and neoplastic (Figure 3 A, B) . GFAP was the first intermediate filament to be detected by IHC [16]. In general, gliomas are GFAP-positive, and since the 1970s, Eng and Rubinstein stated the major function for performing GFAP reactions in gliomas and its value on five diagnostic issues [17]: "*1) to determine the astrocytic nature of extremely primitive or highly anaplastic central nervous system (CNS) primary tumors; 2) the study of mixed tumors of the CNS (gangliogliomas and oligoastrocytomas); 3) demonstration of the glial nature of CNS tumors in which fibril formation is either scant or absent, for instance in ependymomas and astroblastomas; 4) the diagnosis of leptomeningeal dissemination or metastasizing gliomas; 5) exclusion of non-glial tumors that may superficially resemble astrocytomas in routine histological exam.*"

It has been shown that the expression of GFAP is mutually exclusive with that of fibronectin, an extracellular matrix (ECM) protein [18], consequently as the tumor becomes more invasive, GFAP expression tend to decrease, but maintains the positivity in its periphery [1]. This could explain the variable stainning in GBMs, with some specimens showing only focal reaction [2] (Figure 3C) . Despite the loss of GFAP expression during malignancy progression, GFAP expression is not associated with GBM prognosis [2]. The mechanism by which GFAP can be downregulated in GBMs is not completly elucidated. *GFAP* gene mutation is not reported to occur, but recent study showed that silencing of *GFAP* gene by methylation of its promoter region as one of the mechanism responsible for loss of GFAP expression in these tumors [19].

In GBM variants, as GSM, GFAP is also heterogeneously positive, mainly in the spindle cells of the glioma component. The sarcomatous cell component is GFAP-negative (Figure 3D) , but positive for reticulin and mesenquimal markers (*e.g.* vimentin and muscle markers) . On the other hand, a GBM composed by spindle-cells displays immunopositivity for GFAP [2].

In the setting of GBM, the use of GFAP has an extreme importance in the differential diagnosis with other primary and metastatic CNS tumors [2;9]. For instance, in less differentiated tumors, like small-cell GBM, immunopositivity for GFAP, in an adequate panel, helps to discriminate it from lymphomas, small-cell carcinomas and primitive neuroectodermal tumors (PNETs) , which are all GFAP-negative. In addition, as rarely GBM may present "epithelial structures" [1;2], with cribriform, trabecular or pseudoacinar patterns [20], the immunopositivity for GFAP helps to discriminate GBM from metastatic carcinomas (Figure 3E) . Considering meningiomas as a differential diagnosis of GBM, the classical pattern of expression is GFAP negative and Epithelial Membrane Antigen (EMA) positive for meningiomas. However, it is worth to note that EMA may be positive in gliomas, especially when the WHO grade becomes higher [21]. An important issue to avoid false-positive results, is that in metastatic carcinoma and some parenchyma-invading meningiomas and sarcomas, GFAP positivity may be focal, at the periphery and in the center of the lesion, that can be interpreted as entrapped reactive astrocytes [17].

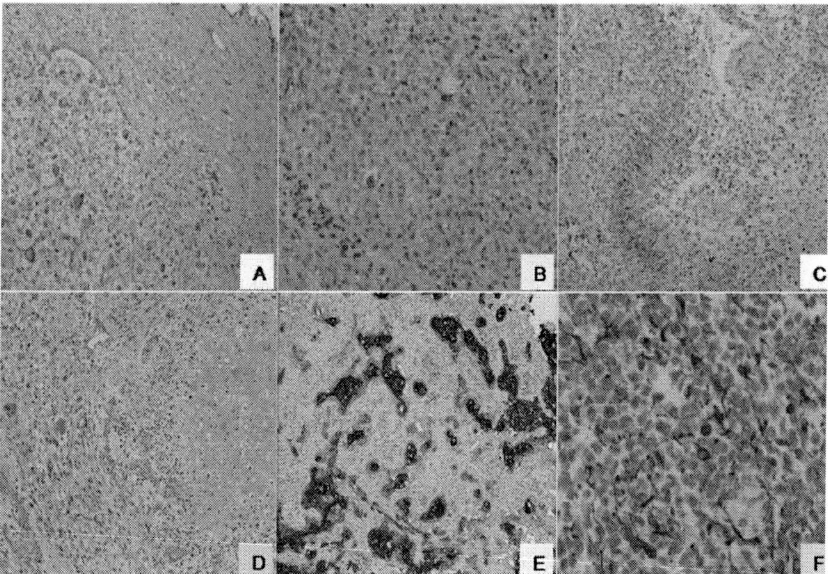

Figure 3. Patterns of immunopositivity for GFAP.A) Diffuse positivity in the tumor (left) and non-neoplastic cortex (right) -40×.B) Endothelia is negative for GFAP-100×. C) Immunoreaction may be focal-in this case, in the neoplastic cells around tumor necrosis (pseudopalisade) -40×. D) In gliosarcoma, the positivity is seen in the glial component-the mesenquimal chondroid area is GFAP negative-40×. E) Epithelial differentiation in a GBM is GFAP positive(same case show in figure 1D) -40×. F) Oligodendroglial areas in a GBM are usually GFAP-negative-400×.

As previously noted, the recognition of oligodendroglial differentiation in a GBM is extremely important. Previously, oligodendrogliomas were referred as negative tumors in GFAP reaction [17] (Figure 3F); however, this concept has changed, with the recognition of the protoplasmatic oligodendrocytes, which can be GFAP positive, in a perinuclear localization [2]. In the study of Ikota *et al*, almost 80% of the oligodendroglial tumors were positive for GFAP [21], either focally or diffusely. As this differential diagnosis is essential, some other antibodies have been tested to adequate define the histogenesis of the high-grade gliomas, such as vimentin, olig-2 and galectin-3, which will be discussed in further sections. Recently, the importance of GFAP has overturned the field of IHC and has also been described as a serum marker for GBM diagnosis in patients with single supratentorial space-occupying lesion [8;16].

In summary, GFAP is the main immunohistochemical marker for GBM diagnosis, but it must be used in a strong correlation with the neurorradiological and histopathological features for adequate diagnosis and correct interpretation of the positive cells.

3.2. Vimentin

Vimentin is also a class III intermediate filament, described in 1978 by Franke *et al.* [22], present in the cytoplasm of glial cells. Contrary to GFAP, vimentin is mainly expressed in the precursor cells of astrocytes, but it is re-expressed by undifferentiated neoplastic astrocytes [23;24]. There are reports of vimentin overexpression both by cDNA (gene level) and IHC (protein level) in the majority of GBMs [25], as well as in all grades of astrocytoma, which could indicate that vimentin is important in early steps of astrocytes transformation [23]. The understanding of the correlation between vimentin and GFAP immunoexpression in astrocytes has brought important contribution to the knowledge of the histogenesis and tumor progression of GBM, in *in vitro* studies [23]. It was demonstrated, for example, that the relationship between the pattern of expression of GFAP, vimentin and cytoplasmatic p53 is similar in undifferentiated glial cells and in primary GBMs [24]. Another diagnostic function of vimentin is the characterization of the spindle cell and mesenquimal component of GSM. Independently of the differentiation (chondral, muscle, etc) , the mesenquimal cells are generally vimentin-positive [1;2].

At last, in routine, vimentin can also help to identify oligodendroglial cells, once there is a different expression of this marker in astrocytic and in oligodendroglial tumors [21;25]. As vimentin is expressed more frequently in astrocytomas, it can help in the diagnosis of GBM-O and anaplastic oligodendroglioma.

3.3. Galectins

Galectins belong to the large family of lectins - carbohydrates-binding proteins - that bind specifically to β-galactosides sugars [26-28]. Currently, there are 15 characterized galectins [28;29]. The structure of the galectins is quite variable. They are proteins with one or two carbohydrate-recognition domain (CRD) in a single polypeptide chain [28]. The mono-CRD galectins can perform functions as monomers (galectins 5, 7 and 10) or homodimers (galectins 1, 2, 11, 13, 14 and 15) [27;28]. Galectin-3 (Gal-3) , has an especial content of proline, glycine and tyrosine, which can be fused onto the CRD, forming oligomers, known as "chimeric galectin" [29].

Galectins are widely distributed both in the extra- and intracellular compartments, and can interact with other proteins in the cell surface, in the ECM, in the cytoplasm and in the nucleus [28], which explains why these lectins are variably involved in various biological processes, such as cellular proliferation, apoptosis, transcriptional regulation, intracellular signalization, adhesion and migration [29]. In neuropathology, galectins 1 and 3 have been the most extensively studied [10;26-37].

3.3.1. Galectin-1

The overexpression of galectin-1 was first detected at mRNA level, with rising levels with increasing astrocytoma grade [28]. Latter, this finding was confirmed with IHC by Rorive *et al.* [33]. This group did not find differences in galectin-1 expression between astrocytic, oligodendroglial and ependimal tumors, yet, they described an important role of galectin-1 in the prognosis: the highest levels of galectin-1 were inversely proportional to patient's survival [33].

Galectin-1 is associated to more invasive tumors, due to its interaction with integrins, which lead to modifications in the actin cytoskeleton, facilitating therefore adhesion to the ECM [33;34]. There are currently various studies on galectin-1, concerning its role in hypoxia, angiogenesis, invasion and drug resistance; however, the majority refers to *in vitro* or experimental studies [33]. The role of galectin-1 in the routine is still limited, but there is a wide field for more research on this subject.

3.3.2. Galectin-3

Various groups have described the expression of galectin-3 (gal-3) in astrocytomas, with conflicting results: Bresalier *et al,* described an increasing expression of gal-3 with the progression of astrocytomas [30]; Gordower *et al,* on the other hand, observed the opposite result two years later [31], however, this group also recognized that some highly malignant tumor cell clones expressed high amounts of galectin [31]. A possible explanation of these conflicting finding is that the gal-3 positivity is found not only in neoplastic cells, but also in microglia, endothelial cells and macrofages and this could make interpretation difficult [27;28].

Bresalier *et al,* also described that other lineages of brain tumors, such as oligodendrogliomas and ependymomas did not express gal-3 [30]. Concerning oligodendroglial tumors, that study was further confirmed: Neder *et al* reported a significant higher cytoplasmatic expression of gal-3 in GBM and pylocitic astrocytomas than in astrocytomas grades II and III and oligodendroglial tumors [10] (Figure 4A, B) . This finding was further confirmed by other authors [35], and states gal-3 immunoexpression as an important feature in the differential diagnosis of pure GBM from GBM-O and anaplastic oligodendroglioma [10;35].

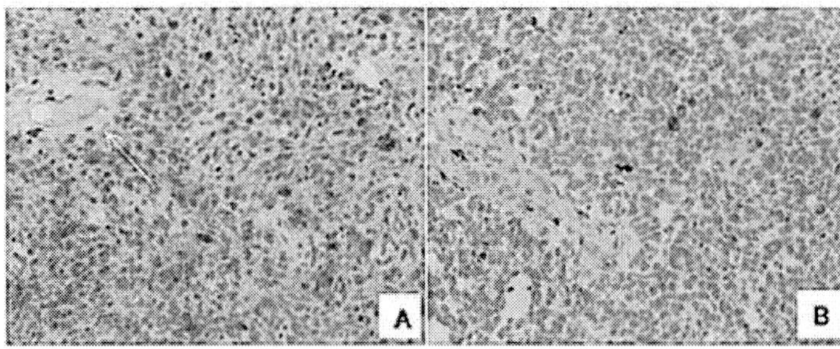

Figure 4. Immunohistochemistry for Galectin-3 in a GBM with oligodendroglial component. A) Astrocytic area, showing diffuse positivity for Gal-3. Note negativity for this marker in the endothelium (arrow) . B) Oligodendroglial component, with negative reaction.

Gal-3 expression was further observed in ependymomas by other authors [35;37]. This is important in the diagnostic practice because some anaplastic ependymomas can simulate the histological appearance of GBM [9], so gal-3 expression would not help in the distinction of these tumors. This can be a dilemma on the subject of pediatric tumors. In these cases, vaguely ependymal tumors are better classified as anaplastyc ependymoma [9].

Another diagnostic issue is pilocytic astrocytoma. The WHO grade I astrocytoma can present some radiological and histopathological characteristics in common with GBM [1;2;9]: contrast-enhancement on neurorradiological exams and nuclear atypia, necrosis and microvascular proliferation at cellular level [1;2;36]. In this same manner, Gal-3 is positive in the neoplastic astrocytes in GBM, especially in the astrocytes that form the pseudopalisade around the necrosis [10], and in virtually all pilocytic astrocytomas [10;35-37]. Moreover, the endothelial cells in both tumors are usually negative [10;35]. Since this pattern is different from grade II and III astrocytomas, which are gal-3 negative in astrocytes and positive in the endothelia, it is hypothesized that reduced gal-3 expression is associated with endothelial cells proliferation [10;35]. It is important to note that the similarities between the angiogenesis in GBM and pylocitic astrocytoma are an unexplored field [35].

Besides this practical importance, many studies in cultured cells have been performed in order to explain the role of gal-3 in various biological processes. The binding of gal-3 to $\alpha 1\beta 1$ integrin, for example, would prevent the interaction of integrins with the ECM proteins, and, therefore, the invasion and migration of neoplastic cells [28]. On the other hand, the interaction between gal-3 and $\alpha 3\beta 1$, NG2 and HIF-1 (hypoxia inducible factor-1) would be responsible by endothelial cells motility and angiogenesis [28].

In summary, the studies have proved that galectin-3 is a useful tool to help in GBM diagnosis. Moreover, the better comprehension about the role of this galectin in the biological processes can be the base for developing new target-therapies.

3.4. Olig-2

The transcription factors olig-1 and olig-2 are involved in the oligodendroglial differentiation and have been investigated as potential markers of oligodendrogliomas [38-40]. In a large study concerning the immunoexpression of olig-2, it has been shown strong positivity in grade II and III oligodendrogliomas [40]. In GBM-Os, there was negative or only weak and focal immunopositivity in less than 10% of the neoplastic cells in the GBM component and strong in the oligodendroglial component [40]. These data could indicate olig-2 as an auxiliary tool in the differential diagnosis of GBM and oligodendroglial tumors or components [1;41;42]. However, careful interpretation of this data must be made, since in TMA studies, olig-2 has been demonstrated in more than 70% of the astrocytic tumors [21].

4. Immunohistochemistry in Prognosis and Predicitive Response to Therapy in Glioblastoma

4.1. Ki67

The protein Ki67 is a non-histone nuclear protein, composed by two polypeptide chains, whose corresponding genes are located in the chromosome 10 [43;44]. It is expressed in the nuclei of cells in all but G0 and early G1 phases of the cellular cycle [45] (Figure 5A) .

Usually, the proliferative activity in GBMs is high and the demonstration of mitotic rate through the expression of the Ki67 protein is highly variable in the tumor, ranging from 15-20% [1], and small cell- and spindle cell GBM frequently exhibit higher proliferative activity [1]. Although some studies have described the correlation between proliferative activity and tumor grade [46;47], this feature does not have a clear prognostic importance in GBMs [1]. Recently, some authors have related the proliferative index with the expression of DNA mismatch repair proteins (MLH1, MSH2 and MSH6) in recurrent lesions [48]

4.2. Epidermal Growth Factor Receptor (EGFR)

The EGFR (HER1 or erbB1) protein plays a central role in gliomagenesis, being the first oncogene amplification described in brain tumors [1;2]. It controls major cellular processes such proliferation, migration, maturation, angiogenesis and differentiation [49]. *EGFR* gene is located on chromosome 7 [2], a chromosome frequently altered in GBM, and *EGFR* gene amplification is observed in approximately 40% of primary GBM cases, and rarely in secondary GBMs. There is a sharp correlation between EGFR overexpression

(Figure 5B) and gene amplification. Besides gene amplification, *EGFR* can be mutated. The most frequent mutation of EGFR is the deletion of exons 2 to 7, resulting in a constitutively activated variant, EGFRvIII [1;8;50], which is present in 20-50% of the cases with EGFR amplification [2;51]. This variant can enhance cell proliferation by activation of the phosphatidylinositol 3-kinase (PI3K) /Akt pathway [4] and via the Ras/mitogen-activated protein Kinase (MAPK) signal transduction pathway [50], and is involved in resistance to both radiotherapy and chemotherapy [50]. EGFR protein overexpression can also occurs independently of gene amplification mechanism, and is detected in more than 1/3 of all GBMs [1].

From the diagnostic point-of-view, it is important to note that although EGFR amplification and overexpression is characteristic of primary GBM, the variant gliosarcoma does not present this genetic pattern [52]. Surprisingly, this was the only noted difference between GBM and GSM at molecular level by Reis *et al* [53]. Since GBM and GSM share some clinical features and sometimes the mesenquimal component is only achieved in subsequent biopsies, IHC can be helpful in distinguishing these entities.

In population-based studies, GBMs in patients younger than 35 years-old did not show *EGFR* amplification [1;54]. Later, it was proved that there is a positive relation between EGFR expression and patient´s age [55]. However, as patient´s age is an independent predictive factor for survival in GBM, it must be carefully interpreted whether the EGFR amplification/overexpression is a worse prognostic factor or not [56;57]. Multivariate analysis did not prove a positive relation between EGFR amplification/overexpression and survival in GBMs [55;58]. Yet, many authors refer that the relation between the alterations of EGFR and p53 is complex and must be related to patient´s age [2;55-57;59;60].

Several studies have also addressed the importance of detecting EGFR overexpression and its mutant EGFRvIII form in the prediction of anti-EGFR therapies, such as Erlotinib, Gefitinib and Cetuximab [50]. Despite the efforts, no clear association was found between the presence of EGFR alterations and the clinical response of GBMs patients to such therapies. An antibody against EGFRvIII was recently described [8]; however, there is cross-reactivity with wild-type EGFR, and besides, it is not commercially available yet [8].

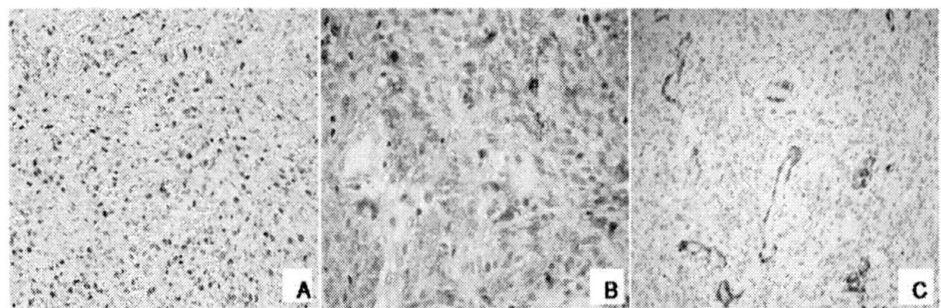

Figure 5. Immunohistochemical markers for glioblastoma. A) Proliferative index by Ki67 expression-nuclear positivity in about 40% of neoplastic cells. B) Diffuse positivity for EGFR, in cytoplasm and membrane localization. C) Negativity for PTEN protein, more frequent in primary GBMs-the endothelial cells remain positive.

4.3. PTEN

The PTEN (phosphatase and tensin homology) gene is a tumor suppressor gene located at the short arm of chromosome 10 [1], which is involved in the growth regulation, apoptosis and, possibly angiogenesis and migration [2]. This gene is mutated in 10-40% of GBMs [2] and when it occurs, the mutated protein inhibits cell proliferation through the inhibition of PIP3 in the PI3K/Akt pathway [2;4].

Mutations of *PTEN* are common events in primary GBM, but rare in the secondary tumors [1;2;4;61]; however, the detection of these mutations are more importantly detected by molecular methods. There are available antibodies for PTEN detection (Figure 5C); however, there are not sufficient studies for establishing it as a useful IHC marker for GBM.

4.4. P53

The *TP53* tumor suppressor gene is located at chromosome 17q and it codifies a 53 KDa protein (p53) , which is involved in the cell cycle control, response do DNA damage, cell death, cell proliferation and neovascularization [4]. The inactivation of the p53 protein predisposes individuals to several types of tumor, since 50% of human tumors are associated with mutations of *TP53* [24].

Mutation of *TP53* is the main genetic mutation in secondary GBM, observed in about 60% of the cases; on the contrary, less than 20% of primary

GBM present this mutation [1;2]. Several type of mutations can occur in *TP53* gene. The wild-type p53 protein has a short half-life (5–30 minutes) because of its rapid turnover; the presence of missense mutations may result in biologically altered proteins with increased stability, which can then be detected by IHC. However, deletion or truncated proteins resulted from nonsense or frameshift mutations are usually negative in the IHC [62]. On the other hand, p53 immunostaining is sometimes present in the absence of gene mutations, due to several mechanisms, including the binding of wild-type p53 by various oncoproteins, such as MDM2 [63]. Therefore, IHC can be less sensitive in detecting tumors harboring *TP53* mutations.

Despite the abovementioned limitations, p53 IHC is used in glioma evaluation. Positive IHC staining can be detected both at nucleus and cytoplasm [2;24]. The cytoplasmatic p53 location may be associated to specific patterns of expression of vimentin and GFAP, which may indicate an arresting in early stages of development [24].

Concerning the prognostic value of the expression of p53 in GBM, it is well accepted that there is a positive relation between the immunoexpression of p53 and survival in multivariate analysis [57;61], in association with other features like EGFR expression and patient′s age, but not as an independent factor. This is also true for pediatric GBM, although Antonelli *et al,* described a tendency for worse prognosis (shorter overall survival and progression-free survival) in patients with p53 overexpression [64].

4.5. Bcl2 And Caspases

Apoptosis is one type of programmed cell death. Although necrosis is the main kind of cell death observed in GBM, apoptosis of neoplastic cells is seen in pseudopalisading, secondary to increased expression or ligation of death receptors of the tumor necrosis factor (TNF) family [1]. The apoptotic rates do not correlate with the prognosis in GBM [1].

Bcl2 belongs to a protein family involved in the intrinsic (mitochondrial) pathway of apoptosis, which include pro-apoptotic proteins as Bax, Bad and Bim, and anti-apoptotic proteins, as Bcl2 and BCLX [65;66]. Bcl2 prevents cells from apoptosis by inhibiting release of citochrome C from the mitochondria [65], and this provides a survival advantage of the neoplastic cells. At IHC, the immunopositivity for Bcl2 is observed in the cytoplasm of tumor cells. It is well known that Bcl2 is highly expressed by more aggressive tumors, especially the hematological ones [49;66]. In brain tumors the expression of Bcl2 is not related to the tumor type or grade and can be detected even in low grade astrocytomas [49], though in low levels [1]. However, immunopositivity for Bcl-2, by conferring resistance to apoptosis, leads to poor response to chemotherapy and radiotherapy [51;67].

The action of Bcl2 is intrinsically related to an enzymatic protein family named caspases, which are the executioners of apoptosis [68]. These proteins can act as initiators or effectors of the intrinsic pathway of apoptosis and are expressed in cells committed to apoptosis [66]. Caspase-3 is the main effector caspase involved in both apoptotic pathways [68]. Some authors refer high expression (50% of neoplastic cells) of caspase-3 and -6 and, to a lesser extent (10%) , caspase-8 and -9 in GBMs, analogous to what happens for instance, in breast and gastric cancer [68], when compared to non-neoplastic samples from these organs. The comprehension of the components of the apoptotic death in GBM is a wide field for more extensive studies, particularly in order to better understand the drug resistance mechanism.

4.6. MGMT

MGMT (O-6-methylguanine-DNA methyltransferase) gene encodes a DNA-repair enzyme that has been shown to contribute to GBM resistance to alkylating chemotherapeutic agents [69]. Specifically, a study from Hegi et al. showed that glioblastoma patients treated whose tumors had a methylated *MGMT* promoter presented a significantly longer median overall survival (21.7 months) and 2-year survival rate (46%) when treated with temozolomide-based chemoradiation, than patients without *MGMT* promoter methylation who were treated similarly (median survival of 12.7 months and 2-year survival rate of 13.8%) [70], indicating MGMT as a promising molecular marker of prognosis in GBMs.

Thus, MGMT IHC is one of the most attractive assay in neuro-oncology. Several studies reported an association between MGMT expression determined by IHC and response to alkylating drugs [71-73]. However, various factors limited the value of IHC for MGMT. Non-neoplastic cells such as microglia, reactive astrocytes, endothelial cells and lymphocytes within the tumor microenvironment also express MGMT, hampering a correct IHC assessment [74]. A high inter-laboratory and inter-observer variability resulted in published threshold levels ranging from <10% up to >50% positive cells, to distinguish positive MGMT-GBM from negative MGMT-GBM [75]. Additionally, many studies failed to observe an association between MGMT expression based on IHC and promoter methylation status [75-77]. Therefore, evaluation of the MGMT status by IHC appears not to be the current most appropriate methodology.

4.7. IDH1

Recent large-scale genomic studies identified *IDH1* as major gene in gliomas, including GBMs [78;79]. *IDH1* is much more frequently mutated in secondary (>80%) than in primary (5-10%) GBM [80-82]. The *IDH1* gene is located on chromosome 2q and codifies the enzyme isocitrate dehydrogenase (IDH1) , localized in the cytoplasm and peroxisomes of tumor cells. The great majority of *IDH1* mutations affect a single codon at the position 132 of the amino acid sequence, being the R132H mutation the most prevalent (93%) [83]. Nevertheless, other substitution mutations can occur in codon 132 in approximately 7% of cases [83, 84].

IDH1 mutations were earlier detected only by molecular genetic analysis. Some groups have developed sensitive and specific antibodies for detection of this mutation suitable for FFPE tissue, which immediately made IDH1 analysis in routine specimens accessible and relatively simple even for modestly-sized pathology laboratories: MIDH1R132H, by Capper *et al* [80], and IMab-1, by Takano *et al* [81]. These antibodies are highly specific for mutated IDH1, and do not detect its wild-type counterpart. A limitation of these antibodies is that they do not recognize other amino acid substitutions in codon 132. The expression of any one of the antibodies is in the cell cytoplasm [80-82;85]. Currently, the expression of IDH1 is useful in the differential diagnosis of gliomas, but also is related to better prognosis, younger age and longer overall survival, not only in GBM, but in astrocytomas grades II and III, oligodendrogliomas of low and high grade and oligoastrocytomas [80;81].

4.8. CD133

CD133- Prominin-1 antigen, has been identified as a potential marker of neural stem cell, and its expression was reported in GBM, with frequencies that varies from 1-30% of cases [86;87]. Several authors showed that CD133 expression is significantly associated with adverse patient outcome [88-90], making CD133 evaluation an important prognostic tool. Currently, several CD133 antibodies are commercially available, however recent studies have reported inconsistent expression pattern among them, hampering clear comparative analysis [91].

4.9. VEGFA

It is recognized that angiogenesis is a key event in the natural progression of gliomas, and contributes to the peritumoral edema and increased the risk of spontaneous hemorrhage [2]. It has been well established that the degree of vascularity correlates with increasing malignancy in astrocytic brain tumors, so that GBMs show the most significant angiogenesis among astrocytic tumors, which is an important independent indicator of poor prognosis [1]. Tumor angiogenesis is orchestrated by a plethora of molecules, including VEGF, acidic and basic fibroblast growth factor (FGF) , IL-8 and -6, hypoxia-inducible factor 1 alpha (HIF-1α) and the angiopoietins, with downregulation of endogenous angiogenesis inhibitors, such as thrombospondins, angiostatin, endostatin and interferons [92].

The six dominant VEGF isoforms (VEGF-A, VEGF-B, VEGF-C, VEGF-D, VEGF-E and placental growth factor) are the main fuel of this process, and together with their receptors have been the major targets in antiangiogenic therapies [93]. VEGF expression in malignant gliomas is most concentrated adjacent to areas of necrosis and hypoxia, including cellular pseudopalisades at the tumor leading edge [94;95]. It is believed that expression of these molecules contribute the GBM prognosis and potentially to its response to anti-angiogenic therapies, however, hitherto there are no studies that evaluated in a comprehensive way all these players, and assessed their combination in GBM management.

5. Conclusions

In the present chapter, we presented several IHC markers for supporting the morphological diagnosis of GBM, and helping to determine prognosis and prediction of therapy response, which obviously do not preclude a careful assessment of routine microscopic features with sufficient clinical and radiological information. IHC has played a major role in differential diagnosis and in improving the diagnostic accuracy in neuropathology. The easy availability of this method associated with its effectiveness makes it crucial in many situations and accessible for the majority of laboratories world-wide.

Acknowledgment

The authors thank the Surgical Pathology Service from the Hospital das Clínicas da Faculdade de Medicina de Ribeirão Preto – Universidade de São Paulo for some of the microphotographs in this chapter.

References

[1] P. Kleihues, P. C. Burger, K. D. Aldape *et al.* Glioblastoma. In: David N.Louis, Hiroko Ohgaki, Otmar D.Wiestler, Webster K.Cavenee, eds. *WHO Classification oftumors of the Central Nervous System.* Lyon: International Agency for Research onCancer (IARC) , 2007:33-49.

[2] D. N. Louis, G. Reifenberger, D. J. Brat, D. W. Ellison. Tumors: introduction and neuroepithelial tumors - Glioblastoma. In: Seth Love, David N. Louis, David W. E. llison, eds. *Greenfield's Neuropathology.* London: Edward Arnold Publishers, 2008:1821-2000.CBTRUS Statistical report: primary brain and central nervous system tumorsdiagnosed in the United States in 2004-2006. CBTRUS Statistical report. 2010. 2-7-2011.Ref Type: Electronic Citation

[3] Ohgaki H., Kleihues P. Genetic pathways to primary and secondary glioblastoma.*Am. J. Pathol.* 2007;170:1445-53.

[4] Fujisawa H., Kurrer M., Reis R. M., Yonekawa Y., Kleihues P., Ohgaki H. Acquisitionof the glioblastoma phenotype during astrocytoma progression is associated with loss ofheterozygosity on 10q25-qter. *Am. J. Pathol.* 1999;155:387-94.

[5] Tran B., Rosenthal M. A. Survival comparison between glioblastoma multiforme and other incurable cancers. *J. Clin. Neurosci.* 2010;17:417-21.

[6] Stupp R., Mason W. P., van den Bent M. J. *et al.* Radiotherapy plus concomitant and adjuvant temozolomide for glioblastoma. *N Engl. J. Med.* 2005;352:987-96.

[7] C. S. jung, A. W. Unterberg, and C. Hartmann. Diagnostic markers for glioblastoma. *Histology and Histopathology.* 2011. Ref Type: In Press

[8] P. C. Burger, B. W. Scheithauer. Tumors of neuroglia and choroid plexus epithelium - Glioblastoma multiforme. In: P. C. Burger, B. W. Scheithauer, eds. *Tumors ofthe central nervous system.* Washington: Armed Forces Institute of Pathology.,1994:25-161.

[9] Neder L, Marie S. K., Carlotti C. G., Jr. *et al.* Galectin-3 as an immunohis.tochemical tool to distinguish pilocytic astrocytomas from diffuse astrocytomas, and glioblastomas from anaplastic oligodendrogliomas. *Brain Pathol.* 2004;14:399-405.

[10] C. R. Taylor, S. R. Shi, N. J. Barr, N. Wu. Techniques of immunohistochemistry: principles, pitfalls and standardization. In: D. J. Dabbs, ed. *Diagnostic Immunohistochemistry.* Philadelphia: Elsevier, 2006:1-42.http://www.piercenet.com/browse.cfm?fldlD=F95B91A9-3DC1-4B56-8E8D-59CA044A8BA7. *Thermo Scientific.* 2011. 2-7-2011.Ref Type: Electronic Citation

[11] Huang S. N., Minassian H., More J. D. Application of immunofluorescent staining on paraffin sections improved by trypsin digestion. *Lab. Invest.* 1976;35:383-90.

[12] Shi S. R., Key M. E., Kalra K. L. Antigen retrieval in formalin-fixed, paraffinembedded tissues: an enhancement method for immunohistochemical staining based on microwave oven heating of tissue sections. *J. Histochem. Cytochem.* 1991;39:741-8.

[13] Jaffer S., Bleiweiss I. J. Beyond hematoxylin and eosin--the role of immunohistochemistry in surgical pathology. *Cancer Invest.* 2004;22:445-65.

[14] C. S.Jung, C.Foerch, A.Schänzer *et al.* Serum GFAP is a diagnostic markerfor glioblastoma multiforme. *Brain* 2007;130:3336-41.

[15] Eng L. F, Rubinstein L. J. Contribution of immunohistochemistry to diagnostic problems of human cerebral tumors. *J. Histochem. Cytochem.* 1978;26:513-22.

[16] Bongcam-Rudloff E., Nister M., Betsholtz C. *et al.* Human glial fibrillary acidic protein: complementary DNA cloning, chromosome localization, and messenger RNA expression in human glioma cell lines of various phenotypes. *Cancer Res.* 1991;51:1553-60.

[17] Restrepo A., Smith C. A., Agnihotri S. *et al.* Epigenetic regulation of glial fibrillary acidic protein by DNA methylation in human malignant gliomas. *Neuro Oncol.* 2011;13:42-50.

[18] Akimoto J., Namatame H., Haraoka J., Kudo M. Epithelioid glioblastoma: a case report. *Brain Tumor Pathol.* 2005;22:21-7.

[19] Ikota H., Kinjo S., Yokoo H., Nakazato Y. Systematic immunohistochemical profiling of 378 brain tumors with 37 antibodies using tissue microarray technology. *Acta Neuropathol.* 2006;111:475-82.

[20] Oshima R. G. Intermediate filaments: a historical perspective. *Exp. Cell Res.* 2007;313:1981-94.

[21] Sultana S., Zhou R., Sadagopan M. S., Skalli O. Effects of growth factors and basement membrane proteins on the phenotype of U-373 MG glioblastoma cells as determined by the expression of intermediate filament proteins. *Am. J. Pathol.*1998;153:1157-68.

[22] Sembritzki O., Hagel C., Lamszus K., Deppert W., Bohn W. Cytoplasmic localization of wild-type p53 in glioblastomas correlates with expression of vimentin and glial fibrillary acidic protein. *Neuro Oncol.* 2002;4:171-8.

[23] Sallinen S. L., Sallinen P. K., Haapasalo H. K. *et al.* Identification of differentially expressed genes in human gliomas by DNA microarray and tissue chip techniques. *Cancer Res.* 2000;60:6617-22.

[24] Zanetta J. P., Badache A., Maschke S., Marschal P., Kuchler S.Carbohydrates and soluble lectins in the regulation of cell adhesion and proliferation.*Histol. Histopathol.* 1994;9:385-412.

[25] Perillo N. L., Marcus M. E., Baum L. G. Galectins: versatile modulators of cell adhesion, cell proliferation, and cell death. *J. Mol. Med. (Berl)* 1998;76:402-12.

[26] Le Mercier M., Fortin S., Mathieu V., Kiss R., Lefranc F. Galectins and gliomas. *Brain Pathol.* 2010;20:17-27.

[27] Stillman B. N., Mischel P. S., Baum L. G. New roles for galectins in brain tumors--from prognostic markers to therapeutic targets. *Brain Pathol.* 2005;15:124-32.

[28] Bresalier R. S., Yan P. S., Byrd J. C., Lotan R., Raz A. Expression of the endogenous galactose-binding protein galectin-3 correlates with the malignant potential of tumors in the central nervous system. *Cancer* 1997;80:776-87.

[29] Gordower L., Decaestecker C., Kacem Y. *et al.* Galectin-3 and galectin-3-binding site expression in human adult astrocytic tumours and related angiogenesis.*Neuropathol. Appl. Neurobiol.* 1999;25:319-30.

[30] Lahm H., Andre S., Hoeflich A. *et al.* Comprehensive galectin fingerprinting in a panel of 61 human tumor cell lines by RT-PCR and its implications for diagnostic and therapeutic procedures. *J. Cancer. Res. Clin. Oncol.* 2001;127:375-86.

[31] Rorive S., Belot N., Decaestecker C. *et al.* Galectin-1 is highly expressed in human gliomas with relevance for modulation of invasion of tumor astrocytes into the brain parenchyma. *Glia* 2001;33:241-55.

[32] Camby I., Belot N., Lefranc F. *et al.* Galectin-1 modulates human glioblastoma cell migration into the brain through modifications to the actin cytoskeleton and levels of expression of small GTPases. *J. Neuropathol. Exp. Neurol.* 2002;61:585-96.

[33] Park S. H., Min H. S., Kim B., Myung J., Paek S. H. Galectin-3: a useful biomarker for differential diagnosis of brain tumors. *Neuropathology* 2008;28:497-506.

[34] Paixao B. A., de Oliveira R. S., Saggioro F. P., Neder L., Chimelli L. M., Machado H. R. In pursuit of prognostic factors in children with pilocytic astrocytomas. *Childs Nerv. Syst.* 2010;26:19-28.

[35] Borges C. B., Bernardes E. S., Latorraca E. F. *et al.* Galectin-3 expression: a useful tool in the differential diagnosis of posterior fossa tumors in children. *Childs Nerv. Syst.* 2011;27:253-7.

[36] Marie Y., Sanson M., Mokhtari K. *et al.* OLIG2 as a specific marker of oligodendroglial tumour cells. *Lancet* 2001;358:298-300.

[37] Aguirre-Cruz L., Mokhtari K., Hoang-Xuan K. *et al.* Analysis of the bHLH transcription factors Olig1 and Olig2 in brain tumors. *J. Neurooncol.* 2004;67:265-71.

[38] Mokhtari K., Paris S., Aguirre-Cruz L. *et al.* Olig2 expression, GFAP, p53 and 1p loss analysis contribute to glioma subclassification. *Neuropathol. Appl. Neurobio.l* 2005;31:62-9.

[39] Kraus J. A., Lamszus K., Glesmann N. *et al.* Molecular genetic alterations in glioblastomas with oligodendroglial component. *Acta Neuropathol.* 2001;101:311-20.

[40] Homma T., Fukushima T., Vaccarella S. *et al.* Correlation among pathology, genotype, and patient outcomes in glioblastoma. *J. Neuropathol. Exp. Neurol.* 2006;65:846-54.

[41] Schonk D. M., Kuijpers H. J., van Drunen E. *et al.* Assignment of the gene(s) involved in the expression of the proliferation-related Ki-67 antigen to human chromosome 10. *Hum. Genet.* 1989;83:297-9.

[42] Gerdes J., Li L., Schlueter C. *et al.* Immunobiochemical and molecular biologic characterization of the cell proliferation-associated nuclear antigen that is defined by monoclonal antibody Ki-67. *Am. J. Pathol.* 1991;138:867-73.

[43] Burger P. C., Shibata T., Kleihues P. The use of the monoclonal antibody Ki-67 in the identification of proliferating cells: application to surgical neuropathology. *Am. J. Surg. Pathol.* 1986;10:611-7.

[44] Torp S. H. Diagnostic and prognostic role of Ki67 immunostaining in human astrocytomas using four different antibodies. *Clin. Neuropathol.* 2002;21:252-7.

[45] Neder L., Colli B. O,. Machado H. R. , Carlotti C. G., Jr., Santos A. C., Chimelli L. MIB-1 labeling index in astrocytic tumors--a clinicopathologic study. *Clin. Neuropathol.*2004;23:262-70.

[46] Stark A. M., Doukas A., Hugo H. H., Mehdorn H. M.. The expression of mismatch repair proteins MLH1, MSH2 and MSH6 correlates with the Ki67 proliferation index and survival in patients with recurrent glioblastoma. *Neurol. Res.* 2010.

[47] Ambroise M. M., Khosla C., Ghosh M., Mallikarjuna V. S., Annapurneswari S.The role of immunohistochemistry in predicting behavior of astrocytic tumors. *Asian Pac. J. Cancer Prev.* 2010;11:1079-84.

[48] Lo H. W.. EGFR-targeted therapy in malignant glioma: novel aspects and mechanisms of drug resistance. *Curr. Mol. Pharmacol.* 2010;3:37-52.

[49] Viana-Pereira M., Lopes J. M., Little S. *et al.* Analysis of EGFR overexpression, EGFR gene amplification and the EGFRvIII mutation in Portuguese high-grade gliomas. *Anticancer Res.* 2008;28:913-20.

[50] Coulibaly B., Nanni I., Quilichini B. *et al.* Epidermal growth factor receptor in glioblastomas: correlation between gene copy number and protein expression. *Hum. Pathol.* 2010;41:815-23.

[51] Reis R. M., Konu-Lebleblicioglu D., Lopes J. M., Kleihues P., Ohgaki H. Genetic profile of gliosarcomas. *Am. J. Pathol.* 2000;156:425-32.

[52] Ohgaki H., Dessen P., Jourde B. *et al.* Genetic pathways to glioblastoma: a population-based study. *Cancer Res.* 2004;64:6892-9.

[53] Srividya M. R., Thota B., Arivazhagan A. *et al.* Age-dependent prognostic effects of EGFR/p53 alterations in glioblastoma: study on a prospective cohort of 140 uniformly treated adult patients. *J. Clin. Pathol.* 2010;63:687-91.

[54] Smith J. S., Tachibana I., Passe S. M. *et al.* PTEN mutation, EGFR amplification, and outcome in patients with anaplastic astrocytoma and glioblastoma multiforme. *J. Natl. Cancer Inst.* 2001;93:1246-56.

[55] Simmons M. L., Lamborn K. R., Takahashi M. *et al.* Analysis of complex relationships between age, p53, epidermal growth factor receptor, and survival in glioblastoma patients. *Cancer Res.* 2001;61:1122-8.

[56] Das P., Puri T., Jha P. *et al.* A clinicopathological and molecular analysis of glioblastoma multiforme with long-term survival. *J. Clin. Neurosci.* 2011;18:66-70.

[57] Batchelor T. T., Betensky R. A., Esposito J. M. *et al.* Age-dependent prognostic effects of genetic alterations in glioblastoma. *Clin. Cancer Res.* 2004;10:228-33.

[58] Korshunov A., Sycheva R., Golanov A. The prognostic relevance of molecular alterations in glioblastomas for patients age < 50 years. *Cancer* 2005;104:825-32.

[59] Umesh S., Tandon A., Santosh V. *et al.* Clinical and immunohistochemical prognostic factors in adult glioblastoma patients. *Clin. Neuropathol.* 2009;28:362-72.

[60] Greenblatt M. S., Bennett W. P., Hollstein M., Harris C. C. Mutations in the p53 tumor suppressor gene: clues to cancer etiology and molecular pathogenesis. *Cancer Res.* 1994;54:4855-78.

[61] Haupt Y., Maya R., Kazaz A., Oren M. Mdm2 promotes the rapid degradation of p53. *Nature* 1997;387:296-9.

[62] Antonelli M., Buttarelli F. R., Arcella A. *et al.* Prognostic significance of histological grading, p53 status, YKL-40 expression, and IDH1 mutations in pediatric high-grade gliomas. *J. Neurooncol.* 2010;99:209-15.

[63] T. P.Stricker, V. Kumar. Neoplasia. *Robbins and Cotran Pathologic Basis of Disease.* Philadelphia: Elsevier, 2010:259-330.

[64] Tirapelli L. F., Bolini P. H., Tirapelli D. P. *et al.* Caspase-3 and Bcl-2 expression in glioblastoma: an immunohistochemical study. *Arq. Neuropsiquiatr.* 2010;68:603-7.

[65] Nagane M., Levitzki A., Gazit A., Cavenee W. K., Huang H. J. Drug resistance of human glioblastoma cells conferred by a tumor-specific mutant epidermal growth factor receptor through modulation of Bcl-XL and caspase-3-like proteases. *Proc. Natl. Acad. Sci. U S A* 1998;95:5724-9.

[66] Bodey B., Bodey V., Siegel S. E. *et al.* Immunocytochemical detection of members of the caspase cascade of apoptosis in high-grade astrocytomas. *In Vivo* 2004;18:593-602.

[67] Esteller M., Garcia-Foncillas J., Andion E. *et al.* Inactivation of the DNArepair gene MGMT and the clinical response of gliomas to alkylating agents. *N Engl. J. Med.* 2000;343:1350-4.

[68] Hegi M. E., Diserens A. C., Gorlia T. *et al.* MGMT gene silencing and benefitfrom temozolomide in glioblastoma. *N Engl. J. Med.* 2005;352:997-1003.

[69] Belanich M., Pastor M., Randall T. *et al.* Retrospective study of the correlation between the DNA repair protein alkyltransferase and survival of brain tumor patients treated with carmustine. *Cancer Res.* 1996;56:783-8.

[70] Jaeckle K. A., Eyre H. J., Townsend J. J. *et al.* Correlation of tumor O6 methylguanine-DNA methyltransferase levels with survival of malignant astrocytoma patients treated with bis-chloroethylnitrosourea: a Southwest Oncology Group study. *J. Clin. Oncol.* 1998;16:3310-5.

[71] Chinot O. L., Barrie M., Fuentes S. *et al.* Correlation between O6-methylguanine-DNA methyltransferase and survival in inoperable newly diagnosed glioblastoma patients treated with neoadjuvant temozolomide. *J. Clin. Oncol.* 2007;25:1470-5.

[72] Felsberg J., Rapp M., Loeser S. *et al.* Prognostic significance of molecular markers and extent of resection in primary glioblastoma patients. *Clin. Cancer. Res.* 2009;15:6683-93.

[73] Preusser M., Charles J. R., Felsberg J. *et al.* Anti-O6-methylguaninemethyltransferase (MGMT) immunohistochemistry in glioblastoma multiforme: observer variability and lack of association with patient survival impede its use as clinical biomarker. *Brain Pathol.* 2008;18:520-32.

[74] Grasbon-Frodl E. M., Kreth F. W., Ruiter M. *et al.* Intratumoral homogeneity of MGMT promoter hypermethylation as demonstrated in serial stereotactic specimens from anaplastic astrocytomas and glioblastomas. *Int. J. Cancer* 2007;121:2458-64.

[75] Lavon I., Fuchs D., Zrihan D. *et al.* Novel mechanism whereby nuclear factor kappaB mediates DNA damage repair through regulation of O(6) -methylguanine-DNA-methyltransferase. *Cancer Res.* 2007;67:8952-9.

[76] Parsons D. W., Jones S., Zhang X. *et al.* An integrated genomic analysis of human glioblastoma multiforme. *Science* 2008;321:1807-12.

[77] Stegh A. H., Brennan C., Mahoney J. A. *et al.* Glioma oncoprotein Bcl2L12 inhibits the p53 tumor suppressor. *Genes Dev.* 2010;24:2194-204.

[78] Capper D., Weissert S., Balss J. *et al.* Characterization of R132H mutationspecific IDH1 antibody binding in brain tumors. *Brain Pathol.* 2010;20:245-54.

[79] Takano S., Tian W., Matsuda M. *et al.* Detection of IDH1 mutation in human gliomas: comparison of immunohistochemistry and sequencing. *Brain Tumor Pathol.* 2011;28:115-23.

[80] Krell D., Assoku M., Galloway M., Mulholland P., Tomlinson I., Bardella C. Screen for IDH1, IDH2, IDH3, D2HGDH and L2HGDH mutations in glioblastoma. *PLoS ONE* 2011;6:e19868.

[81] Hartmann C., Meyer J., Balss J. *et al.* Type and frequency of IDH1 and IDH2 mutations are related to astrocytic and oligodendroglial differentiation and age: a study of 1,010 diffuse gliomas. *Acta Neuropathol.* 2009;118:469-74.

[82] Thol F., Damm F., Ludeking A. *et al.* Incidence and Prognostic Influence of DNMT3A Mutations in Acute Myeloid Leukemia. *J. Clin. Onco.l* 2011;29:2889-96.

[83] Uno M., Oba-Shinjo S. M., Silva R. *et al.* IDH1 mutations in a Brazilian series of Glioblastoma. *Clinics (Sao Paulo)* 2011;66:163-5.

[84] Bao S., Wu Q., McLendon R. E. *et al.* Glioma stem cells promote radioresistance by preferential activation of the DNA damage response. *Nature* 2006;444:756-60.

[85] Beier D., Hau P., Proescholdt M. *et al.* CD133(+) and CD133(-) glioblastoma-derived cancer stem cells show differential growth characteristics and molecular profiles. *Cancer Res.* 2007;67:4010-5.

[86] Zeppernick F., Ahmadi R., Campos B. *et al.* Stem cell marker CD133 affects clinical outcome in glioma patients. *Clin. Cancer Res.* 2008;14:123-9.

[87] Yan X., Ma L., Yi D. *et al.* A CD133-related gene expression signature identifies an aggressive glioblastoma subtype with excessive mutations. *Proc. Natl. Acad. Sci. U S A* 2011;108:1591-6.

[88] Pallini R., Ricci-Vitiani L., Montano N. *et al.* Expression of the stem cell marker CD133 in recurrent glioblastoma and its value for prognosis. *Cancer* 2011;117:162-74.

[89] Hermansen S. K., Christensen K. G., Jensen S. S., Kristensen B. W.. Inconsistent immunohistochemical expression patterns of four different CD133 antibody clones in glioblastoma. *J. Histochem. Cytochem.* 2011;59:391-407.

[90] Hanahan D., Folkman J. Patterns and emerging mechanisms of the angiogenic switch during tumorigenesis. *Cell* 1996;86:353-64.

[91] Reardon D. A., Wen P. Y., Desjardins A., Batchelor T. T., Vredenburgh J. J. Glioblastoma multiforme: an emerging paradigm of anti-VEGF therapy. *Expert Opin. Biol. Ther.* 2008;8:541-53.

[92] Plate K. H., Breier G., Weich H. A., Mennel H. D., Risau W. Vascular endothelial growth factor and glioma angiogenesis: coordinate induction of VEGF receptors, distribution of VEGF protein and possible in vivo regulatory mechanisms. *Int. J. Cancer* 1994;59:520-9.

[93] Fischer I., Gagner J. P., Law M., Newcomb E. W., Zagzag D. Angiogenesis in gliomas: biology and molecular pathophysiology. *Brain Pathol.* 2005;15:297-310.

In: Glioblastoma ISBN: 978-1-62100-858-3
Editors: M. F. Bezerra et.al, pp. 201-226© 2012 Nova Science Publishers, Inc.

Chapter 10

Anticoagulants as a Therapeutic Alternative for Glioblastoma Treatment

T. C. Carneiro-Lobo[1], S. Konig[2], R. Q. Monteiro[1]
[1]Institute of Medical Biochemistry at the Federal University of Rio de Janeiro, Brazil
[2]Departament of Anatomy at the Federal University of Rio de Janeiro, Brazil

Abstract

An association between cancer and thrombosis has long been described. Abnormal elevated expression of tissue factor (TF) , the physiological initiator of blood coagulation, has been well documented in several tumor types, including glioblastoma (GBM) , and seems to be directly correlated with thromboembolic complications in cancer patients. In the last few years, it has become clear that the processes responsible for the progression of cancer are highly dependent on components of the blood coagulation cascade and TF has been pointed as a key determinant of the coagulation/cancer interaction. Actually, TF expression, that has been shown to correlate with the histological grade of malignancy of glioma, is involved in modulation of several intracellular pathways relevant for malignant angiogenesis and tumor growth. GBM is one of the most vascularized malignant tumors and intense angiogenesis is a distinguishing pathological hallmark relative to lower-grade glioma.

Moreover, there is a high incidence of thrombotic events throughout the course of malignant glioma. In fact, the prothrombotic properties of GBM cells seem to contribute to the appearance of hypoxic regions within the tumor and, ultimately, to the formation of the GBM-typical necrotic foci that are well-recognized predictors of poor prognosis. Most remarkable, TF is overexpressed in cells around these necrotic foci found in GBM, known as pseudopalisading cells. These regions are highly hypoxic and seem to play a key role in GBM aggressiveness, presenting an increased production of vascular endothelial growth factor (VEGF) , interleukin-8 (IL-8) and metalloproteases. In addition to prothrombotic role, TF enables the activation of the G protein-coupled protease-activated receptors (PARs) . These receptors might be activated through proteolytic cleavage by blood coagulation enzymes thus eliciting the production of several pro-tumoral factors including cytokines, angiogenic factors and metalloproteases among others. Given the importance of coagulation activation in human gliomas, it has been proposed that TF, as well as other clotting proteins, could serve as a therapeutic target. It has already been shown that argatroban, a specific thrombin inhibitor, reduced tumor mass and tumor induced behavioral deficits and prolongs survival time in animal models. We showed that Ixolaris, a potent anticoagulant that does not produce major bleeding when injected subcutaneously in different animal models, potently decreases tumor growth in a human GBM model. Notably, inhibition of tumor growth was accompanied by downregulation of VEGF and vessel density in tumor mass. Our results provide strong evidence that TF may be regarded as an important therapeutic target for GBM.

INTRODUCTION

The evidence of a clinical association between thrombosis and cancer was first described for almost two centuries by two French physicians, Jean-Baptiste Bouillard and Armand Trousseau. Both noted that patients who present with idiopathic venous thromboembolism (VTE) frequently harbor an occult malignancy, while VTE appeared to be a common clinical complication in patients with known cancer [Bouillard and Bouillaud, 1823; Trousseau, 1865]. After the publication of his seminal book in 1865, this two-way clinical association between VTE and cancer turned to be referred as Trousseau's syndrome. Over the years, deep vein thrombosis, pulmonary embolism, migratory thrombophlebitis and disseminated intravascular coagulopathy have been described to be the most common associated thrombotic complications [Sack, 1977; Noble and Pasi, 2010]. The multiplicity of pathophysiologic mechanisms that apparently contribute to the excessive blood coagulation associated with cancer led the definition of this syndrome to be refined and extended to unexplained thrombotic events that precede the diagnosis of an occult visceral malignancy or appear concomitantly with the tumor [Varki, 2007]. Only more recently, large, population-based, case-control studies attempted to quantify the propensity of this association and clearly indicate that patients with cancer have a significant increased risk for VTE, particularly during the few months after diagnosis and in the presence of distant metastasis [Levitan, 1999; Prandoni, 2002; Blom, 2005; Blom, 2006; Wun and White, 2009]. This thromboembolic risk was estimated to be 7-fold elevated across all patients with cancer, with the most impressive increase in risk seen in patients with haematological malignancies (up to 28-fold) [Blom, 2005]. Malignancies associated with the highest incidence of VTE include kidney, stomach, pancreas, ovary and brain [Levitan, 1999]. Cancer therapy, whether it be chemotherapy, anti-angiogenic or hormonal therapy, and surgical procedures have themselves been shown to increase the risk for VTE [Blom, 2004; Blom, 2006; Barlogie, 2001; Zangari, 2001; Saphner, 1991; White, 2005]. Recognized as the principal clinical complication in cancer, VTE is the second leading cause of death of these patients [Hoffman, 2001; Furie and Furie, 2006]. Beyond mortality, complications among patients with cancer who survive an episode of VTE can severely compromise their quality of life. Anticoagulation therapy of patients with cancer was therefore originally developed to prevent potentially lethal evolution of thrombosis.

Malignant Glioma and Thrombosis

An especially high risk for VTE has been found in patients with primary cerebral malignancy, in particular in those with high-grade glioma. Unlikely to others malignancies, this risk has been evaluated to extend beyond the post-operative period, remaining constant until death [Marras, 2000; Walsh and Kakkar, 2001; Wen, 2006; Simanek, 2007; Semrad, 2007; Jenkins, 2010]. Most commonly accepted to be in the range of 20-30% over the course of the disease, the estimated incidence of post-operative deep venous thrombosis has been reported to be as high as 72%. A retrospective review of 96 patients also showed the predominance of women in the group of patients who developed thrombotic events, therefore suggesting that hormonal factors may predispose this risk in the setting of glioblastoma (GBM) [Prayson, 2009]. VTE thromboprophylaxis is utilized with caution in glioma patients because of the concern for intracranial hemorrhage [Perry, 2010]. Age greater than 75 has been confirmed as a specific risk factor for VTE in GBM patients, beyond the more generic risk factors such as prolonged immobility or indwelling central venous catheter devices [Semrad, 2007]. Therapy-specific risks factors have also been suggested. Preliminary studies based on the analysis of small cohorts of patients already suggested that treatment with thalidomide or administration of chemotherapy seem to increase the risk for VTE in glioma patients [Dhami, 1993; Simanek, 2007]. Although known to predispose patients for VTE in other cancers, the risks associated with radiotherapy and corticosteroids treatment (used to manage the vasogenic edema) , two essential approaches in glioma therapy, have not yet been clearly defined for these patients. Attention has also been paid to the effects of Bevacizumab, an anti-vascular endothelial growth factor (VEGF) monoclonal antibody, which recently received U.S. Food and Drug Administration approval in recurrent GBM. While this anti-angiogenic agent has been reported to be associated with intratumoral bleeding in extra-central nervous system (CNS) cancer types [Gordon, 2005; Elice, 2008] and to increase the risk for VTE in non-primary CNS malignancies [Nalluri, 2008], recent studies suggested that this risk may also be extended to GBM patients [Friedman, 2009; Norden, 2011].

If the risk for VTE in malignant glioma was clearly identified, data that could support that in GBM, like in other cancers, the development of VTE is predictive of poor survival remain controversial. While the analysis of a neurosurgical cohort reported that patients with VTE had a 30% higher risk of death within two years compared to those without VTE [Semrad, 2007], other studies failed to observe an association between thrombosis and significant reduced survival [Shet, 2003; Simanek, 2007; Prayson, 2009]. This may be due, in part, to the high aggressiveness of GBM and overall poor survival of the patients. Beyond the extraordinarily high risk of VTE, it is also well-documented that intravascular thrombosis can often be identified during the resection of GBMs and that the presence of these thrombi is highly suggestive to the surgeon of GBM as opposed to other primary tumors of the brain [Raza, 2002]. While the incidence of microscopic thrombi within the tumor has been evaluated in the range of 68,8-94% in GBM patients, no correlation of microscopic tumor thrombi with the development of VTE or a worse outcome was evidenced in these patients [Brat, 2004b; Tehrani, 2008; Prayson, 2009]. However, the association between these thrombotic events and the prognosis of patients diagnosed with primary anaplastic astrocytoma led investigators to suggest that the presence of microthrombi may serve as a marker for a more aggressive behaviour [Tehrani, 2008].

Thrombosis: More than a Side-Effect in Cancer Progression

VTE has long been thought largely to be an epiphenomenon in cancer that complicate the course of patients and anticoagulation therapy therefore originally adopted to prevent potentially lethal evolution of thrombosis. However, large clinical studies also demonstrated that, in many types of malignancies, idiopathic VTE is conversely associated with a significantly increased risk of malignancy, suggesting that, more than an side-effect, blood coagulation disorders might themselves play a determinant role in oncogenesis [Prandoni, 1992; Sorensen, 2000; Rickles, 2001]. The idea that tumors could take some advantage of hemostasis activation emerged with Theodor Billroth, a contemporary of Trousseau, who already interpreted the pathological finding of tumor cells embedded in a thrombus as evidence for the role of venous thrombosis in the metastatic process [Billroth, 1878].

More recently, studies evidenced elevated amount of fibrin, indicative of thrombin generation, is a common clotting abnormality in patients with cancer [Walz, 1994]. Experimental evidence demonstrated that fibrin can be easily detected within the first 15 min after tumor cell injection into the venous circulation [Hilgard, 1983]. Local fibrin scaffold was reported to form a provisional matrix for the tumor and to induce the incoming of new vessels [Dvorak, 1987]. Frequently observed at the sites of tumor cell arrest in the microvasculature, fibrin clots were proposed to facilitate and strengthen tumor cell lodgement to the microvasculature, thus contributing to metastatic processes [Rickles, 1983; Dvorak, 1983, 1987]. These observations have led to try the use of anticoagulants in the control of metastasis. Among the anticoagulants used, warfarin and heparin were demonstrated to indeed interfere with metastasis process in different models [Dvorak, 1987; Al-Mondhiry, 1984; Zacharski, 1979; Hilgard, 1983; Neubauer, 1986; McCulloch and George, 1987, 1989; Smith, 1986; Millar, 1974; Beuth, 1987]. In order to clarify the underlying mechanisms of this interference, a study focusing on the specific and exclusive inhibition of thrombin by recombinant desulfatohirudin, also reported a successful and significant reduction in experimental metastasis in a murine melanoma model [Esumi, 1991]. Beyond procoagulant activities, cancer cells are also known to promote coagulation through suppression of fibrinolytic activities. By preventing the generation of plasmin, that degraded fibrin, the Plasminogen activator inhibitor type-1 (PAI-1) promotes persistence of blood clots (Sidenius, 2003) . Association of high levels of PAI-1 with poor prognosis has been extensively documented in some cancers, including GBM [Kinder, 1993; Foekens, 1994]. The suppression of PAI-1 expression in host mice has been showed to prevent local invasion and tumor vascularization of transplanted malignant keratinocytes [Bajou, 1998]. Upregulation of PAI-1 was also associated with metastasis in hypoxic tumor environments [Denko and Giaccia, 2001].

In 2005, 3 studies linked more closely malignant transformation to thrombus formation by demonstrating that activation of clotting can be a direct result of the molecular transforming events [Boccacio, 2005; Yu, 2005; Rong, 2005]. Boccacio and colleagues obtained a genetically modified mouse in which the activated *MET* oncogene was specifically targeted to rare hepatic cells within an otherwise normal tissue [Boccacio, 2005]. These animals develop slowly, progressive hepatocarcinogenesis and a hemostatic disturbance that is reminiscent of Trousseau's syndrome. This syndrome was characterized by elevated blood levels of fibrin d-dimer, a prolonged prothrombin time and a marked reduction of the platelet count, with venous thrombosis occurring early and being followed by a progressive coagulopathy and fatal internal hemorrhage. Genome-wide expression profiling of hepatocytes expressing the *MET* oncogene demonstrated that, among the 70 hemostasis-associated genes represented in the microarray, PAI-1 and cyclooxygenase-2 (COX-2) genes were strongly induced, linking directly activation of hemostasis with tumor progression [Boccacio, 2005]. The other studies published in the same year presented evidences that oncogenic events can regulate the expression of the protein Tissue Factor (TF) , a major initiator of blood coagulation [Yu, 2005; Rong, 2005]. Moreover, TF expression was observed to be evident within cancer cells and at cell surface, but also as a soluble extracellular form that was as well capable of promoting plasma coagulation. Extracellular TF has indeed been previously documented as possible full-length protein, an alternatively spliced variant and a microvesicles-associated form (MVs) [Bogdanov, 2003; Aras, 2004]. Procoagulant TF-containing membrane microvesicles have been proposed to be the cause of thrombotic events at a distance [Tesselaar, 2007b], thus providing a possible mechanism for the yet observed association between TF upregulation and the development of cancer coagulopathy [Kakkar, 1995,]. MVs release from cancer cells including GBM cells show potent procoagulant activity in vitro and in vivo [Yu and Rak, 2004; Davila et al, 2008; Lima, 2011]. Several studies have demonstrated that TF-associated MVs may detected in plasma from a variety of cancer patients and could correlate with the risk of thrombosis in these patients (Tesselaar, 2007a and b; Jenkins, 2009; Zwicker, 2009) . Clinical studies with GBM patients have shown an elevated procoagulant activity associated with circulating MVs which may contribute to prothrombotic state and leads to VTE complications [Sartori, 2011]. In addition, several lines of evidence demonstrated MVs from cancer cells have an important role in intercellular communication in the tumor microenvironment. A communication could influence the behavior of microenvironment during angiogenesis, invasion and metastasis [Skog, 2008; Al-Nedawi, 2009; Cocucci, 2009; Mathivanan, 2010]. Belting and colleagues proposed that TF-associated MVs provided by GBM cells modulated a procoagulant signaling in endothelial cells, resulting in increased angiogenesis and accelerated tumor growth [Svensson, 2011]. These studies provide evidence that the detection of TF expression in MVs may be an important approach to identify cancer patients at increased risk for prothombotic effects in cancer.

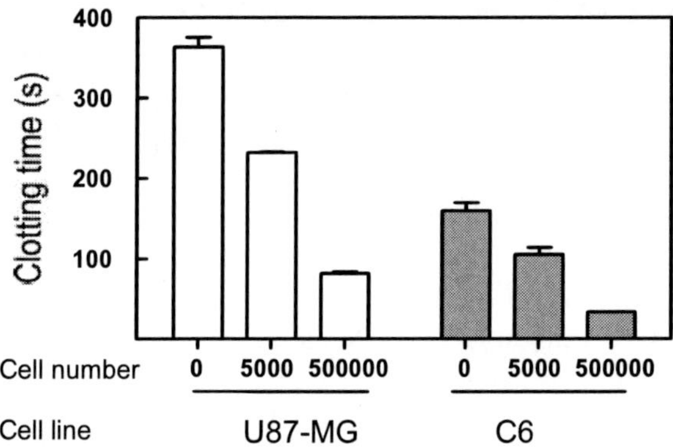

Figure 1. Procoagulant activity of tumor cells. As a result of simultaneous TF expression and phosphatidylserine exposure, GBM cell lines accelerate plasma coagulation. Figure shows the procoagulant response of human U87-MG and rat C6 cell lines upon addition to citrated human and rat plasma, respectively, and further recalcification with $CaCl_2$.

PROCOAGULANT PROPERTIES OF GBM CELLS

Several lines of evidence suggest that coagulation proteins play significant roles in cancer biology. TF, the primary initiator of the coagulation cascade, under physiological conditions is usually a transmembrane receptor that, upon disruption of vascular integrity, functions as a cofactor for circulating blood factor VIIa (FVIIa) , which in turn causes thrombin activation, platelet aggregation, fibrin deposition, and local hemostasis [Kalafatis, 1994; Monroe,

2002]. Furth ermore, TF has long been shown to be constitutively expressed in tumor cells, tumor-associated stroma and cancer-associated inflammatory cells [Contrino, 1996; Amirkhosravi, 1998; Rickles, 2001; Tesselaar, 2007a; Rak, 2009] and display important roles in tumor initiation, tumor growth and angiogenesis in glioma [Milsom, 2008].

In fact, high levels of TF in GBM cells correlate with potent procoagulant activity *in vitro* (figure 1) [Fernandes, 2006; Carneiro-Lobo, 2009]. Moreover, a strong correlation between TF expression and grade of malignancy has also been reported, in particular in human glioma (Hamada, 1996; Guan, 2002; Carneiro-Lobo, unpublished observations) .

The transition from anaplastic astrocytoma to GBM is characterized by necrotic foci surrounded by typical hypercellular configurations, referred as "pseudopalisading necrosis", and increased angiogenesis [Baker, 1996; Rong, 2006]. Cancer cells that form these pseudopalisades have been demonstrated to be under hypoxic conditions and to be associated to increased production of VEGF, IL-8 and metalloproteases, and are therefore proposed to play a key role in GBM aggressiveness [Zagzag, 2000; Semenza, 2001; Brat, 2003; Brat, 2004; Rong, 2005]. It is noteworthy that these pseudopalisading cells were also shown to express high levels of TF (Rong, 2005) . The increase of cell density associated with the high proliferative rate of GBM might explain the arising of intratumoral hypoxic areas in high-grade gliomas.

However, recent investigations alternatively proposed that hypoxia might result from preliminary vascular injury (Brat, 2004a and b) . In this model, proliferating tumors cells first gain access to oxygen and nutrients by "co-opting" of host's blood vessels [Holash, 1999; Zagzag, 2000].

In response, vascular endothelial cells upregulate Angiopoietin-2 (Ang-2) , a factor known to be expressed by high-grade gliomas but not low-grade gliomas or normal brain [Stratmann, 1998; Zagzag, 1999]. Possibly acting on tumoral blood vessels as a Tie-2 receptor antagonist, Ang-2 causes vascular destabilization, as illustrated by structural changes of endothelial cells, such as hypertrophy, discohesion and eventually apoptosis [Holash, 1999; Zagzag, 2000; Semenza, 2003]. These structural changes have been demonstrated to be required for the induction of angiogenesis that will in turn support the accelerated growth of tumor mass. The elevated incidence of intratumoral microscopic thrombi in GBM, occurring in particular within a subset of pseudopalisading cells surrounding necrosis, has led Brat's group to suggest that these typical hypercellular configurations arose from the hypoxic migration of tumor cells from central vaso-occlusion and toward a viable vasculature [Brat, 2004a]. The authors thus proposed that, more than an uninteresting side-effect, vaso-occlusion secondary to thrombosis within GBM could cause or at least accentuate the development of hypoxia, a critical driving force in GBM biology [Zagzag, 2000; Semenza, 2003].

TISSUE FACTOR EXPRESSION IS MODULATED BY ONCOGENIC EVENTS

Diverse oncogenic signaling pathways have been linked with constitutive TF expression in several cancer types including GBM [Rak and Klement, 2000; Yu, 2005].

Yu and colleagues showed that activation of K-Ras and loss of *p53* were both necessary to achieve full expression of TF in a colorectal cancer model [Yu, 2005].

In human GBM cell lines, loss of the *PTEN* tumor suppressor gene, together with hypoxia, leads to AKT activation and upregulation of the Ras/MEK/ERK signaling cascade. This signaling coincides with up-regulation of TF gene expression [Rong, 2005]. In addition, the mechanisms evidenced by Rong and colleagues in glioma model to underlie the increased expression of TF by cancer cells, and its ability to promote plasma coagulation appeared of particular interest since *PTEN* loss and hypoxia are both events occurring at the transition from anaplastic astrocytoma to GBM. Further, analysis demonstrated that the highest TF expression was present within cells that from the hypoxic pseudopalisades surrounding necrosis [Rong, 2005]. Indeed, the tumor suppressor *PTEN* is inactivated by mutations, promoter methylation or other mechanisms in almost 80% of human GBM and TF is expressed in >90% of such tumors [Haas-Kogan, 1998; Luo, 2003; Di Cristofano, 2000; Furnari, 2007]. Conversely, evidence of *PTEN* inactivation is rarely found in astrocytomas, that expressed only low levels of TF [Hamada, 1996; Guan, 2002]. *PTEN* inactivation also leads to the upregulation of the Ras/MEK/ERK signaling pathway, reported in most GBMs [Yart, 2002; Furnari, 2007].

Epidermal growth factor receptor (EGFR) has an important role in normal development and oncogenesis [Citri and Yarden, 2006]. EGFR amplification or mutation (EGFRvIII) is a genetic event associated with GBM [Huang, 2007] and has been involved with tumor growth, invasion, and angiogenesis [Pore, 2006]. In 2009, Rong and colleagues show that EGFR induced TF expression by up-regulation JunD/activator protein-1 (AP-1) transcriptional activity on the TF promoter and was regulated by c-Junc NH_2-terminal Kinase

(JNK) . In addition, reconstitution of *PTEN* in *PTEN*-deficient GBM cells attenuated EGFR-induced TF expression by antagonizing phosphatidylinositol 3-kinase (PI3K) , which leads to reduction both Akt and JNK activities. Importantly, these studies suggest that oncogenic mechanisms may up-regulate TF expression in GBM cells independently of hypoxia. Together, these data suggest that mutation may be the first event leading to thrombosis and that the ensuing hypoxia and necrosis may amplify this process [Rong, 2009].

Recently, Magnus, (2010) described that expression of oncogene EGFR mutants in a panel of GBM cell lines not only induce TF, but also the related elements of the TF/PAR pathway, including PAR-1, PAR-2 and ectopic expression of its protease ligand FVIIa. Thus, EGFR mutants may promote procoagulant activity and TF/PAR signaling in GBM cells with up-regulation of angiogenic factors (VEGF and IL-8) .

In conclusion, oncogenic transformation and hypoxia are sufficient to sensitize cancer cells to procoagulant activity and signaling through simultaneous up-regulation of TF and PARs.

PAR Signaling in Tumor Progression

Pro-tumoral effects of TF and blood clotting enzymes (FVIIa, FXa and thrombin) are intimately related to a small family of G protein-coupled receptors named Protease Activated Receptor (PARs 1-4) . These receptors are a group of seven-transmembrane domain receptor with a unique way of activation [Vu, 1991; Couhglin, 2005]. Different to the common ligant binding system for receptor activation, TF and blood clotting enzymes lead to a proteolytic cleaving of the N-terminal extracellular receptor sequence of the PAR. By this it creates a new specific amino terminus. Remaining tethered to the receptor, it binds to the second extracellular loop of the transmembrane receptor to initiate signaling. Each of these PARs has a unique N-terminal tethered ligand sequence [Coughlin, 2000; Elste and Petersen, 2010]. In addition, short synthetic peptides based on the "tethered ligand" sequence of the PARs can selectively activate PAR 1, 2 and 4 and initiate to a specific cellular signaling [Hansen , 2008].

PAR-1, PAR-3 and PAR-4 can be activated most strongly by thrombin and FVIIa and FXa can activate both PAR-1 and PAR-2. PARs expression is not limited to abnormal cells and, in fact, participate in numerous physiological and pathophysiological process including endothelial activation, embryonic development, platelet aggregation, inflammation, cancer progression and other processes. They are expressed at low levels in normal epithelial, but in contrast they are overexpression in a variety of carcinomas, including GBM [Okamoto, 2001; Jiang, 2004; Shi, 2004; Magnus, 2010]. In addition, the expression of PAR-1 in human tumor samples has been associated with malignancy grade as well as expression of PAR-2 in human tumor samples showed no difference between malignancy grade [Carneiro-Lobo, unpublished observations].

Activation of PAR-1 and PAR-2 have been studied in many cell types *in vitro* and have been shown to promote migration, invasion, proliferation, metastasis, prevent apoptosis, and induce a broad repertoire of pro-angiogenics factors such as VEGF, interleukin-8 (IL-8) , and CXCL-1, and immune regulators such as granulocyte-macrophage colony stimulating factor (M-CSF or CSF1) . Although, TF/FVIIa/PAR-2 appears to be a more potent stimulus for the up-regulation of the immune and angiogenesis regulators in breast cancer cells [Hjortoe, 2004; Veersteg, 2004; Morris, 2006; Albrektsen, 2007].

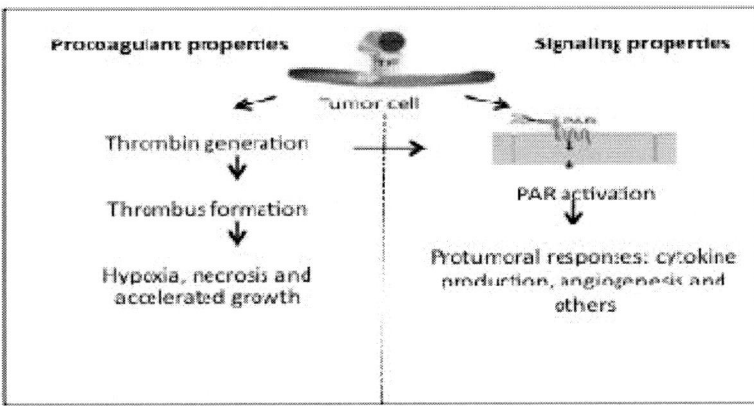

Figure 2. Proposed role for TF in GBM progression. Association of tumor-derived TF with FVIIa leads to coagulation activation and further thrombin generation. Local thrombin generation leads to fibrin deposition and subsequent thrombus formation in tumor vessels. It is proposed that intratumoral thrombosis may generate hypoxic conditions leading to necrosis and accelerated growth. Alternatively, thrombin and TF/FVIIa complex may activate PAR1 and PAR2, respectively, leading to signaling events that evoke protumoral responses such as cytokine production, angiogenesis, increased proliferation and others.

It has been shown that A172 and U87-MG human GBM cell lines constitutively express PAR-1 and PAR-2. Activation of these receptors with specific agonist peptides demonstrated that PAR-2 but not PAR-1 activation induces VEGF expression in both cell lines [Mariano-Oliveira, unpublished observation].

These data indicate that PAR-2 activation in tumor cells could enhance tumor growth *in vivo* and contribute to up-regulation of VEGF expression. In fact, it has been recently demonstrated that PAR-2 contributes to the angiogenic switch during mammary tumor development [Versteeg, 2008a]. Furthermore, the identification of a monoclonal antibody called 10H10, which selectively blocks TF/FVIIa/PAR-2 signaling without affecting its pro-coagulant activity, inhibit tumor growth and angiogenesis in MDA-MB-231 model, consistent with the crucial role of pro-angiogenic TF/FVIIa/PAR-2 signaling established by in vitro studies [Versteeg, 2008b]. Moreover Gessler et al. (2010) have shown that inhibition of TF signaling by monoclonal antibody 10H10 reduces migration and invasion in high-grade glioma cell lines, under both normoxic or hypoxic conditions. These data indicated an important role for the TF-PAR-2 signaling in cancer progression.

Recently, has been shown that deregulated tumor cell PAR-2 signaling is associated with increased phosphorylation of the TF cytoplasmic domain. Based on the analysis of human breast cancer samples, invasive breast cancer showed marked increased of TF, PAR-2 and TF phosphorylation, in contrast to non-invasive ductal cancinoma. Upregulation of the TF-PAR-2 signaling pathway was correlated with increased expression of VEGF, confirming the link to tumor angiogenesis. Thus, TF phosphorylation in breast cancer may be a useful biomarker to identify patients that can benefit from therapeutic interventions in TF signaling pathways, but additional studies are required to establish whether this prognostic marker is present in GBM [Rydén, 2010].

In 1998, results obtained by Bar-Shavit's group demonstrated the involvement of thrombin receptor, also known as protease-activated receptor 1 (PAR-1) , in tumor cell invasion [Even-Ram, 1998]. Further, PAR-1 has been found to be involved in the progression of several cancer types. PAR-1 is activated by thrombin, which is recognized as a potent mitogenic in cancer and tumor metastasis through sustained ERK1/2 activation [Bahou, 2003]. This receptor may also signal in response to proteases from tumor and the tumor microenvironments such as MMP-1 [Boire, 2005]. Several studies have shown that thrombin plays an important role in the growth of gliomas. In 2002, Yamahata demonstrated that thrombin receptor expression was detectable in a number of human glioma cell lines. In addition, thrombin or PAR-1 agonist peptide induced the VEGF mRNA expression and secretion of VEGF protein. Recently, Magnus et al. (2010) , shown that glioma cell lines stimulated with FVIIa, PAR-1 or PAR-2 activating peptides lead to increased levels of proangiogenic factors such as IL-8 and VEGF in culture supernatants. These data indicate that TF, PAR-1 and PAR-2 display a role in the glioma progression.

ANTICOAGULANT AS ANTITUMOR DRUGS

Several studies suggest that thrombin plays an important role in GBM growth [Hua, 2005; Rong, 2005;]. In this case, Argatroban could be a useful for the treatment of high-grade gliomas. Argatroban is a small molecule and synthetic direct thrombin inhibitor that binds to the enzyme's catalytic site. Previous studies have found that anti-thrombin treatment with Argatroban reduced cell proliferation, tumor mass, edema formation, neurological deficits and prolongs survival time in glioma models [Hua, 2005]. In fact, these studies provide evidence that thrombin could be a therapeutic target for malignant gliomas.

As discussed previously, there is a direct correlation between TF levels and tumor grade for multiple tumor types [Kakkar, 1995; Nakasaki, 2002; Rak, 2009], including gliomas [Hamada et al., 1996; Guan et al., 2002]. Potent TF inhibitors have been isolated from nematode (NAPc2) [Stassens, 1996] and tick (Ixolaris) [Francischetti, 2002].

Nematode anticoagulant proteins (NAPc2) from the hematophagous nematode *Ancylostoma caninum*, like Ixolaris is a potent inhibitor of TF/FVIIa complex upon binding to FX/FXa. In this study, NAPc2 inhibited the metastasis of CT26 colon carcinoma to mouse lung. In addition, NAPc2 showed therapeutic effects on colon cancer xenograft tumor growth when combined with other therapeutic agents. This study suggests that the antitumor effect of TF inhibitors rely on TF expression by tumor cells [Zhao, 2009]. Moreover, it seems that inhibition of primary tumor growth and angiogenesis are strongly dependent on blockade of FVIIa/TF proteolytic activity on the tumor cell rather than inhibition of FVIIa/TF procoagulant reactions. In this context, NAPc2 but not NAP5 (potent inhibitor of FXa) decreased primary tumor growth *in vivo*, in the B16 melanoma model [Hembrough, 2003]. Consistent with these data, NAPc2 can be thus effective in both the early and late stages of tumor progression.

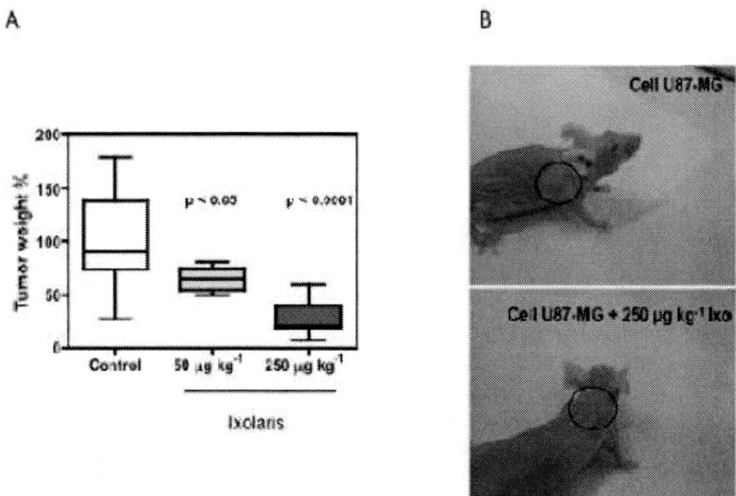

Figure 3. Ixolaris, a potent TF/FVIIa inhibitor, blocks in vivo growth of human GBM (U87-MG) cells in a xenograft model. (A) Animals were treated with PBS (white bar) or 50 µg kg-1 (light gray bar) or 250 µg kg-1 (gray bar) Ixolaris. (B) Pictures show a representative control (upper panel) and treated (250 µg kg-1 Ixolaris, lower panel) animal. Full description in Carneiro-lobo et al, 2009.

Ixolaris is a tick salivary 140 amino acid protein containing 10 cysteines and 2 Kunitz-like domains, binds to FXa or FX as a scaffold for inhibition of the TF/FVIIa complex, in which the FVIIa catalytic site is inactivated, as previously demonstrated by inhibition of synthetic or macromolecular FX substrate, forming an inhibited quaternary complex similar to TF pathway inhibitor (TFPI) [Francischetti, 2002]. Recently, we demonstrate that inhibition of the TF-FVIIa complex by Ixolaris blocks *in vivo* growth of humam GBM (U87-MG) cells in a xenograft model (figure 3) without increasing bleeding [Carneiro-Lobo, 2009]. This phenomenon is accompanied by a significant decreased in VEGF expression and angiogenesis in tumor mass. The antitumor effect of Ixolaris has been also observed in a murine melanoma model, in which Ixolaris blocks both primary tumor growth and induced metastasis [Monteiro, unpublished observation]. Given the known antithrombotic properties of Ixolaris [Nazareth, 2006], it is possible that suppression of angiogenesis derives at least in part, from reduction of intratumoral thrombosis, which could in turn decrease the hypoxic regions within tumor mass and hypoxia-driven VEGF production. In conclusion, we have proposed that Ixolaris blocks primary tumor growth through inactivation of FVIIa/TF complex on the tumor cell surface, with subsequent interruption of PAR-2 signaling. On the other hand, inactivation of FVIIa/TF complex n the tumor cell surface also blocks downstream coagulation reaction, thus reducting the procoagulant ability of the tumor cell and decreasing its metastatic potential. Thus, Ixolaris may attenuate the procoagulant state of cancer patients on one hand and prevent angiogenesis on the other, thus interfering with two important components that contribute to tumor growth and metastasis in vivo.

CONCLUSION

Despite the development of novel therapeutics for the treatment of GBM, no significant improvement of the prognosis of patients diagnosed with this highly aggressive subtype of glioma was observed in the past decades. Anticoagulants have been originally used to improve patients' quality of life and prevent potentially lethal evolution of associated thrombosis. Recent evidences demonstrate that cancer cell-derived TF play a central role in glioma progression and aggressiveness, contribute to both clotting-dependent and clotting-independent PAR-driven events. These observations pointed out the use of inhibitors of the coagulation pathway as an attractive resource for GBM coadjuvant treatment, beyond the attenuation of the procoagulant state of patients. Therefore the better understanding of the contribution of TF as well as protease receptors to GBM biology are of particular therapeutic interest requiring further investigations.

REFERENCES

Albrektesen T.; Sorensen B. B.; Hjortoe G. M.; Fleckner J.; Rao L. V. M.; Petersen L. C. Transcriptional program induced by factor VIIa-tissue-factor, PAR-1 and PAR-2 in MDA-MB-231 cells. *J. Theomb. Haemost.*, 2007 5, 1588-97.

Al-Mondhiry H. Tumor interaction with hemostasis: the rationale for the use of platelet inhibitors and anticoagulants in the treatment of cancer. *Am. J. Hematol.*, 1984 16 2, 193-202.

Al-Nedawi K.; Meehan B.; Kerbel R. S.; Allison A. C.; Rak J. Endothelial expression of autocrine VEGF upon the uptake of tumor-derived microvesicles containing onco- genic EGFR. *Proc. Natl. Acad. Sci.* USA, 2009 106, 3794–3799.

Amirkhosravi A.; Meyer T.; Warnes G.; Amaya M.; Malik Z.; Biggerstaff J. P.; Siddiqui F. A.; Sherman P.; Francis J. L. Pentoxifylline inhibits hypoxia-induced upregulation of tumor cell tissue factor and vascular endothelial growth factor. *Thromb. Haemost.*, 1998 80 4, 598-602.

Aras O.; Shet A.; Bach R. R.; Hysjulien J. L.; Slungaard A.; Hebbel R. P.; Escolar G.; Jilma B.; Key N. S. Induction of microparticle- and cell-associated intravascular tissue factor in human endotoxemia. *Blood*, 2004 103 12, 4545-53.

Bahou W. F. Protease-activated receptors. Curr Top Dev Biol, 2003 54, 343-69.

Bajou K.; Noël A.; Gerard R. D.; Masson V.; Brunner N.; Holst-Hansen C.; Skobe M.; Fusenig N. E.; Carmeliet P.; Collen D.; Foidart J. M. Absence of host plasminogen activator inhibitor 1 prevents cancer invasion and vascularization. *Nat. Med.*, 1998 4 8, 923-8.

Barker F. G. II; Davis R. L.; Chang S. M.; Prados M. D. Necrosis as a prognosis factor in glioblastoma multiforme. *Cancer*, 1996 77, 1161-1166.

Barlogie B.; Desikan R.; Eddlemon P.; Spencer T.; Zeldis J.; Munshi N.; Badros A.; Zangari M.; Anaissie E.; Epstein J.; Shaughnessy J.; Ayers D.; Spoon D.; Tricot G. Extended survival in advanced and refractory multiple myeloma after single-agent thalidomide: identification of prognostic factors in a phase 2 study of 169 patients. *Blood*, 2001 98 2, 492-4.

Beuth J.; Ko H. L.; Uhlenbruck G.; Pulverer G. Combined immunostimulation (Propionibacterium avidum KP 40) and anticoagulation (heparin) prevents metastatic lung and liver colonization in mice. *J. Cancer Res. Clin. Oncol.*, 1987 113 4, 359-62.

Billroth T. *Lectures on surgical pathology and therapeutics: a handbook for students and practictioners*. 8th ed. London: The New Sydenham Society 1878.

Blom J. W.; Doggen C. J.; Osanto S.; Rosendaal F. R. Malignancies, prothrombotic mutantions, and the risk of venous thrombosis. *JAMA*, 2005 293 6, 715-22.

Blom J. W.; Doggen C. J.; Osanto S.; Rosendaal F. R. Old and new risk factors for upper extremity deep venous thrombosis. *J. Thromb. Haemost.*, 2003 11, 2471-8.

Blom J. W.; Osanto S.; Rosendaal F. R. High risk of venous thrombosis in patients with pancreatic cancer: a cohort study of 202 patients. *Eur. J. Cancer*, 2006 42 3, 410-4.

Boccaccio C.; Medico E. Cancer and blood coagulation. *Cell Mol. Life Sci.*, 2005 63 9, 1024-7.

Bogdanov V. Y.; Balasubramanian V.; Hathcock J.; Vele O.; Lieb M.; Nemerson Y. Alternatively spliced human tissue factor: a circulating, soluble, thrombogenic protein. *Nat. Med.,* 2003 4, 458-62.

Boire A.; Covic L.; Agarwal A.; Jacques S.; Sherifi S.; Kuliopulos A. PAR-1 is a matrix metalloprotease-1 receptor that promotes invasion and tumorigenesis of breast cancer cells. *Cell*, 2005 120, 303-313.

Bouillard J. B.; Bouillaud S. De l'Obliteration des veines et de son influence sur La formation dês hydropisies partielles: consideration sur La hydropisies passive et general. *Arch. Gen. Med.*, 1823 1, 188-204.

Brat D. J.; Mapstone T. B. Malignant glioma physiology: Cellular response to hypoxia and its role in tumor progression. *Ann. Intern. Med.*, 2003 138, 659-658.

Brat D. J.; Castellano-Sanchez A. A.; Hunter S. B.; Pecot M.; Cohen C.; Hammond E. H.; Devi S. N.; Kaur B.; Van Meir E. G. Pseudopalisades in glioblastoma are hypoxic, express extracellular matrix proteases, and are formed by an actively migrating cell population. *Cancer Res.*, 2004a 64 3, 920-7.

Brat D. J.; Van Meir E. G. Vaso-occlusive and prothrombotic mechanisms associated with tumor hypoxia, necrosis, and accelerated growth in glioblastoma. *Lab. Invest.*, 2004b 84 4, 397-405.

Carneiro-Lobo T. C.; Konig S.; Machado D. E.; Nasciutti L. E.; Forni M. F.; Francischetti I. M.; Sogayar M. C.; Monteiro R. Q. Ixolaris, a tissue factor inhibitor, blocks primary tumor growth and angiogenesis in a glioblastoma model. *J. Thromb. Haemost.*, 2009 7, 1-10.

Citri A.; Yarden Y. EGF-ERBB signaling: towards the systems levels. *Nat. Rev. Mol. Cell Biol.,* 2006 7, 505-16.

Cocucci E.; Racchetti G.; Meldolesi J. Shedding microvesicles: Artefacts no more. *Trends Cell Biol.*, 2009 19, 43–51. Cotrino J.; Hair G.; Kreutzer D. L.; Rickles F. R. In situ detection of tissue factor in vascular endothelial cells: correlation with the malignant phenotype of human breast disease. *Nat. Med.*, 1996 2, 209-15.

Coughlin S. R. Protease-activated receptors and platelet function. *Thromb. Haemost.*, 1999 82 2, 353-356.

Coughlin SR. Protease-activated receptors in hemostasis, thrombosis and vascular biology.
J Thromb Haemost. 2005 Aug;3(8):1800-14.

Davila M.; Amirkhosravi A.; Coll E.; Desai H.; Robles L.; Colon J.; Baker C. H.; Francis J. L. Tissue factor-bearing microparticles derived from tumor cells: impact on coagulation activation. *J. Thromb. Haemost.*, 2008 6, 1517–1524.

Denko N. C.; Giaccia A. J. Tumor hypoxia, the physiological link between Trousseau's syndrome (carcinoma-induced coagulopathy) and metastasis. *Cancer Res.* 2001 61 3, 795-8.

Dhami M. S.; Bona R. D.; Calogero J. A.; Hellman R. M. Venous thromboembolism and high grade gliomas. *Thromb. Haemost.*, 1993 170 3, 393-6.

Di Cristofano A.; Pandolfi PP. The multiple roles of PTEN in tumor suppression. *Cell*, 2000 100 4, 387-90.

Dvorak H. F. Thrombosis and cancer. *Hum. Pathol.*, 1987 18 3, 275-84.

Dvorak H. F.; Senger D. R.; Dvorak A. M. Fibrin as a component of the tumor stroma: origins and biological significance. *Cancer Metastasis Rev.*, 1983 1, 41-73.

Elice F.; Rodeghiero F.; Falanga A.; Rickles F. R. Thrombosis associated with angiogenesis inhibitors. *Best Pract. Res. Clin. Haematol.*, 2009 22 1, 115-28.

Elste A. P.; Petersen I. Expression of proteinase-activated receptor 1-4 (PAR 1-4) in human cancer. *J. Mol. Histol.*, 2010 41, 89-99.

Esumi N.; Fan D.; Fidler I. J. Inhibition of murine melanoma experimental metastasis by recombinant desulfatohirudin, a highly specific thrombin inhibitor. *Cancer Res.*, 1991 51 17, 4549-56.

Even-Ram S.; Uziely B.; Cohen P.; Grisaru-Granovsky S.; Maoz M.; Ginzburg Y.; Reich R.; Vlodavsky I.; Bar-Shavit R. Thrombin receptor overexpression in malignant and physiological invasion processes. *Nat. Med.*, 1998 4, 909-914.

Fernandes R. S.; Kirszberg C.; Rumjanek V.M.; Monteiro R. Q. On the molecular mechanisms for the highly procoagulant pattern of C6 gli- oma cells. *J. Thromb. Haemost.*, 2006 4, 1546–1552.

Foekens J. A.; Schmitt M.; Van Putten W. L.; Peters H. A.; Kramer M. D.; Jänicke F., Klijn J. G. Plasminogen activator inhibitor-1 and prognosis in primary breast cancer. *J. Clin. O*ncol., 1994 12 8, 1648-58.

Francischetti I. M.; Valenzuela J. G.; Andersen J. F.; Mather T. N.; Ribeiro J. M. Ixolaris, a novel recombinant tissue factor pathway inhibitor (TFPI) from the salivary gland of the tick, Ixodes scapularis: identification of factor X and factor Xa as scaffolds for the inhibition of factor VIIa/tissue factor complex. *Blood*, 2002 99, 3602-12.

Friedman H. S.; Prados M. D.; Wen P. Y.; Mikkelsen T.; Schiff D.; Abrey L. E.; Yung W. K.; Paleologos N.; Nicholas M. K.; Jensen R.; Vredenburgh J.; Huang J.; Zheng M.; Cloughesy T. Bevacizumab alone and in combination with irinotecan in recurrent glioblastoma. *J. Clin. Oncol.*, 2009 27 28, 4733-40.

Furie B., Furie B. C. Cancer-associated thrombosis. *Blood Cells, Molecules, and Diseases,* 2006 36, 177-181.

Furnari F. B.; Fenton T.; Bachoo R. M.; Mukasa A.; Stommel J. M.; Stegh A.; Hahn W. C.; Ligon K. L.; Louis D. N.; Brennan C.; Chin L.; DePinho R. A.; Cavenee W. K. Malignant astrocytic glioma: genetics, biology, and paths to treatment. *Genes Dev.*, 2007 21 21, 2683-710.

Gessler F.; Voss V.; Dutzmann S.; Seifert V.; Gerlach R.; kogel D. Inhibition of tissue factor/protease-activated receptor-2 signaling limits proliferation, migration and invasion of malignant glioma cells. *Neuroscience*, 2010 165 4, 1312-1322.

Gordon M. S.; Cunnuingham D. Managing patients treated with bevacizumab combination therapy. *Oncology*, 2005 69 3, 25-33.

Guan M.; Jinb J.; Sua B.; Liua W. W.; Lua Y. Tissue factor expression and angiogenesis in human glioma. *Clinical Biochemistry*, 2002 35, 321-325.

Haas-Kogan D.; Shalev N.; Wong M.; Mills G.; Yount G.; Stokoe D. Protein kinase B (PKB/Akt) activity is elevated in glioblastoma cells due to mutation of the tumor suppressor PTEN/MMAC. *Curr. Biol.*, 1998 8 21, 1195-8.

Hamada K.; Kuratsu J.; Saitoh Y.; Takeshima H.; Nishi T.; Ushiy. Expression of tissue factor correlates with grade of malignancy in human glioma. *Cancer*, 1996 77, 1877-83.

Hembrough T. A.; Swartz G. M.; Papathanassiu A.; Vlasuk G. P.; Rote W. E.; Green S. J.; Pribluda V. S. Tissue factor/factor VIIa inhibitor block angiogenesis and tumor growth through a nonhemostatic mechanism. *Cancer Res.*, 2003 63, 2997-3000.

Hilgard P. Anticoagulants and tumor growth: pharmacological considerations. Symp Fundam *Cancer Res.*, 1983 36,353-60.

Holash J.; Maisonpierre P. C.; Compton D.; Boland P.; Alexander C. R.; Zagzag D.; Yancopoulos G. D.; Wiegand S. J. Vessel cooption, regression, and growth in tumor mediated by angiopointins and VEGF. *Science*, 1999 284 5422, 994-998.

Hua Y.; Tang L.; Keep R. F.; Schallert T.; Fewel M. E.; Muraszko K. M.; Hoff J. T.; Xi G. The role of thrombin in glioma. *J. Thromb. Haemost.*, 2005 3, 1917-23.

Hoffman R.; Haim N.; Brenner B. Cancer and thrombosis revisited. *Blood,* 2001 15, 61-67.

Huang P. H.; Mukasa A.; Bonavia R.; Flynn R. A.; Brewer Z. E.; Cavenee W. K.; Furnari F. B.; White F. M. Quantitative analysis of EGFRvIII celular signaling networks reveals a combinatorial therapeutic strategy for glioblastoma. *Proc. Natl. Acad. Sci. USA*, 2007 104, 12867-72.

Jenkins E. O.; Schiff D.; Mackman N.;Key N. S. Venous thromboembolism in malignant glioma. *J. Thromb. Haemost.* 2009; 8(2): 221-7.

Jiang X.; Bailly M. A.; Panetti T. S.; Cappllom; Konigsberg W. H.; Bromberg M. E. Formation of tissue factor-factor VIIa-factor Xa complex promotes cellular signaling and migration of human breast cancer cells. *J. Thromb. Haemost.*, 2009 2, 93–101.

Kakkar A. K.; Lemoine N. R.; Scully M. F.; Tebbutt S.; Williamson R. C. Tisue factor expression correlates with histological grade in human pancreatic cancer. *Br. J. Surg.*, 1995 82, 1101-4.

Kalafatis M.; Swords N. A.; Rand M. D.; Mann K. G. Membrane-dependent reaction in blood coagulation: role of the vitamin K-dependent enzyme complexes. *Biochemical ET Biophysica Acta*, 1994 1227, 113-129.

Levitan N.; Dowlati A.; Remick S. C.; Tahsildar H. I.; Sivinski L. D.; Beyth R.; Rimm A. A. Rates of initial and recurrent thromboembolic disease among patients with malignancy versus those without malignancy. Risk analysis using Medicare claims data. *Medicine* (Baltimore) , 1999 78 5, 285-291.

Lima G. L.; Oliveira S. A.; Campos C. L.; Bonamino M.; Chammas R.; Werneck C. C.; Vicente P. C.; Barcinski A. M.; Petersen C. L.; Monteiro Q. R. Malignant transformation in melanocytes is associated with increased production of procoagulant microvesicles. *Thrombosis and Haemostasis*, 2011 106 4, 1-12.

Luo J.; Manning B. D.; Cantley L. C. Targeting the PI3K-Akt pathway in human cancer: rationale and promise. *Cancer Cell*, 2003 4 4,257-62.

Magnus N.; Garnier D.; Rak J. Oncogenic epidermal growth factor receptor up-regulated multiple elements of the tissue factor signaling pathway in human glioma cells. *Blood*, 2010 116 5, 815-8.

Marras L. C.; Geerts W. H.; Perry J. R. The risk of venous thromboembolism in increased throughout the course of malignant glioma: an evidence-based review. *Cancer*, 2000 89 3, 640-6.

Mathivanan S.; Ji H.; Simpson R. J. Exosomes: Extracellular organelles important in intercellular communication. *J. Proteomics*, 2010 73, 1907–1920.

McCulloch P.; George W. D. Warfarin inhibition of metastasis: the role of anticoagulation. *Br. J.Surg.*, 1987 74 10, 879-83.

McCulloch P.; George W. D. Warfarin inhibition of metastasis: the role of anticoagulation. *Br. J. Surg.*, 1987 74 10, 879-83.

Millar R. C.; Ketcham A. S. The effect of heparin and warfarin on primary and metastatic tumors. *J. Med.* (Westbury) . 1974 5 1, 23-31.

Milson C. C.; Yu J. L.; Mackman N.; Micallef J.; Anderson G. M.; Guha A.; Rak J. W. Tissue factor regulation bu epidermal growth factor receptor and epithelial-to-mesenchymal transitions: effect on tumor initiation and angiogenesis. *Cancer Res.*, 2008 68, 100068-76.

Monroe D. M.; Hoffman M.; Roberts H. R. Platelets and thrombin generation. *Arterioscler Thromb. Vasc. Biol.*, 2002 22 9, 1381-1389.

Morris D. R.; Ding Y.; Ricks T. K.; Gullapalli A.; Wolfe B. L.; Trejo J. Protease-activated receptor-2 is essential for factor VIIa and Xa-induced signaling, migration, and invasion of breast cancer cells. *Cancer Res.*, 2006 66, 307-14.

Nakasaki T.; Wada H.; Shigemori C.; Miki C.; Gabazza E. C.; Nobori T.; Nakamura S.; Shiku H. Expression of tissue factor and vascular endothelial growth factor is associated with angiogenesis in colorectal cancer. *Am. J. Hematol.*, 2002 69, 247–254.

Nalluri S. R.; Chu D.; Keresztes R.; Zhu X.; Wu S. Risk of venous thromboembolism with the angiogenesis inhibitor bevacizumab in cancer patients: a meta-analysis. *JAMA*, 2008 300 19, 2277-2285.

Nazareth R. A.; Tomaz L. S.; Ortiz-Costa S.; Atella G. C.; Ribeiro J. M.; Franciscetti I. M.; Monteiro R. Q. Antithrombotic properties of Ixolaris, a potent inhibitor of the extrinsic pathway of the coagulation cascade. *Thromb. Haemost.*, 2006 96, 7-13.

Neubauer B. L.; Bemis K. G.; Best K. L.; Goode R. L.; Hoover D. M.; Smith G. F.; Tanzer L. R.; Merriman R. L. Inhibitory effect of warfarin on the metastasis of the PAIII prostatic adenocarcinoma in the rat. *J. Urol.*, 1986 135, 1, 163-6.

Noble S.; Pasi J. Epidemiology and pathophysiology of cancer-associated thrombosis. *Br. J. Cancer*, 2010 102 Suppl 1, S2-9.

Norden A. D.; Bartolomeo J.; Tanaka S.; Drappatz J.; Ciampa A. S.; Doherty L. M.; Lafrankie D. C.; Rulant S.; Quant E. C.; Beroukhim R.; Wen P. Y. Safety of concurrent bevacizumab therapy and anticoagulation in glioma patients. *J. Neurooncol.* 2011 in press.

Okamoto T.; Nishibori M.; Sawada K.; Iwagaki H.; Nakaya N.; Jikuhara A.; tanaka N.; Saeki K. The effects of stimulating protease-activated receptor-1 and 2 in A172 human glioblastoma. *J. Neural. Transm.*, 2001 108 2, 125-40.

Prandoni P.; Lensing A. W.; Buller H. R.; Cogo A.; Prins M. H.; Cattelan A. M.; Cuppini S.; Noventa F.; Ten Cate J. M. Deep-vein thrombosis and the incidence of subsequent symptomatic cancer. *N Engl. J. Med.*, 1992 327 16, 1128-33.

Prandoni P.; Lensing A. W.; Prism M. H.; Bernardi E.; Marchiori A.; Bagatella P.; Frulla M.; Mosena L.; Tormene D.; Picciolli A.; Simioni P.; Giroiami A. Residual venous thrombosis as a predictive factor of recurrent venous thromboembolism. *Ann. Itern. Med.*, 2002 137 12, 955-960.

Prayson N. F.; Angelov L.; Prayson R. A. Microscopic thrombi in glioblastoma multiforme do not predict the development of deep venous thrombosis. *Ann. Diagn. Pathol.*, 2009 13 5, 291-6.

Rak J.; Klement G. Impact of oncogenes and tumor suppressor genes on deregulation of hemostasis and angiogenesis in cancer. *Cancer Metastasis Rev.*, 2000 19 1-2, 93-6.

Rak J.; Milsom C.; Magnus N.; yu J. Tissue factor in tumour progression. *Best Pract. Res. Clin. Haematol.,* 2009 22, 71-83.

Raza S. M.; Lang F. F.; Aggarwal B. B.; Fuller G. N.; Wildrick D. M.; Sawaya R. Necrosis and glioblastoma: a friend or a foe? A review and a hypothesis. *Neurosurgery*, 2002 51, 2-12.

Rickles F. R.; Edwards R. L.; Barb C.; Cronlund M. Abnormalities of blood coagulation in patients with cancer. Fibrinopeptide A generation and tumor growth. *Cancer*, 1983 51 2, 301-7.

Rickles F. R.; Falanga A. Molecular basis for the relationship between thrombosis and cancer. *Thromb. Res.*, 2001 102 6, 215-224.

Rong Y.; Belozerov E. V.; Tucker-Burden C.; Chen G.; Durden L. D.; Olson J. J.; Van meir G. E.; Mackman N.; Brat J. D. Epidermal growth factor receptor and PTEN modulate tissue factor expression in glioblastoma through JunD/activator protein-1 transcriptional activity. *Cancer Res.*, 2009 69, 2540-2549.

Rong Y.; Durden L. D.; Van Meir G. E.; Brat J. D. Pseudopalisading Necrosis in Glioblastoma: A familiar Morpho;ogic feature that links vascular pathology, hypoxia, and angiogenesis. *J. Neuropathol. Exp. Neurol.*, 2006 65, 529-539.

Rong Y.; Post D. E.; Pieper R. O.; Durden D. L.; Van Meir E. G.; Brat D. J. PTEN and hypoxia regulates tissue factor expression and plasma coagulation by glioblastoma. *Cancer Res.*, 2005 65; 1406-13.

Ruf W, Disse J, Carneiro-Lobo TC, Yokota N, Schaffner F. Tissue factor and cell signalling in cancer progression and thrombosis. J Thromb Haemost. 2011 Jul;9 Suppl 1:306-15.

Rydén L.; Grabau D.; Schaffner F.; Jonsson P. E.; Ruf W.; Belting M. Evidence for tissue factor phosphorylation and its correlation with protease-activated receptor expression and the prognosis of primary breast cancer. *Int. J. Cancer*, 2010 126, 2330-2340.

Sack G. H.; Levin J.; Bell W. R. Trousseau's syndrome and other manifestation of chronic disseminated coagulopathy in patients with neoplasms: clinical, pathophysiologic, and therapeutic features. *Medicine* (Baltimore) , 1977 56, 1-37.

Saphner T.; Tormey D. C.; Gray R. Venous and arterial thrombosis in patients Who received adjuvant for breast cancer. *J. Clin. Oncol.*, 1991 9 2, 286-294.

Sartori M. T.; Della Puppa A.; Ballin A.; Saggiorato G.; Bernardi D.; Padoan A.; Scienza R.; D'Avella D.; Cella G. Prothrombotic state in glioblastoma multiforme: an evaluation of the procoagulant activity of circulating microparticles. *J. Neurooncol.*, 2011 104 1, 225-31.

Semenza G. L. Angiogenesis in ischemic and neoplastic disorders. *Annu. Rev. Med.*, 2003 54, 17-28.

Semrad T. J.; O'Donnell R.; Wun T.; Chew H.; Harvey D.; Zhou H.; White R. H. Epidemiology of venous thromboembolism in 9489 payients with malignat glioma. *J. Neurosurg.*, 2007 106 4, 601-8.

Shet A.; Schorer A. E.; Kuskowski M. A. Venous thromboembolism is common but does not alter survival in glioblastoma multiforme. *Proc. Am. Soc. Clin. Oncol.*, 2003 abstract [432].

Shi X.; Gangadharan B.; Brass L. F.; Ruf W.; Muller B. M. Protease-activated receptor (PAR-1 and PAR-2) contribute to tumor cell motility and metastasis. *Mol. Cancer Res.*, 2004 2, 395-402.

Simanek R.; Vormittag R.; Hassler K.; Schwarz M.; Zielinski C.; Pabinger I.; Marosi C. Venous thromboembolism and survival in patients with high-grade glioma. *Neuro. Oncol.*, 2007 2, 89-95.

Skog J.; Würdinger T.; Van Rijn S.; Meijer D. H.; Gainche L.; Sena-Esteves M.; Curry W. T. Jr; Carter B. S.; Krichevsky A. M.; Breakefield X. O.

Glioblastoma microvesicles transport RNA and proteins that promote tumour growth and provide diagnostic biomarkers. *Nat. Cell Biol.*, 2008 10, 1470– 1476.

Smith G. F.; Neubauer B. L.; Sundboom J. L.; Best K. L.; Goode R. L.; Tanzer L. R.; Merriman R. L.; Frank J. D.; Herrmann R. G. Correlation of the in vivo anticoagulant, antithrombotic, and antimetastatic efficacy of warfarin in the rat. *Thromb. Res.*, 1988 50 1, 163-74.

Sorensen H. T.; Mellemkjaer L.; Olsen J. H.; Baron J. A. Prognosis of cancers associated with venous thromboembolism. *N Engl. J. Med.*, 2000 343 25, 1846-50.

Stassens P.; Bergum P. W.; Gansemans Y.; Jespers L.; Laroche Y.; Huang S.; Maki S.; Messens J.; Lauwereys M.; Cappello M.; Hotez P. J.; Lasters I.; Vlasuk G. P. Anticoagulant repertoire of the hookworm Ancylostoma caninum. *Proc. Natl. Acad. Sci. USA*, 1996 93, 2149-54.

Stratmann A.; Risau W.; Plate K. H. Cell type-specific expression of angiopoietin-1 and angiopoietin-2 suggests a role in glioblastoma angiopoietin. *Am. J. Pathol.*, 1998 153, 1459-66.

Svensson K. J.; Kucharzewska P.; Christianson H. C.; Sköld S.; Löfstedt T.; Johansson M. C.; Mörgelin M.; Bengzon J.; Ruf W.; Belting M. Hypoxia triggers a proangiogenic pathway involving cancer cell microvesicles and PAR-2-mediated heparin-binding EGF signaling in endothelial cells. *Proc. Nalt. Acad. Sci.,* USA 2011 9 suppl 1, 306-15.

Tehrani M.; Friedman T. M.; Olson J. J.; Brat D. J. Intravascular thrombosis in central nervous system malignancies: a potencial role in astrocyroma progression to glioblastoma. *Brain Pathol.*, 2008 18 2, 164-71.

Tesselaar M. E.; Osanto S. Risk of venous thromboembolism in lung cancer. *Curr. Opin. Pulm Med.*, 2007a 13 5, 362-7.

Tesselaar M. E.; Romijn F. P.; Van Der Linden I. K.; Prins F. A.; Bertina R. M.; Osanto S. Microparticle-associated tissue factor activity: a link between cancer and thrombosis? *J. Thromb. Haemost.*, 2007b 5 3, 520-7.

Trousseau A. *Phlegmasia Alba dolens*. Clinique Medicale de I'Hotel-Dieu de Paris 1865; 3 (94): 654-712.

Varki A. Trousseau's syndrome: multiple definitions and multiple mechanisms. *Blood*, 2007 110 6, 1723-1729.

Versteeg HH, Schaffner F, Kerver M, Petersen HH, Ahamed J, Felding-Habermann B, Takada Y, Mueller BM, Ruf W. Inhibition of tissue factor signaling suppresses tumor growth. Blood. 2008 Jan 1;111(1):190-9. (a)

Versteeg H. H.; Schaffner F.; Kerver M.; Ellies L. G.; Andrade-Gordon P.; Mueller B. M.; Ruf W. Protease-activated receptor (PAR) 2, but not PAR-

1, signaling promotes the development of mammary adenocarcinoma in polyoma middle T mice *Cancer Res.*, 2008 68, 7219-27. (b)

Vu T. K.; Hung D. T.; Wheaton V. I.; Coughlin S. R. Molecular cloning of a funcional thrombin receptor reveals a novel proteolytic mechanism of receptor activation. *Cell*, 1991 64, 1057-1068.

Walsh D. C.; Kakkar A. K. Thromboembolism in brain tumors. *Curr. Opin. Pulm Med.*, 2001 7 5, 326-31.

Wen P. Y.; Schiff D.; Kesari S.; Drappatz J.; Giga D. C.; Doherty L. Medical management of patients with brain tumors. *J. Neurooncol.*, 2006 80 3, 313-32.

White R. H.; Chew H. K.; Zhou H.; Parikh-Patel A.; Harris D.; Harvey D.; Wun T. Incidence od venous thrombolism in the year the diagnosis od cancer in 528,693 adults. *Arch. Intern. Med.*, 2005 165 15, 1782-7.

Yamahata H.; Takeshima H.; Kuratsu J.; Sarker K. P.; Tanioka K.; Wakimaru N.; Nakata M.; Kitajima I.; Maruyama I. The role of thrombin in the neo-vascularization of malignant gliomas: an intrinsic modulator for the up-regulation of vascular endothelial growth factor. *In. J. Oncol.*, 2002 20, 921-8.

Yart A.; Roche S.; Wetzker R.; Laffargue M.; Tonks N.; Mayeux P.; Chap H.; Raynal P. A function for phosphoinositide 3-kinase beta lipid products in coupling beta gamma to Ras activation in response to lysophosphatidic acid. *J. Biol. Chem.*, 2002 277 24, 21167-78.

Yu J. L.; May L.; Lhotak V.; Shahrzad S.; Shirasawa S.; Weitz J. I.; Coomber B. L.; Mackman N.; Rak J. W. Oncogenic events regulate tissue factor expression in colorectal cancer cells: implications for tumor progression and angiogenesis. *Blood*, 2005 105, 1734–41.

Zacharski L. R.; Donati M. B.; Rickles F. R. Registry of clinical trials of antithrombotic drugs in câncer: seconde report. The Scientific and Standardization Committe of the international Society on Thrombosis and Haemostasis Subcommitte on Hemostasis and Malignancy. *Thromb. Haemost.* 1993 70, 357-360.

Zacharski L. R.; Henderson W. G.; Rickles F. R.; Forman W. B.; Cornell C. J. Jr; Forcier R. J.; Harrower H. W.; Johnson R. O. Rationale and experimental design for the VA Cooperative Study of Anticoagulation (Warfarin) in the Treatment of Cancer. *Cancer* (Phila.) 1979 44 2, 732-41.

Zagzag D.; Hooper A.; Friedlander D. R.; Chan W.; Holash J.; Wiegand S. J.; Yancopoulos G. D.; Grumet M. In situ expression of angiopoietins in astrocytomas identifies angiopoietin-2 as an early marker of tumor angiogenesis. *Exp. Neurol.*, 1999 159, 391-400.

Zagzag D.; Zhong H.; Scalzitti J. M.; Laughner E.; Simons J. W.; Semenza GL. Expression of hypoxia-inducible factor 1 alpha in brain tumors: association with angiogenesis, invasion, and progression. *Cancer*, 2000 88, 2606-2618.

Zhao J.; Aguilar G.; Palencia S.; Newton E.; Abo A. rNAPc2 inhibits colorectal câncer in mice through tissue factor. *Clin. Cancer Res.*, 2009 15, 208-16.

Zwicker JI, Liebman HA, Neuberg D, Lacroix R, Bauer KA, Furie BC, Furie B. Tumor-derived tissue factor-bearing microparticles are associated with venous thromboembolic events in malignancy. Clin Cancer Res. 2009 Nov 15;15(22):6830-40.

In: Glioblastoma ISBN: 978-1-62100-858-3
Editors: M. F. Bezerra et.al, pp. 227-240© 2012 Nova Science Publishers, Inc.

Chapter 11

BRAF IN GLIOBLASTOMAS: CLINICAL IMPLICATIONS

***Naiara Correa Nogueira-de-Souza*[1], *José Reinaldo Almeida*[2], *Sergio Vicente Serrano*[3], *and Rui Manuel Reis*[1,4]**

[1]Molecular Oncology Research Center; [2]Department of Neurosurgery; [3]Department of Clinical Oncology, Barretos Cancer Hospital, Barretos, São Paulo, Brazil

[4]Life and Health Sciences Research Institute (ICVS) , Health Sciences School, University of Minho, Braga, Portugal

ABSTRACT

Glioblastomas are the most common and malignant primary central nervous system tumors. The current management of patients with glioblastomas is surgery, followed by concomitant radiotherapy with temozolomide–based chemotherapy. Despite this integrated approach, the prognosis of these patients is very dismal, with a median overall survival of 16 months. Therefore, new and more effective therapeutic options are needed to change this dark scenario. Over the past decade, significant advances have been made in understanding the molecular pathogenesis of malignant gliomas. In general, malignancy results from consecutive genetic mutations and alterations of growth-factor signaling. The increased knowledge of the molecular pathways underlying glioblastomas development is creating a new avenue of potential therapeutic targets.

The BRAF protooncogene, codifies a serine/threonine kinase important in the MAPK signaling cascade. A hotspot mutation of BRAF (V600E) , was identified in several tumor types, mainly, in melanomas and papillary thyroid cancer, which leads to hyperstimulation of the MAPK pathway and cellular transformation. Several drugs have been developed to target BRAF oncogene, and recently, exciting results have been achieved in phase I/II clinical trials of metastatic melanoma patients harboring BRAF V600E mutation treated with such class of tyrosine inhibitors. In this chapter we will summarized the current knowledge of BRAF alterations in glioblastomas biology and will address the potential therapeutic impact of the novel BRAF inhibitors in the treatment of these patients.

1. INTRODUCTION

Glioblastoma (GBM) is the most prevalent primary brain tumor found in adults and it is also the most aggressive and lethal neoplasm of the central nervous system. It accounts for 16.7% of all histological types of primary brain neoplasms, and for 53.7% of all gliomas. The male to female incidence ratio is 1.58.[1, 2] GBM affects over 17,000 persons in the United States each year and has an estimated age adjusted overall incidence of 3.0 per 100,000 in the population. Surgery is the primary treatment option, however due to its highly infiltrative nature, complete resection is virtually impossible.[3] Radiotherapy and chemotherapy are current standard therapies, yet the median overall survival with multimodality combined treatment remains in the range of 12 to 18 months.[4, 5]

Clinical features of GBM are nonspecific inasmuch as any kind of neurological disturbance can be present, depending on age of the patient, anatomical location of the tumor and tumor growth rate. Neurological clinical manifestations can be localized, related to functional activity of the affected region in the brain, such as language difficulty, sensation loss, focal seizures, visual field abnormalities. General neurological symptoms are also common, mainly due to intracranial hypertension caused by the mass effect of the tumor, which include headache, nausea, vomiting, consciousness impairment, papilledema. Only a small percentage of patients with GBM (7%) report clinical manifestations with duration over one year prior to diagnosis.[6] Some clinical outcome predictors have being described, among which age, Karnofsky Performance Scale (KPS) score and extent of resection are the most frequent. Younger patients with good performance in which a macroscopic total resection of the tumor was achieved have a significant survival advantage.[7, 8]

Glioblastomas can be clinically classified as primary (or *de novo*) glioblastomas, which arise without the evidence of precursor lesions, whereas, secondary GBM arise from lower grade gliomas (grade II or III) .[9] This classification system remains unsatisfactory owing to its lack of reproducibility. There is a high rate of inter- and even intra-observer discrepancies[10] and also a lack of precision in terms of prognosis.

2. Systemic Treatment for Glioblastoma

Limitations for each of the current treatment options are due to factors intrinsic to the tumor's biology and the microenvironment within the brain. Thus, surgical resection is limited by the non-circumscribed borders of the tumor, which are undetectable intraoperatively. As for radiation therapy, neurotoxicity to adjacent normal tissues is an issue when trying to achieve doses effective for tumor control. Furthermore, chemotherapy is constrained by the blood-brain barrier (BBB) . Many times substantial toxicity occurs with minimal benefit in order to administer therapeutic dosages.[11]

Due to these factors until recently clinical trials designed to discover effective adjuvant chemotherapy regimens have been disappointing. A meta-analysis of data from 12 randomized trials (with a total of 3,004 patients) demonstrated that adjuvant nitrosoureas, either alone or in combination regimens, generated slightly longer median survival times with considerable myelosuppression and no difference in the long-term survival rate.[12-14] Although nitrosourea-based chemotherapy is modestly effective for patients with GBM, its use has recently been supplanted by the oral alkylating agent, temozolomide.

Toxicity with temozolomide is relatively mild and it has a good central nervous system penetration. The pivotal study conducted jointly by the European Organization for Research and Treatment of Cancer (EORTC) trial 22981–26981, and the National Cancer Institute of Canada (NCIC) trial CE.3 confirmed the usefulness of temozolomide and radiation in newly diagnosed glioblastomas.[15] This study randomized 573 patients to receive either 60 Gy of standard fractionated radiation alone or daily temozolomide at 75 mg/m^2 concurrently with the same radiation regimen, followed by six cycles of adjuvant temozolomide (150 to 200 mg/m^2 for 5 days during each 28-day cycle) . The patients in the radiation plus temozolomide arm had a statistically significant improvement in survival over those in the radiation only arm ($P < 0.001$) . At follow-up evaluation after a median time of 28 months, the median survival periods in the two arms were 12.1 and 14.6 months, respectively. The 2-year overall survival rates were 10.4% and 26.5%, respectively. Despite the survival benefit associated with adjuvant RT and temzolomide-based chemotherapy, virtually all patients with GBM eventually relapse following initial therapy.

It is becoming increasingly clear that tumors that share identical histopathologic features can actually represent multiple distinct molecular phenotypes.[16] A more detailed molecular understanding of these tumors is thus crucial in order to improve classification, to better predict outcome, to better stratify patients included in clinical trials and, finally, to tailor specific treatments to individual tumor types or patients.

3. Mitogen-Activated Protein Kinase (MAPK) Signaling Pathway

The discovery of the MAPK signaling pathway in the 1980's has led to many and fundamental insights into tumor biology.[17-19] This signaling cascade is extremely complex and is involved in a number of upstream activation factors, such as cytokine, growth factors and G-protein, which upon ligation to their transmembrane receptors, activate a downstream signaling cascade, where RAS, RAF, MEK and ERK – constituting the MAPK - play a central role in transmiting the extracellular signals to the nucleus. Abnormal activation of the MAPK pathway leads to signal imbalance and can potentially result in cancer formation. This irregular stimulation is due to mutations at upstream membrane receptors and RAS/RAF signaling pathway, or downregulation of inhibitors of the cascade, such as NF1 or RKIP. The MAPK pathway also influences chemotherapeutic drug resistance and is currently an important pathway to target for therapeutic intervention.[20, 21] (Figure 1)

Ras

The RAS superfamily, an important component of the MAPK signaling network, consists of several members including RAS, RAB, RHO, ARF, and RAN sub-families.

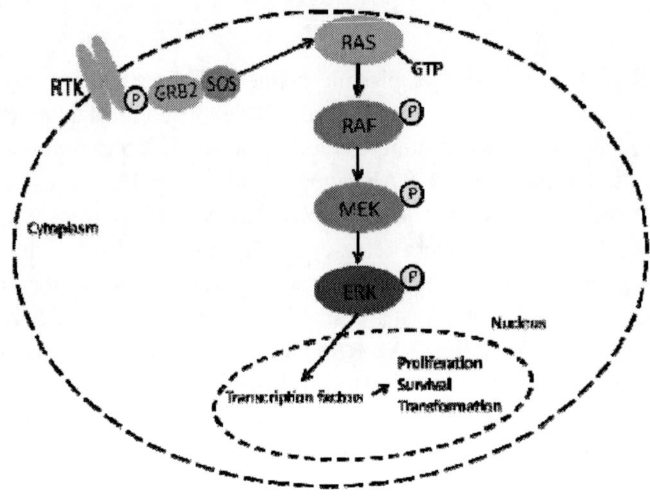

Figure 1. The MAPK signalling pathway.

The proteins K-RAS, H-RAS, and N-RAS are the major components of the RAS family.[22] The RAS proteins, participate in the regulation of essential cell physiological functions such as proliferation and survival.

They are monomeric 21-kDa proteins that have a high degree of homology, especially in their amino-terminal and carboxyl-terminal domains.[22]

The unique function of the RAS proteins is characterized by their transition between inactive GDP-bound (guanosine diphosphate, one G-proteins) and active GTP-bound (guanosine triphosphate, other G-proteins) to achieve cell signaling, resulting in the GTP/GDP-binding signal transducing molecules from the cell surface to the nucleus. RAS is normally present in the inactive GDP-bound form and external stimuli, such as the presence of mitogens, cytokines, and growth factors are necessary for activation. The binding of these ligands at RTKs (receptor tyrosine kinases) , results in dimerization of the receptor which in turn binds to GRB2 protein (growth factor receptor-bound protein 2) , either directly or through other mediator proteins to recruit the intracellular SOS (son of sevenless) protein to the cell surface through interaction with GRB2. The RTK-GRB2-SOS complex then binds to RAS-GDP resulting in the dissociation of GDP that preferentially binds to GTP to activate downstream RAF molecules.[23]

Raf

The RAF proteins are cytoplasmic serine/threonine kinases and include three main isoforms ARAF, BRAF, and CRAF. In contrast to RAS family molecules, RAF proteins can dimerize and the inactive forms are bound to 14-3-3 proteins. Recruitment of RAF signaling at the cell surface starts after RAS-GTP interaction with RAF molecules which cause a series of phosphorylation events which release the inhibition of RAF by 14-3-3. Activation of RAF leads to heterodimerization among the RAF isomers which in turn recruit, binds, and activates a scaffolding protein called KSR1 (kinase suppressor of RAS1) . After RAS/RAF activation, and interaction of KSR1 with RAF heterodimers, two kinases, extracellular signal-regulated kinase (ERK) and mitogen-activated or extracellular signal-related protein kinase kinase (MEK) are recruited to interact with KSR1. Consequently the downstream substrates/activators of RAF kinases phosphorylation, MEK (MEK1 and MEK2) and ERK (ERK1 and ERK2) are activated and phosphorylated. ERK is then sent to the nucleus where it plays a critical role in regulating gene expression, proliferation, and cell survival.[24-26] These stages are necessary for the activation of CRAF and ARAF. In contrast, BRAF phosphorylation appears to be constitutive and independent of RAS activation. BRAF is a stronger inducer of MEK phosphorylation, and this prominent role may account for the fact that somatic mutations associated with cancer are relatively frequent in BRAF but rare in the ARAF and CRAF.[27, 28] Additionally, in normal conditions, the MEK/ERK signaling pathway can be repressed by SPRY2, a protein identified as an inhibitor of MAPK signaling in epithelial and fibroblast cell lines.[29]

BRAF Mutation

A seminal study by Davies *et al*, evaluated the presence and frequency of mutation in *BRAF* gene in wide-range of human neoplasms.[30] The authors observed that the great majority of *BRAF* mutations occur as a single amino acid substitution of glutamic acid for valine at codon 600 (V600E) within the kinase domain. V600E mutations are found in different human cancers, with a particularly high frequency in melanoma (43%) and thyroid cancer (39%) . They are also present at lower frequencies in a wide range of cancers, such as colorectal, lung, and ovarian carcinoma (data were extracted from COSMIC database - http://www.sanger.ac.uk/genetics/CGP/cosmic/) .[30] The

BRAF V600E mutant has enhanced kinase activity and consequently stimulates the downstream MEK/ERK signaling pathway independently of RAS-GTP. Additionally, it no longer repressed by SPRY2. It has been shown that SPRY2 only binds to wild-type BRAF to initiate inhibition of MEK/ERK signaling, but this event does not occur with the BRAF V600E protein.[29, 31-33]

Different *BRAF* mutations have been mapped to various regions of the BRAF protein; however, the mutations at the abovementioned 600 residue in BRAF appear to be the most frequent among human cancers.[30] Some of the other *BRAF* mutations have been described to result in BRAF molecules with compromised BRAF activity, which must signal through RAF-1. Other mutations, such as D593V, may activate alternative signal transduction pathways.[34, 35]

4. BRAF Alterations in Glioblastomas

In the original study by Davies, *et al*, V600E *BRAF* mutations occur at a low frequency in glioma cell lines.[30] Further studies, addressed the presence of *BRAF* mutations in a more comprehensive manner. In 2005, Basto and colleagues analyzed a series of 82 gliomas of distinct WHO malignant grade for exon 11 and exon 15 (V600E) regions, and reported the presence of the V600E mutation in two cases.[36] Similarly, Knobbe and colleagues, analyzed 94 GBM for mutations in *BRAF*, *NRAS*, *KRAS* and *HRAS*, and reported the presence of the V600E mutation in 3 cases.[37] In conclusion, it seems that the *BRAF* V600E mutation is present, yet is an uncommon event in GBM, with mutation rates ranging from 0 to 18% of cases (Table 1) .

Besides gene activation by mutations, *BRAF* has been shown to be disrupted in gliomas through other genetic events, such as gene amplification and gene fusion. *BRAF* gene is located at the 7q35 region. Since gains of chromosome 7 are a frequent event in GBM,[38, 39] it is not surprising to see *BRAF* gene anormalities in these tumors. Using conventional comparative genomic hybridization (CGH) , gains of *BRAF* region were identified in 63% of GBM cases.[40] Yet, it is still arguable whether these amplification/gains lead to BRAF activation, as has been reported for pilocytic astrocitomas.[41, 42] Recently, it has been shown that the *BRAF* gene can also be a target for gene fusion. It is now well recognized that low-grade astrocytomas, mainly pilocytic astrocytomas, are characterized by *BRAF-KIAA1549* fusion gene resulting in constitutive activation of the MAPK pathway.[43-45]

Table 1. Summary of *BRAF* V600E mutations in glioblastomas

Study	N° of GBMs	Percentage of cases with V600E
Knobbe, et al., 2004 [37]	94	3,2
Basto, et al., 2005 [36]	34	5,9
Jeuken et al., 2007 [40]	19	0
Hagemann, et al., 2009 [47]	44	2,3
El-Habr, et al., 2010 [48]	66	0
Schiffman, et al., 2010 [49]	11	18,2
Schindler, et al., 2011 [50]	133	2,2
Dias-Santagata, et al., 2011 [51]	71	2,8

Besides KIAA1549, other genes such as FAM131B, can be involve in BRAF gene fusion events in astrocytomas.[46] In glioblastomas, the presence of these *BRAF* gene fusions have not been reported.[44, 45]

5. BRAF As A Therapeutic Target in GBM

Molecularly targeted therapies are transforming the care of patients with malignant gliomas, including GBM. An arsenal of small molecule inhibitors and antibodies are becoming available for clinical use, which can target key components of the signal transduction machinery that are commonly activated in gliomas.[52] In this setting, several drugs have been developed to target BRAF oncogene.

Sorafenib (Nexavar, Bayer) , was one of the first RAF kinase inhibitors to be tested, however several studies showed that it lacks potency and selectivity for the RAF kinases.[53] Surprisingly, in melanoma, which has a high frequency of *BRAF* mutations, sorafenib lacks significant clinical activity [54]. Currently, growing experience shows that its primary mechanism of action is anti-angiogenic rather than RAF inhibition [55, 56]. Vemurafenib (PLX4032, Plexxikon/Roche) is a second generation selective RAF inhibitor with strong *in vitro* activity against all three isoforms of RAF.[57] Interestingly, vemurafenib demonstrates potent inhibition of MAPK in tumors harboring the V600E *BRAF* mutations.[58] In contrast, in cells which are *BRAF* wild-type, vemurafenib showed little inhibition in the MAPK pathway.[59] Impressively, vemurafenib phase 1 and 2 clinical trials, showed response rates of more than 50% in patients with metastatic melanomas harboring *BRAF* V600E mutations.[60, 61] Recently a randomized phase 3 clinical trial compared vemurafenib with dacarbazine in 675 patients with previously untreated, metastatic melanoma with the *BRAF* V600E mutation.[62] At 6 months, overall survival was 84% (95% confidence interval [CI], 78 to 89) in the vemurafenib group and 64% (95% CI, 56 to 73) in the dacarbazine group. Major clinical responses have also been reported using a second, selective RAF inhibitor, GSK2118436. In a phase 1 trial of GSK2118436, a 63% response rate was observed in the cohort of patients with V600E *BRAF* mutant melanoma.[63]

These remarkable results of vemurafenib in melanoma patients exhibiting *BRAF* V600E mutation raise some expectations for GBM patients with the same *BRAF* mutation. However, it is still unknown whether patients with GBM would respond to treatment using BRAF inhibitors. Based on the successful treatment of selected patients with metastatic melanoma to the brain, it is presumed that BRAF inhibitors have the capability to cross the brain-blood barrier. More preclinical and initial clinical trials are needed to evaluate its relevance in GBM treatment.

6. Conclusion

Any hope of improving the dismal prognosis of GBM patients depends on the possibility to correctly identify and target molecular signaling events important for the continued tumor survival and maintenance. Despite the low frequency of *BRAF* mutations in GBMs, the outstanding efficacy of BRAF inhibitors, in the presence of *BRAF* V600E mutation in other type of tumors, particularly cutaneous melanoma, raise great expectations toward the application of such pharmaceutic agents in *BRAF* mutated GBM patients.

7. References

[1] Lim, S. K., et al., Glioblastoma multiforme: a perspective on recent findings in human cancer and mouse models. *BMB reports*, 2011. 44(3): p. 158-64.

[2] CBTRUS Statistical Report: Primary Brain and Central Nervous System Tumors Diagnosed in the United States in 2004-2007. 2011 February

2011 August 22, 2011] Available from: http://www.cbtrus.org/2011-NPCR-SEER/WEB-0407-Report-3-3-2011.pdf.

[3] Grossman, S. A., et al., Survival of patients with newly diagnosed glioblastoma treated with radiation and temozolomide in research studies in the United States. Clinical cancer research: *an official journal of the American Association for Cancer Research,* 2010. 16(8): p. 2443-9.

[4] Easaw, J. C., et al., Canadian recommendations for the treatment of recurrent or progressive glioblastoma multiforme. *Curr. Oncol.*, 2011. 18(3): p. e126-e136.

[5] Stupp, R., M. J. van den Bent, and M. E. Hegi, Optimal role of temozolomide in the treatment of malignant gliomas. *Current neurology and neuroscience reports,* 2005. 5(3): p. 198-206.

[6] Cobb, C. A. Y., J. R., *Glial and neuronal tumors of the brain in adults, in Neurological Surgery,* J. R. Youmans, Editor 1982, WB Saunders Co: Philadelphia, PA, USA. p. 2759-2835.

[7] Lacroix, M., et al., A multivariate analysis of 416 patients with glioblastoma multiforme: prognosis, extent of resection, and survival. *Journal of neurosurgery,* 2001. 95(2): p. 190-8.

[8] Bauchet, L., et al., Oncological patterns of care and outcome for 952 patients with newly diagnosed glioblastoma in 2004. *Neuro-oncology*, 2010.He, J., et al., Glioblastomas with an oligodendroglial component:a pathological and molecular study. Journal of neuropathology and experimental *neurology*, 2001. 60(9): p. 863-71.

[9] Coons, S. W., et al., Improving diagnostic accuracy and interobserver concordance in the classification and grading of primary gliomas. *Cancer*, 1997. 79(7): p. 1381-93.

[10] Salgaller, M. L. and L. M. Liau, Current status of clinical trials for glioblastoma. *Rev. Recent Clin. Trials*, 2006. 1(3): p. 265-81.

[11] Stewart, L. A., Chemotherapy in adult high-grade glioma: a systematic review and metaanalysis of individual patient data from 12 randomised trials. *Lancet*, 2002. 359(9311): p. 1011-8. Chemotherapy for high-grade glioma. *Cochrane Database Syst. Rev.*, 2002(4): p. CD003913. Batchelor, T. Adjuvant chemotherapy for malignant gliomas. UpToDate, Inc. 2011 09/06/2011 07/24/2011]; Available from: http://www.uptodate.com/contents/adjuvantchemotherapyfor malignant gliomas?source=search_resultandselectedTitle=1%7E64#H1.

[12] Stupp, R., et al., Radiotherapy plus concomitant and adjuvant temozolomide for glioblastoma. *The New England journal of medicine*, 2005. 352(10): p. 987-96.

[13] Hanahan, D. and R. A. Weinberg, Hallmarks of cancer: the next generation. *Cell*, 2011.144(5): p. 646-74.

[14] DeFeo, D., et al., Analysis of two divergent rat genomic clones homologous to the transforming gene of Harvey murine sarcoma virus. *Proceedings of the National Academy of Sciences of the United States of America*, 1981. 78(6): p. 3328-32.

[15] Chang, E. H., et al., Human genome contains four genes homologous to transforming genes of Harvey and Kirsten murine sarcoma viruses. *Proceedings of the National Academy of Sciences of the United States of America,* 1982. 79(16): p. 4848-52.

[16] Schubbert, S., K. Shannon, and G. Bollag, Hyperactive Ras in developmental disorders and cancer. Nature reviews. *Cancer*, 2007. 7(4): p. 295-308.

[17] Buday, L. and J. Downward, Many faces of Ras activation. *Biochimica et biophysica acta*, 2008. 1786(2): p. 178-87.

[18] Malumbres, M. and M. Barbacid, RAS oncogenes: the first 30 years. Nature reviews. *Cancer*, 2003. 3(6): p. 459-65.

[19] Cox, A. D. and C. J. Der, Ras family signaling: therapeutic targeting. *Cancer biology and therapy*, 2002. 1(6): p. 599-606.

[20] Mitin, N., K. L. Rossman, and C. J. Der, Signaling interplay in Ras superfamily function. *Current biology*: CB, 2005. 15(14): p. R563-74.

[21] Wellbrock, C., M. Karasarides, and R. Marais, The RAF proteins take centre stage. Nature reviews. *Molecular cell biology*, 2004. 5(11): p. 875-85.

[22] McCubrey, J. A., et al., Roles of the Raf/MEK/ERK pathway in cell growth, malignant transformation and drug resistance. *Biochimica et biophysica acta*, 2007. 1773(8): p. 1263-84.

[23] Wan, P. T., et al., Mechanism of activation of the RAF-ERK signaling pathway by oncogenic mutations of B-RAF. *Cell*, 2004. 116(6): p. 855-67.

[24] Hmitou, I., et al., Differential regulation of B-raf isoforms by phosphorylation and autoinhibitory mechanisms. *Molecular and cellular biology,* 2007. 27(1): p. 31-43.

[25] Emuss, V., et al., Mutations of C-RAF are rare in human cancer because C-RAF has a low basal kinase activity compared with B-RAF. *Cancer research*, 2005. 65(21): p. 9719-26.

[26] Tsavachidou, D., et al., SPRY2 is an inhibitor of the ras/extracellular signal-regulated kinase pathway in melanocytes and melanoma cells with wild-type BRAF but not with the V599E mutant. *Cancer research*, 2004. 64(16): p. 5556-9.

[27] Davies, H., et al., Mutations of the BRAF gene in human cancer. *Nature*, 2002. 417(6892): p. 949-54.

[28] Cohen, Y., et al., BRAF mutation in papillary thyroid carcinoma. *Journal of the National Cancer Institute*, 2003. 95(8): p. 625-7.

[29] Kimura, E. T., et al., High prevalence of BRAF mutations in thyroid cancer: genetic evidence for constitutive activation of the RET/PTC-RAS-BRAF signaling pathway in papillary thyroid carcinoma. *Cancer research*, 2003. 63(7): p. 1454-7.

[30] Vakiani, E. and D. B. Solit, KRAS and BRAF: drug targets and predictive biomarkers. *The Journal of pathology*, 2011. 223(2): p. 219-29.

[31] Garnett, M. J. and R. Marais, Guilty as charged: B-RAF is a human oncogene. *Cancer cell*, 2004. 6(4): p. 313-9.

[32] Garnett, M. J., et al., Wild-type and mutant B-RAF activate C-RAF through distinct mechanisms involving heterodimerization. *Molecular cell*, 2005. 20(6): p. 963-9.

[33] Basto, D., et al., Mutation analysis of B-RAF gene in human gliomas. *Acta neuropathologica*, 2005. 109(2): p. 207-10.

[34] Knobbe, C. B., J. Reifenberger, and G. Reifenberger, Mutation analysis of the Ras pathway genes NRAS, HRAS, KRAS and BRAF in glioblastomas. *Acta Neuropathol*, 2004. 108(6): p. 467-70. Comprehensive genomic characterization defines human glioblastoma genes and core pathways. *Nature*, 2008. 455(7216): p. 1061-8.

[35] Verhaak, R. G., et al., Integrated genomic analysis identifies clinically relevant subtypes of glioblastoma characterized by abnormalities in PDGFRA, IDH1, EGFR, and NF1. *Cancer cell*, 2010. 17(1): p. 98-110.

[36] Jeuken, J., et al., RAS/RAF pathway activation in gliomas: the result of copy number gains rather than activating mutations. *Acta neuropathologica*, 2007. 114(2): p. 121-33.

[37] Bar, E. E., et al., Frequent gains at chromosome 7q34 involving BRAF in pilocytic astrocytoma. *Journal of neuropathology and experimental neurology*, 2008. 67(9): p. 878-87.

[38] Jacob, K., et al., Duplication of 7q34 is specific to juvenile pilocytic astrocytomas and a hallmark of cerebellar and optic pathway tumours. *British journal of cancer*, 2009. 101(4): p. 722-33.

[39] Hawkins, C., et al., BRAF-KIAA1549 Fusion Predicts Better Clinical Outcome in Pediatric Low-Grade Astrocytoma. *Clinical cancer research: an official journal of the American Association for Cancer Research*, 2011. 17(14): p. 4790-8.

[40] Jones, D. T., et al., Tandem duplication producing a novel oncogenic BRAF fusion gene defines the majority of pilocytic astrocytomas. *Cancer research*, 2008. 68(21): p. 8673-7.

[41] Jeuken, J. W. and P. Wesseling, MAPK pathway activation through BRAF gene fusion in pilocytic astrocytomas; a novel oncogenic fusion gene with diagnostic, prognostic, and therapeutic potential. *The Journal of pathology*, 2010. 222(4): p. 324-8.

[42] Cin, H., et al., Oncogenic FAM131B-BRAF fusion resulting from 7q34 deletion comprises an alternative mechanism of MAPK pathway activation in pilocytic astrocytoma. *Acta neuropathologica*, 2011. 121(6): p. 763-74.

[43] Hagemann, C., et al., RAF expression in human astrocytic tumors. *International journal of molecular medicine*, 2009. 23(1): p. 17-31.

[44] El-Habr, E. A., et al., Analysis of PIK3CA and B-RAF gene mutations in human astrocytomas: association with activation of ERK and AKT. *Clinical neuropathology*, 2010. 29(4): p. 239-45.

[45] Schiffman, J. D., et al., Oncogenic BRAF mutation with CDKN2A inactivation is characteristic of a subset of pediatric malignant astrocytomas. *Cancer research*, 2010. 70(2): p. 512-9.

[46] Schindler, G., et al., Analysis of BRAF V600E mutation in 1,320 nervous system tumors reveals high mutation frequencies in pleomorphic xanthoastrocytoma, ganglioglioma and extra-cerebellar pilocytic astrocytoma. *Acta neuropathologica*, 2011. 121(3): p. 397-405.

[47] Dias-Santagata, D., et al., BRAF V600E Mutations Are Common in Pleomorphic Xanthoastrocytoma: Diagnostic and Therapeutic Implications. *PLoS One*, 2011. 6(3): p. e17948.

[48] Huang, T. T., et al., Targeted therapy for malignant glioma patients: lessons learned and the road ahead. *Neurotherapeutics*, 2009. 6(3): p. 500-12.

[49] Wilhelm, S. M., et al., BAY 43-9006 exhibits broad spectrum oral antitumor activity and targets the RAF/MEK/ERK pathway and receptor tyrosine kinases involved in tumor progression and angiogenesis. *Cancer research*, 2004. 64(19): p. 7099-109.

[50] Eisen, T., et al., Sorafenib in advanced melanoma: a Phase II randomized discontinuation trial analysis. *British journal of cancer*, 2006. 95(5): p. 581-6.

[51] Stein, M. N. and K. T. Flaherty, CCR drug updates: sorafenib and sunitinib in renal cell carcinoma. *Clinical cancer research: an official journal of the American Association for Cancer Research*,2007. 13(13): p. 3765-70.

[52] Flaherty, K. T., Sorafenib in renal cell carcinoma. *Clinical cancer research: an official journal of the American Association for Cancer Research*, 2007. 13(2 Pt 2): p. 747s-752s.

[53] Tsai, J., et al., Discovery of a selective inhibitor of oncogenic B-Raf kinase with potent antimelanoma activity. *Proceedings of the National Academy of Sciences of the United States of America*, 2008. 105(8): p. 3041-6.

[54] Joseph, E. W., et al., The RAF inhibitor PLX4032 inhibits ERK signaling and tumor cell proliferation in a V600E BRAF-selective manner. *Proceedings of the National Academy of Sciences of the United States of America*, 2010. 107(33): p. 14903-8.

[55] Hatzivassiliou, G., et al., RAF inhibitors prime wild-type RAF to activate the MAPK pathway and enhance growth. *Nature*, 2010. 464(7287): p. 431-5.

[56] Flaherty, K. T., et al., Inhibition of mutated, activated BRAF in metastatic melanoma. *The New England journal of medicine*, 2010. 363(9): p. 809-19.

[57] Ribas, A., et al. BRIM-2: An open-label, multicenter phase II study of vemurafenib in previously treated patients with BRAF V600E mutation-positive metastatic melanoma. In 2011 ASCO Annual Meeting. 2011. Chicago, Il: *J. Clin. Oncol.*

[58] Chapman, P. B., et al., Improved survival with vemurafenib in melanoma with BRAFV600E mutation. *The New England journal of medicine,* 2011. 364(26): p. 2507-16.

[59] Kefford, R., et al. Phase I/II study of GSK2118436, a selective inhibitor of oncogenic mutant BRAF kinase, in patients with metastatic melanoma and other solid tumors. In 2010 *Annual Meeting ASCO*. 2010. Chicago, MI.

INDEX

A

B

C

E

F

G

H

I

J

K

L

M

N

O

P

T

U

V

W

X

Y